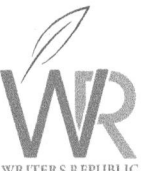

A 24-HOUR HOME REMEDY GUIDE TO YOUR BACK PAIN

DR. MAHMOUD SOUS
BHOOMIKA PATHAK
PRIYANKA YADAV

Copyright © 2021 by Dr. Mahmoud Sous.

All rights reserved. No part of this book may be reproduced in any form or by any electronic or mechanical means, including information storage and retrieval systems, without permission in writing from the publisher, except by reviewers, who may quote brief passages in a review.

This publication contains the opinions and ideas of its authors. It is intended to provide helpful and informative material on the subjects addressed in the publication. The authors and publisher specifically disclaim all responsibility for any liability, loss, or risk, personal or otherwise, which is incurred as a consequence, directly or indirectly, of the use and application of any of the contents of this book.

WRITERS REPUBLIC L.L.C.
515 Summit Ave. Unit R1
Union City, NJ 07087, USA

Website: *www.writersrepublic.com*
Hotline: *1-877-656-6838*
Email: *info@writersrepublic.com*

Ordering Information:
Quantity sales. Special discounts are available on quantity purchases by corporations, associations, and others. For details, contact the publisher at the address above.

Library of Congress Control Number:	2021918445	
ISBN-13:	978-1-63728-815-3	[Paperback Edition]
	978-1-63728-816-0	[Hardback Edition]
	978-1-63728-817-7	[Digital Edition]

Rev. date: 10/14/2021

ABOUT THE AUTHORS

Dr. Mahmoud Sous – Ph.D.

During the period of 1995-1999, I went to the medical school in Poland to research about the various methods of back pain treatment. After finishing my PhD, I took variety of courses including naturopath, acupuncture, and manual techniques. This gave me an idea that exercises, and massage could be helpful in treatment of chronic pain. But my findings didn't stop me here, I also worked as a naturopath practitioner in Canada where I got familiar about treatments with Chinese medicines, osteopath techniques and some other manual therapies which helps in pain management.

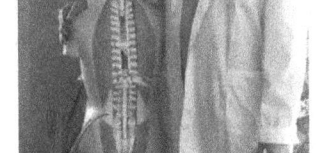

Fixing injuries requires an understanding of anatomy and biomechanics. That is why my research and treatment belong to the holistic approach of using different techniques and remedies for the treatment of back pain. In 1990, I realize that there are some complex spinal aspects and issues which leads to of back pain. So, from my case studies I formulated a guideline which is clear and easy to understand and will fix your issues.

My goal is to help people visualize how the body functions and what happens inside when you experience pain. Healing requires to focus on one's action because pain results due to faulty actions and movements. This thought motivated me to work on a book which will include all home remedies where people can treat themselves to fix their pain. I have included knowledge based on my clinical research using manual massage therapy, food habits, nutrition facts, heat, sauna, hydrotherapy, cold water treatments which overall helps in pain management. It gives me pleasure to introduce this book to the community where I have shared all my experienced treatment plans.

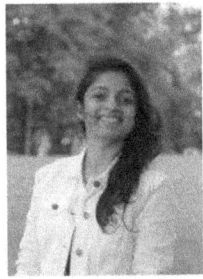

Bhoomika Pathak (Physiotherapist)
After graduating in 2014, I have been working with various clinical conditions like sports injury, musculoskeletal injury, and neurological disorders for 7 years. Along with Dr. Mahmoud, I have worked on treatment and pain management for back pain population. With all the successful outcomes till now, we have designed a home remedy book with 24-hour stepwise guide to treat your back pain.

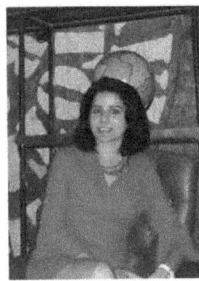

Priyanka Yadav (Physiotherapist)
Since completing my study in Physiotherapy, I always aspired to work for the society. Seeing people suffering motivated me to work for this book. Along with Dr. Mahmoud, I have been constantly working with various use of herbs and its effects in pain management.

Dr. Sous's Team who have contributed with their approaches in this book,
- Dr. Fauzia Ahmed – Chiropractor
- Dr. Youssef Elaridi – Reg. Massage therapist
- Larry Wang – Acupuncturist
- Dr. Alexy Kaganovsky - Naturopath
- Sheena Anand – Resident Physiotherapist
- Navjot Kaur – Physiotherapist
- Doris Valentin – Massage therapist
- Lennix – Massage therapist
- Mandeep Kaur – Physiotherapist
- Payal Vaghani – Physiotherapist
- Adla Hito – Herbalist & Nutritionist

This book will include a complete management of your back pain starting with pain management, correction of posture, self exercises for strengthening, self-massage techniques, incorporation of herbs to reduce inflammation and stiffness, hydrotherapy, heat and cold application, nutritional food to eat during pain. It will be a stepwise guide to treat and monitor your back and restore your functions. Find out what are the factors which are causing you back pain and start healing it today. This could be useful to any individual who is experiencing back pain needs a cure. Hopefully, this book will give you a glimpse into those other areas. So please accept this humble offering of help which represents my current understanding as of today this book is published.

We believe in a Pain-Free Society!

Contents

Chapter No.	Title	Page No.
1	Back pain overview	1
2	Self-assess your back	5
3	Resting positions for spinal alignment	11
4	Heat and Cold Therapy	13
5	General stretching techniques	17
6	General mobility exercises	22
7	General strengthening exercises	26
8	Massage technique for pain relief	30
9	Treatment options for back pain	34
10	Herbs and herb infused oils	39
11	Herbal teas for relaxation and pain relief	60
12	Herbal poultice (paste) recipe for pain relief	63
13	Herbal inhalation and gargling for relaxation	69
14	Body and foot soak recipes for relaxation	78
15	Scrubs and peeling recipes to rejuvenate skin and pain relief	86
16	Nutritional facts and benefits of balance diet to reduce pain	98
17	Cervicogenic headache and its management	106
18	Migraine headache and its management	109
19	Vertigo	111
20	Neck Tendonitis	114
21	Neck pain associated with disk herniation	117
22	Neck pain associated with cervical spinal stemosis	127
23	Cervical spondylosis – Degeneration of bones	130
24	Middle back (thoracic) pain due to disk herniation	133
25	Low back pain due to muscle strain	142
26	Low back pain due to disc herniation	146
27	Low back pain due to lumbar stenosis	154
28	Low back pain due to degenerative changes	158
29	Scoliosis	162
30	Numbness, tingling and paresthesia	167
31	Ankylosing Spondylitis	170
32	Sacro-iliac joint dysfunction	174
33	Tailbone pain	178
34	Back pain during pregnancy	180
35	Post-partum back pain	184
36	Back pain due to irritable bowel syndrome	189
37	Back pain due to acidity	191
38	Back pain due to flat foot	192
39	Back pain due to Erb's palsy or brachial plexus injury	195
40	Back pain due to Kidney stones	198
41	Prophylactics	200

CHAPTER 1: BACK PAIN OVERVIEW

If you ever had pain in your back, you are not alone. It can be anywhere ranging from your neck, pain up between the shoulder blades or lower back to the tailbone, affects so many of us at some point in our life that has made us worry. Back pains are one of the most common reasons people see a doctor or miss their day at work. Even school aged children can have back pain. It is a leading of disability worldwide.

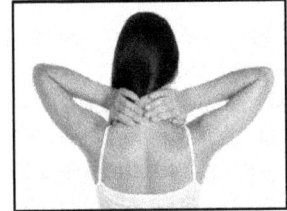

What structures make up the back?

The back is a structure made up of bones, muscles and other tissues that forms the part of the body from the neck to your hips. Stacked on top of one another are more than 30 bones, the vertebrae that forms the spine. Starting from the top it has four regions:

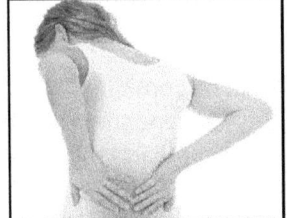

- Seven Neck Vertebrae or Cervical Vertebrae
- Twelve Upper back or Thoracic Vertebrae
- Five Lower back or Lumbar Vertebrae
- Tailbone which is made up of Sacrum and Coccyx as a unit

Each of these bones contains a round hole that, when arranged together with all the others, creates a channel which surrounds the spinal cord. The spaces between these bones are maintained by round, spongy pads called the discs which acts much like shock absorbers when the body moves. There are also bands of tissue known as ligaments and tendons which holds these bones in place and attaches the muscles to spinal column. Nerves emerge from the spinal cord through spaces between the vertebrae.

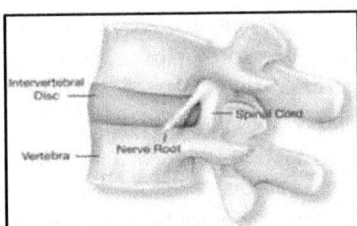

The neck and lower back region are highly prevalent to pain and injury because of its weight-bearing function and involvement in moving, twisting, and bending. Neck holds the weight of head and lower back holds the weight of upper body. There are 31 spinal nerves. Each vertebrae have a spinal nerve. The nerves are categorized by the vertebra which house them. There are: 8 cervical nerves, 12 thoracic nerves, 5 lumbar nerves, 5 sacral nerves, 1 coccygeal nerve. 16 of these 31 nerves has a specific myotome that controls voluntary muscle movement. Most muscles in the limbs receive innervation from more than one spinal nerve root and are hence comprised of multiple myotomes. The list below details which movement(s) has the strongest association with each myotome: C5- shoulder abduction, C6– Elbow flexion Wrist extension, C7 – Elbow extension, C8 – Finger flexion, T1 – Finger abduction, L2 – Hip flexion, L3 – Knee extension, L4 – Ankle dorsiflexion, L5 – Great toe extension, S1 – Ankle plantarflexion.

Myotome testing is an essential part of neurological examination when suspecting radiculopathy. Muscle strength in a particular myotome may help in identifying at which level a nerve root compromised. Testing of myotomes, in the form of isometric resisted muscle testing, gives information about the level in the spine where a lesion may be present. During myotome testing, you are looking for muscle weakness of a particular group of muscles. Results may indicate lesion to the spinal cord nerve root, or intervertebral disc herniation pressing on the spinal nerve roots. The details for myotome testing are described in chapter 2 for self-assessment.

Muscles of back

Muscles make up a large part of the anatomy (structure) of the back. They start at the top of the neck and go down to the tailbone. There are three different types of muscles in the body: the heart muscle, smooth muscles, and skeletal muscles. The back muscles are skeletal muscles. They support bones, in this case, the vertebrae. By tightening and relaxing, the skeletal muscles create movement. As with other parts of the body, the back has several layers of muscles. Some are closer to the surface (called superficial muscles). Moving deeper into the body, there are intermediate muscles and deep muscles.

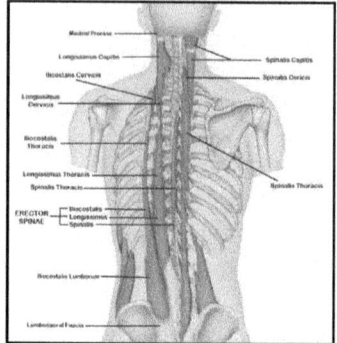

There are three groups of muscles that make up the sacrospinalis. These extend from the neck area to the lower back. The spinalis are muscles that are closest to the spine. There is a set of muscles in the upper back (called the thoracic area) called the spinalis thoracis. The iliocostalis muscles are furthest from the spine. There are three sets of iliocostalis muscles: 1) in the cervical area (iliocostalis cervicis), 2) in the upper back or thoracic area (iliocostalis thoracis), and 3) in the lumbar area (iliocostalis lumborum).

What Is "Core?"

There are many common misconceptions about the "core" even among fitness professionals. Most people probably think that the core is simply the abdominals, aka "6-pack." However, the core is much more than that.

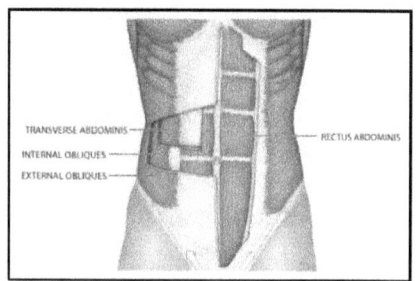

The core is the center of our body, and it functions to stabilize the trunk while the arms and legs move during functional movements. When we view it this way, we see that the core actually includes:
- Muscles that stabilize the hips.
- The system of muscles that make up the torso
- Muscles that stabilize the shoulders.

Why Is the Core so Important?

The core muscles have two main functions 1) to spare the spine from excessive load and 2) to transfer force from the lower body to the upper body and vice versa. Having a strong, stable core helps us to prevent injuries and allows us to perform at our best. The back is one of the most important parts of the human anatomy. It is also one the most neglected. Back muscles give power to the body, that play a major role in all functions. They connect the hips, butt, chest, shoulder and neck. It is a conjunction between major body muscles of human body parts. Strengthening our back muscles should not be treated as a luxury, but rather an obligation. These muscles do not only serve us in spotting activities and power workouts, but they also serve us in our daily lives.

Many people have back pain—whether it's upper back pain or low back pain—and this may be partly caused by weak abdominal muscles. Since your abs are the front anchor of your spine, if they are weak, then the other structures supporting your spine (your back muscles, for example) will have to work harder. By developing stronger core muscles, you'll be less likely to injure or strain your back muscles.

What can cause you pain?

Most of the pain is mechanical in nature, meaning that there is disruption in the way the components of the back (spine, muscles, discs, and nerves). It can result from any injury, activity, or some medical conditions. As people get older, they are more prone to degenerative disc diseases, work related injuries whereas in younger generation it can be because of poor posture, sprains or strains, injury. Some examples of pain are given below:

- **Injuries:** This includes sprains (overstretched or torn ligaments), strains (tears in tendons or muscles), spasms (sudden contraction of a muscle or group of muscles) or traumatic injuries such as from playing sports, car accidents or fall which can injure your muscles, tendons, rupture discs or compress spine.

- **Degenerative problems:** This includes spondylosis the degeneration of spine as people get older, intervertebral disc degeneration where discs wear down and lose their cushioning ability or arthritis or any inflammatory diseases in spine.
- **Nerve and spinal cord problems:** This includes spinal nerve compression, inflammation or injury, sciatica where there is radiating pain from back to legs, spinal stenosis, which is narrowing of the spinal column, spondylolisthesis which happens when vertebrae slip out of place, pinching the nerves, herniated discs, infections, cauda equina syndrome and osteoporosis in which bone density decreases and leads to painful fractures in vertebrae.
- **Congenital (By Birth):** Skeletal irregularities such as scoliosis, lordosis (an abnormally exaggerated arch in lower back), kyphosis and other, Spina bifida which involves incomplete development of the spinal cord.
- **Non-spinal sources:** Kidney stones which causes sharp pain in lower back at one side, fibromyalgia which involves widespread muscle pain and fatigue, tumors that press on or destroy the bone spine and pregnancy which is associated with pain after childbirth.

What are the risk factors for developing back pain?
- Age: It is common with advancing age. Loss of bone strength, intervertebral disc begins to lose fluid and flexibility, risk of spinal stenosis and degeneration of bones.
- Weight gain: Being overweight or obese puts more stress on back and leads to pain.
- Job-related factors: Job duties which requires heavy lifting, pushing, or pulling particularly with twisting or vibrating spine can lead to pain. Poor posture or sitting in chair while doing desk job can also contribute to pain.
- Fitness level: Weak back and abdominal muscles may not support the spine and can create excessive stress on back.
- Smoking: It can restrict blood flow and oxygen to disc, causing them to degenerate faster.
- Backpack overload in children: A backpack overloaded with schoolbooks can strain and cause back muscle fatigue.
- Genetics: Some conditions of back like where there is fusion of spinal joints leading to immobility of spine (Ankylosing spondylitis) includes a genetic component.
- Psychological factors: Mood and depression and stress can influence the likelihood of experiencing back pain.

How the symptoms with back pain look like?
Back pain can range from a muscle aching to a shooting, burning, or stabbing sensation. In addition, the pain may radiate down your leg or worsen with bending, twisting, lifting, standing, or walking. Here is a list of symptoms which includes:
- Stiffness in any area where the pain is felt either it could be neck, upper back or lower back and restricts the range of motion.
- Inability to maintain normal posture due to stiffness and/or pain.
- Muscle spasm either activity or at rest.
- Pain that persists for a maximum of more than 15 days
- Notable loss of muscle function such as ability to tiptoe or heel walk
- Pain with radiates to the extremities like if there is nerve compression at neck, the pain will radiate to the arm, hands, and chest wall and if there is any compression at lower back the pain will radiate to the buttocks and legs.
- Pain in back while doing strenuous activity like coughing, sneezing, farting, passing stool. Usually present with disc lesions.
- Dribbling of urine while coughing or sneezing. This indicates nerve compression at low back.
- Difficulty sitting or standing for long hours.
- Sharp pain while lying down
- Sleep disturbances

When to see your doctor?

The symptoms for most occurrence of back pain is non-emergent and can be traditionally self-treated, but there are some warning signs which need to be looked upon and seeks urgent medical care.

- Lower back pain that radiates to the front of abdomen which occurs in a rare medical condition called abdominal aortic aneurysm. It shows specific symptoms like stabbing pain of severe intensity felt deep in between chest and belly button, shallow breathing, cold sweats, and general weakness.
- Difficulty or inability to control urine and other bowl movements with sensory loss. This can be due to damage to the nerves near your tailbone.
- Back pain caused by benign or metastatic spine tumors. It shows other associated symptoms like unrelenting pain despite rest and medication, fever with chills, night pain, progressive or sudden weakness in legs and unexplained weight loss.
- Spinal infections like osteomyelitis which results in back pain. It will also include fever with chills, pain that is worse at night, swelling and warmth around the infection area, weight loss.
- Back pain associated with acute trauma which include sudden injuries, fall or accident.
- Sudden pain with known risk of fracture, such as osteoporosis.
- A recent increase in pain that does not subside with over-the-counter medicines and associated with nausea and vomiting.

REMEMBER THIS: *"Back pain can be complex and challenging condition to treat and can cause pain despite the best of efforts. The causes of neck pain and back we discussed are very common, but they require definitive and specific treatment. Also, early diagnosis is important in every case, it's important for you to know what to look for and treat accordingly."*

CHAPTER 2: SELF ASSESS YOUR BACK

The following questions are designed to see if you could benefit from treatment to address your back and neck pain.

1. Do you have neck and back pain that limits you performing your activities like dressing, toileting, bathing, grooming?
2. Do you have neck or back pain that restricts you from performing any recreational activities like hiking or sports?
3. Do you have neck or back pain that restricts you from performing any daily household activities like laundry, vacuuming or cleaning?
4. Do you have pain at night that significantly interferes with your sleeping?
5. Do you have any of the following symptoms in your arms or legs like pain, burning, shooting pain, ache/numbness, tingling?
6. Have you noticed weakness in your arms or legs?
7. Have you noticed significant loss of balance or difficulty walking?
8. Do you have a weakness in the foot or "foot drop"?
9. Have you experienced loss of bowel or bladder control?

If you answered **yes** to any of the questions up to five, it can be treated traditionally. But, if you are experiencing the symptoms in questions six through nine, you may need an immediate referral to a specialist. If your pain seems to have occurred *"out of nowhere"* or you have minor pain you attribute to a simple strain, there are some preliminary assessments that may be helpful in helping you to decide what the problem is and what type of treatment would be the most helpful.

<u>Myotome testing technique:</u> Begin by asking the client to perform a movement as per instructions and hold an isometric contraction against therapist resistance for a count of 5.

C5- Shoulder abduction Ask the patient to raise both their arms to the side of them simultaneously as strongly as then can while the examiner provides resistance to this movement. Compare the strength of each arm.

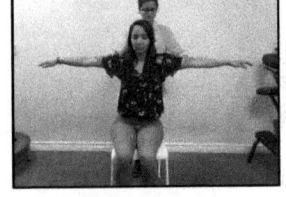

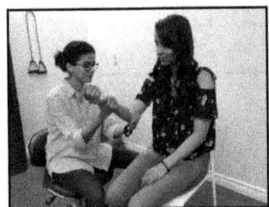

C6- Elbow flexion Test the strength of lower arm flexion by holding the patient's wrist from above and instructing them to "flex their hand up to their shoulder". Provide resistance at the wrist. Repeat and compare to the opposite arm. This tests the biceps muscle. Test the strength of wrist extension by asking the patient to extend their wrist while the examiner resists the movement. This tests the forearm extensors. Repeat with the other arm.

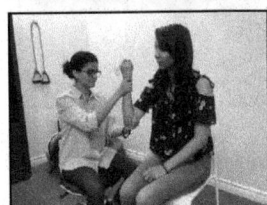

C7- Elbow extension Ask the patient to extend their forearm against the examiner's resistance. Begin their extension from a fully flexed position because this part of the movement is most sensitive to a loss in strength. This tests the triceps. Note any asymmetry in the other arm.

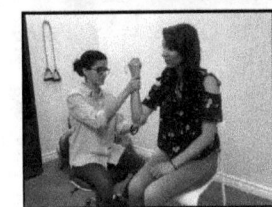

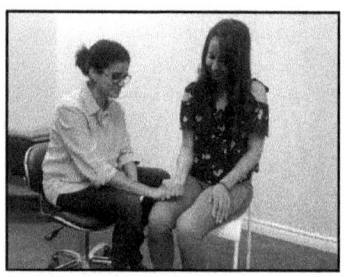 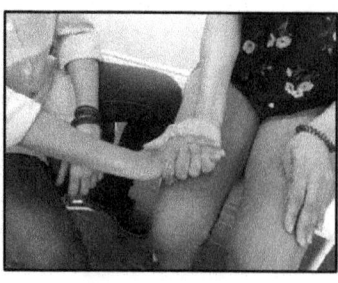

C8- Finger Flexion Examine the patient's hands. Look for intrinsic hand, thenar and hypothenar muscle wasting. Test the patient's grip by having the patient hold the examiner's fingers in their fist tightly and instructing them not to let go while the examiner attempts to remove them. Normally the examiner cannot remove their fingers. This tests the forearm flexors and the intrinsic hand muscles. Compare the hands for strength asymmetry. Finger flexion is innervated by the C8 nerve root via the median nerve.

T1- Finger abduction & adduction Test the intrinsic hand muscles once again by having the patient abduct or "fan out" all their fingers. Instruct the patient to not allow the examiner to compress them back in. Normally, one can resist the examiner from replacing the fingers. Finger abduction or "fanning" is innervated by the T1 nerve root via the ulnar nerve. Thumb Opposition To complete the motor examination of the upper extremities, test the strength of the thumb opposition by telling the patient to touch the tip of their thumb to the tip of their pinky finger. Apply resistance to the thumb with your index finger. Repeat with the other thumb and compare. Thumb opposition is innervated by the C8 and T1 nerve roots via the median nerve.

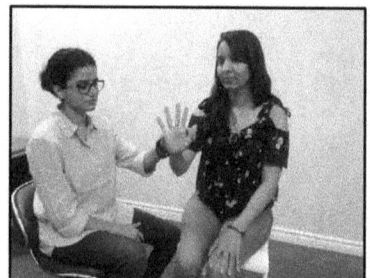

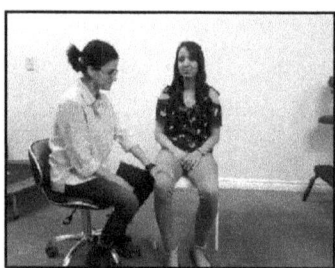 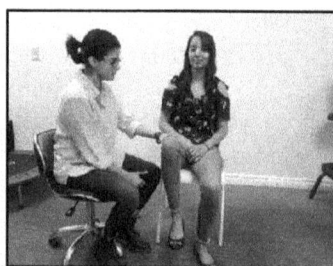

L1 & L2: Hip Flexion Proceeding to the lower extremities, first test the flexion of the hip by asking the patient to lie down and raise each leg separately while the examiner resists. Repeat and compare with the other leg. This tests the iliopsoas muscles.

L3 Test extension at the knee by placing one hand under the knee and the other on top of the lower leg to provide resistance. Ask the patient to "kick out" or extend the lower leg at the knee. Repeat and compare to the other leg. This tests the quadriceps muscle.

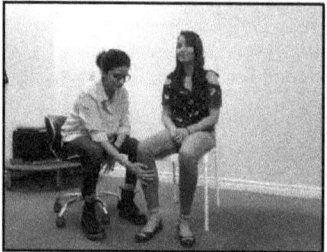 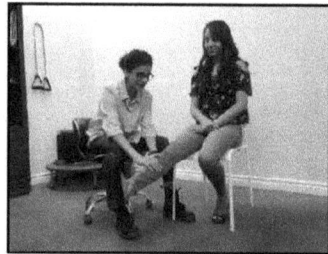

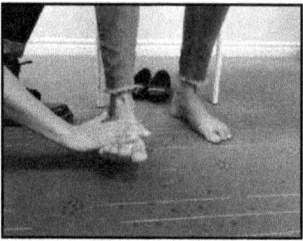 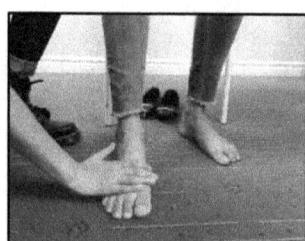

L4: Ankle Dorsiflexion Test dorsiflexion of the ankle by holding the top of the ankle and have the patient pull their foot up towards their face as hard as possible. Repeat with the other foot. This tests the muscles in the anterior compartment of the lower leg.

L5: Great toe extension Ask the patient to move the large toe against the examiner's resistance "up towards the patient's face". This tests the extensor hallucis longus muscle.

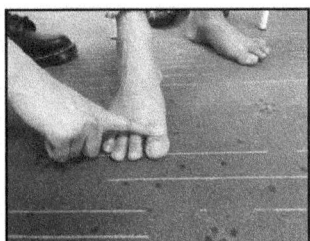 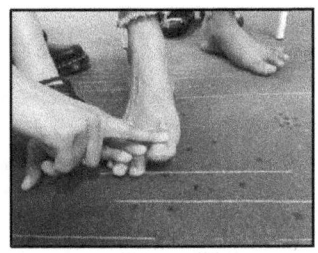

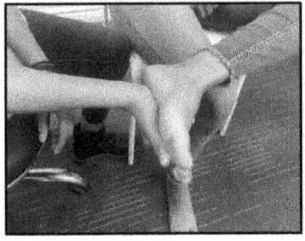 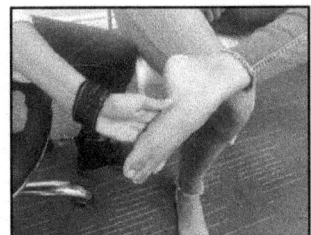

S1: Ankle plantar flexion and eversion/knee flexion holding the bottom of the foot, ask the patient to press down as hard as possible. Or in standing rise up onto the ball of their foot. Repeat with the other foot and compare. This tests the gastrocnemius and soleus muscles in the posterior compartment of the lower leg.

S2: Test flexion at the knee by holding the knee from the side and applying resistance under the ankle and instructing the patient to pull the lower leg towards their buttock as hard as possible. Repeat with the other leg. This tests the hamstrings.

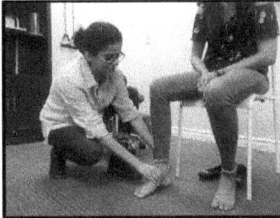 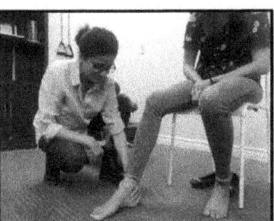

Self-test for neck pain

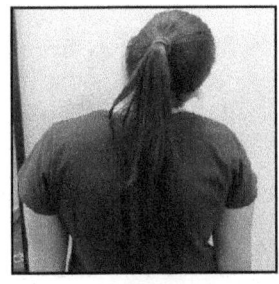 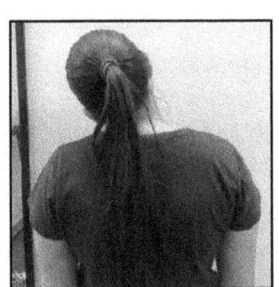

Look in your mirror and tip your ear to your shoulder. No, not bringing your shoulder to your ear; your ear/head are the only body parts that need to be moving. Each side should be equal. If you cannot bend your neck any of the side shows tightness and limited neck mobility.

Pretend that you are checking your blind spots. You need to look over your shoulders using your NECK ONLY. If you find that you are using your eyes only to check or moving your upper body, you are most likely struggling with rotation in your neck.

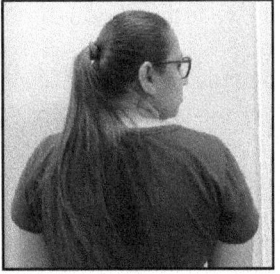 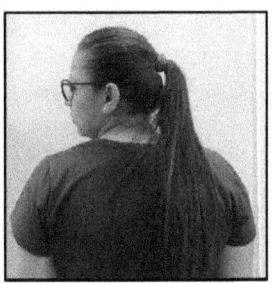

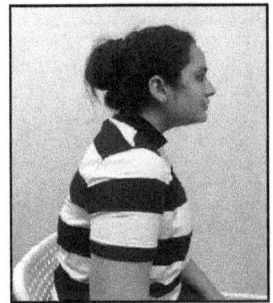

A lot of us suffer from something called 'anterior head carriage', meaning our head is carried out in front of our shoulders. Have someone compare the center of your shoulder with your ear canal. Ideally, the two should line up.

Upper extremity nerve glide test:
- Standing up straight, place the arm to be stretched out to your side with the palm facing up.
- Slowly bend your wrist down towards the ground keeping the palm up.
- Then tilt your head away from the arm being stretched and notice any change in sensation,
- Then tilt your head towards the side being stretched and observe any change.

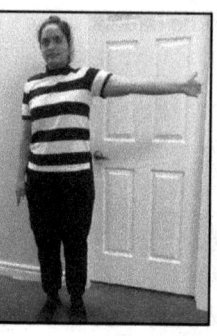 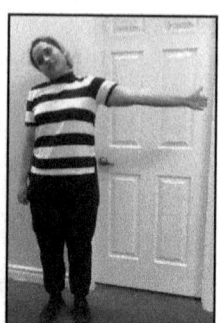

Negative test: No significant change in pulling or symptoms down the arm when moving the neck.
Positive test: If your pain symptoms get worse when tilting the head away from the arm and better when tilting the head to the side of the outstretched arm. It shows the nerve root is under excessive tension at the neck.

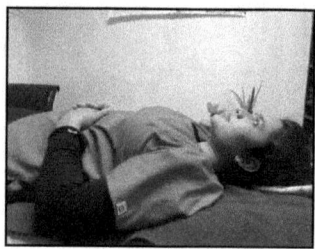 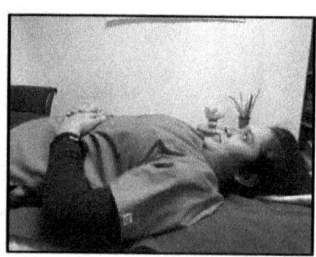

Chin tuck, lift, and hold:
Begin the test by lying flat with nothing under your head. You may bend your knees to allow the natural curve in your lower back. Begin by tucking your chin and then raising the head off the floor about 1 inch maintaining the tucked position. Hold the position, if possible, without letting the chin protrude or the head to drop back the floor. May attempt up to 3 times, taking 3-minute rests between attempts.
Negative test: Able to maintain proper testing position for the duration of the exercise. Men – 38 seconds and women: 30 seconds
Positive test: Unable to maintain testing position for required duration or without pain. It indicates weakness of the deep neck stabilizers muscles placing increased stress on ligaments and disc in the neck.

Self-distraction:
- This can be performed in standing or sitting.
- With your hands feel for the two bony bumps at the back of the skull, place the base of your thumbs on these points and interlace the fingers.
- Gently squeeze your hands around the base of the skull and move the hands up, you may also slightly tilt the chin to your chest while you do this.
- Maintain for up to 30 seconds and take notice of any changes in pain or symptoms.

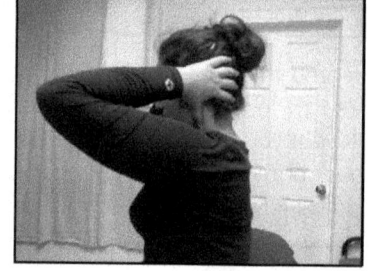

Negative test: This test is negative when lifting your head does not decrease any pain/symptoms in the neck or into the arms.
Positive test: This test is positive when lifting your head up relieves the pain or arm symptoms by at least 50%. This indicates something is compressing the nerve root as they run down your neck.

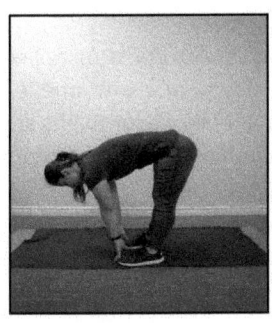 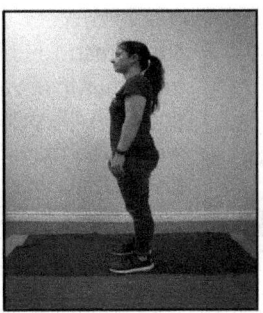

The forward bend test: Stand up straight with your hands at your side. Bend forwards and reach to your toes as far as you can go.

Negative test: Your low back pain does not get worse when you bend over the waist.

Positive test: If your pain gets worse bending over the test is positive. If the pain goes down the back of the leg, your pain might be caused by a disc irritation, a nerve root irritation or facet joint irritation.

Quadrant test:
- Stand up straight with your hands on your waist.
- Bend your spine backwards (extension) then side bend and rotate to the side of your spine that you have pain.
- Repeat this on the opposite side as well.

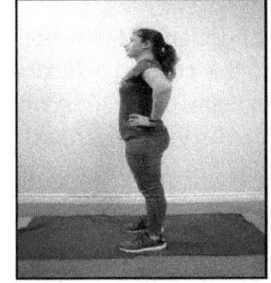 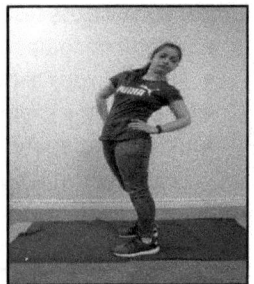

Negative test: This test is negative if the position does not reproduce your pain.

Positive test: If you get into the testing position and the test reproduces your low back pain. It indicates that there is facet joint irritation. If it radiates down the leg, it means that there is likely pressure being put on the nerve roots that are coming out of your spinal cord.

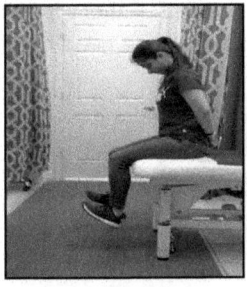 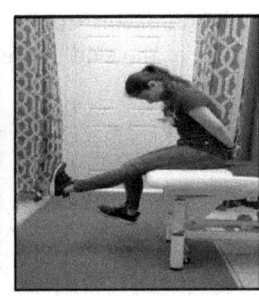

Slump test:
Sit at the edge of a table or chair.
Slouch over and tuck your chin down to your chest.
Bring one of your ankles into dorsiflexion
Straighten your knee until you feel a pull anywhere from your low back to bottom of your foot.
Most people will feel a pull behind the knee.
Once you feel a pull, look up towards the ceiling.

Negative test: This test is negative when lifting your head does not decrease the stretch/ pull/ pain in the back of the leg when you lift your head up.

Positive test: This test is positive when lifting your head up relieves the pain by at least 50%. It indicates the nerve are being pressed and are not moving smoothly in the path.

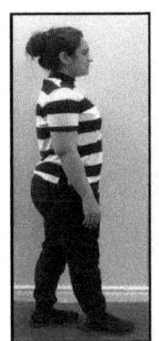 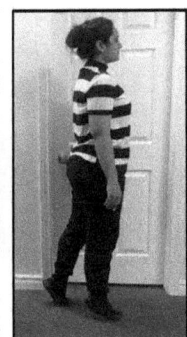

Heel walk: Try walking on your heels, keeping the toes off the floor. If you are unable to keep one of your feet from dropping flat to the floor, you might have damage caused by nerve at L4 and L5 disc level.

Toe walk: Try walking on your toes, keeping the heels of both feet off the floor. If the heel of one-foot falls to the floor and you are unable to walk on your toes, you may have nerve damage due to L5 disc herniation.

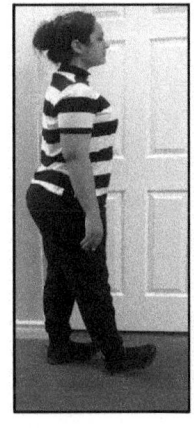 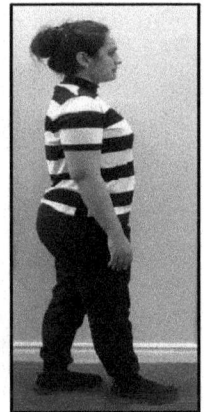

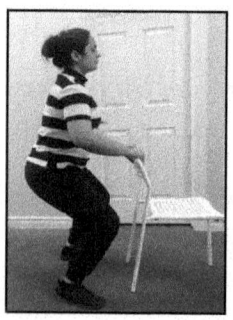 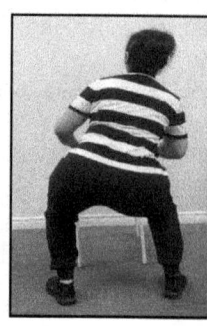 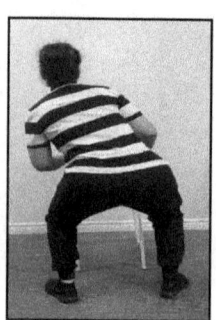

Squat test: Hold on to a bedpost or railing and squat halfway down, first with one leg and then the other. If one of your thighs are weak, you may have nerve damage from a disc herniation in upper back.

Lumbar canal stress test:
- Stand in an upright position and raise your hands above
- Extend your back in this position and come back to starting position.
- Repeat the same movement for 30 seconds.
- If you experience pain in your lower back than there is narrowing of your spinal canal which is putting pressure on your nerves, causing spinal canal stenosis

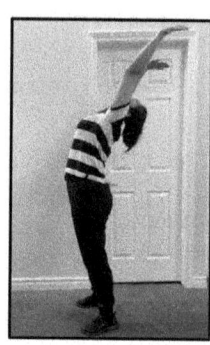

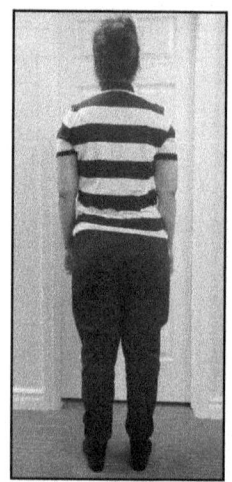 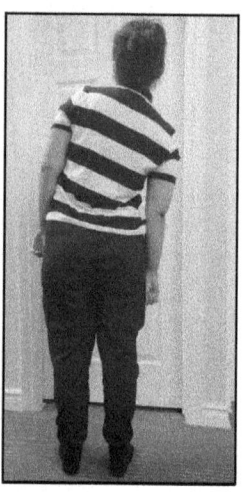

Spinal Curvature examination:
Stand straight in front of the mirror.
Observe your shoulder level. If they are not aligned, then there could be possibility of scoliosis in your upper back.
Also, look to your lateral curvature undressed, if there is any extra fold on either of the side. If present can be bending of spine to that side.

Note: "People generally treat their back with rest and over-the-counter medicines. But back pain usually should include some resting positions, home remedies, exercises, proper food, and nutrition. We will provide you with a complete 24 hours guide stepwise approach to treat your pain and differentiate with other conditions in the following chapters."

CHAPTER 3: RESTING POSITIONS FOR SPINAL ALIGNMENT

Most cases of back pain stem from strain or sprain due to simple overuse, unaccustomed activity, excessive lifting, or an accident. In most cases the best move is to wait and see if the pain resolves on its own. Rest from strenuous activity like heavy lifting, twisting, high intensity workouts, dancing and activities that involves rapid movement of spine.

Why are resting positions important?
- It allows time for recovery which is essential for muscle growth
- Prevent muscle fatigue
- Reduce risk of further injury to muscle
- Resting Positions can help you get better sleep by letting your hormones return to a normal, balanced state.
- It increases energy levels
- It reduces tension of your body muscles
- It reduces muscle pain after exercises
- Keeps your spine aligned
- Reduces tension headaches
- Helps reducing pain caused by chronic condition by reducing pressure and compression
- Relieves sinus buildup
- Putting pillow under knees help balance the body and reduces pressure on lumbar spin

There are some specific positions which can be incorporated and will relieve stress from the spine. It will help the surrounding muscles to relax.

Position 1: Sleep on your back, put a small pillow under the back of your knees and neck. It will reduce stress on your spine and support the natural curve in your lower back. The pillow for your head should support your head, the natural curve of your neck, and your shoulders.

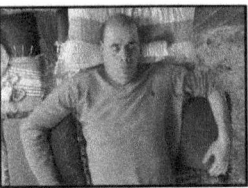 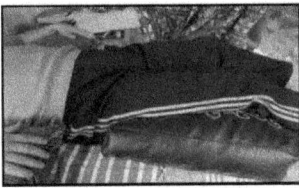 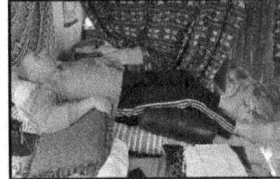 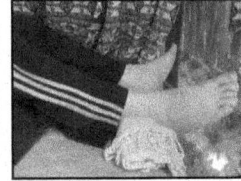

Position 2: Placing a flat pillow under the stomach and pelvis area which will help to keep the spine in better alignment. If you sleep on your stomach, a pillow for your head should be flat, or sleep without a pillow. This will help reduce stress on your spine.

Position 3: Sleep on your side, place a firm pillow between your knees will prevent your upper leg from pulling your spine out of alignment and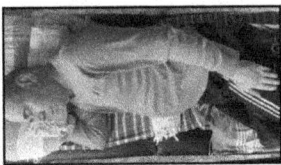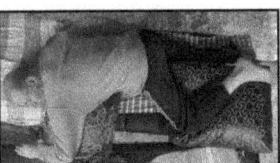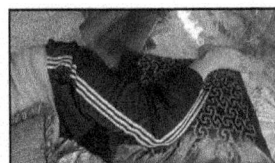
reduce stress on your hips and lower back. Pull your knees up slightly toward your chest. The pillow for your head should keep your spine straight. Putting a rolled towel or small pillow under your waist may also help support your spine.

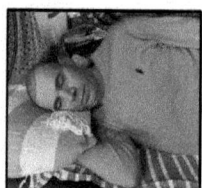 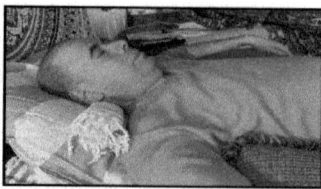

Position 4: Take a small, hand-sized bath towel and fold it lengthwise in half. Roll it up firmly so it has a diameter of 3 to 5 inches and use rubber bands or duct tape to hold it tightly together. Put this roll at the space between your pillow and neck or you can directly put it under your neck. This will reduce stress on your neck

Position 5: Lie down flat on the ground. Put a chair near your legs. Bend you hip and knee to 90 degrees and place your lower legs on the chair. This position will straighten the curvature at lower back and relieve any extra stress.

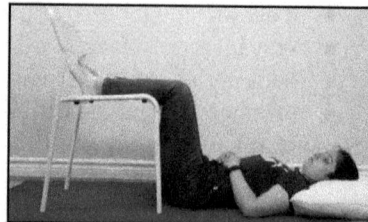

CHAPTER 4: HEAT AND COLD THERAPY

We treat everything from arthritis to muscle soreness to inflammation with icepacks or heating pads. Topical application of ice or heat can bring a surprising level of pain relief for most types of back pain. But the tricky part is knowing what situation calls for hot, and which calls for cold. Sometimes it includes both. As general rule of thumb, use ice for acute injuries or pain, along with inflammation and swelling. Use heat for muscle pain or stiffness.

Cold Therapy

How it works?
It helps improving the reduced blood flow to an injured area. This slows the rate of inflammation and reduces the risk of swelling and tissue damage. Acts as a local anesthetic. It slows down the pain messages being transmitted to the brain. Helps treat a swollen and inflamed joint or muscle. It is most effective within 48 hours of an injury.

Homemade Ice pack
- A frozen towel. To make a towel into a cold pack, place a folded, damp towel in a plastic bag and put it in the freezer for ten to twenty minutes. Then take the towel out of the bag and place it on the affected area.
- Sponge. Wet a sponge and put in the freezer. After it is frozen, take it out and put it in a baggie, then wrap it in a sock or a towel before applying it to the sore back.
- Rice. Another alternative is to fill a sock with rice and place it in the freezer, as rice will get as cold as ice but does not melt when used.
- Gel-type pack. Still another alternative is to fill a bag with liquid dishwasher detergent and freeze it, which gives it a consistency of a gel pack.
- Frozen bag of peas. If ice is needed quickly, it is easy to grab a bag of frozen peas or other vegetables out of the freezer, wrap it in a towel and apply it to the painful area.

Steps to make homemade ice pack at home:
- Place ice cubes in a big bowl and put some cold water in it.
- You can put some herbs like oregano, mint, lemon juice and vinegar to the water for pain relief.
- Take a washcloth or hand towel, and dip it in the ice-cold water.
- Now squeeze the towel with your hands to drain excess water.
- Place the homemade compress on your skin for up to 15 minutes.
- Dry the area with a towel after you're done.
- Reapply: For swelling, reapply the compress after two hours

How can you use ice?

- A cold compress should be applied to the inflamed area for 20 minutes every 4-6 hours for 3 days. Massaging the area with an ice cube or an ice pack in a circular motion from two to five times a day, for a maximum of 5 minutes only, to avoid ice burns.
- Helpful during the first 48 hours following an injury or stress that strains the muscles.
- Always check the area every 5 minutes to avoid ice burns.

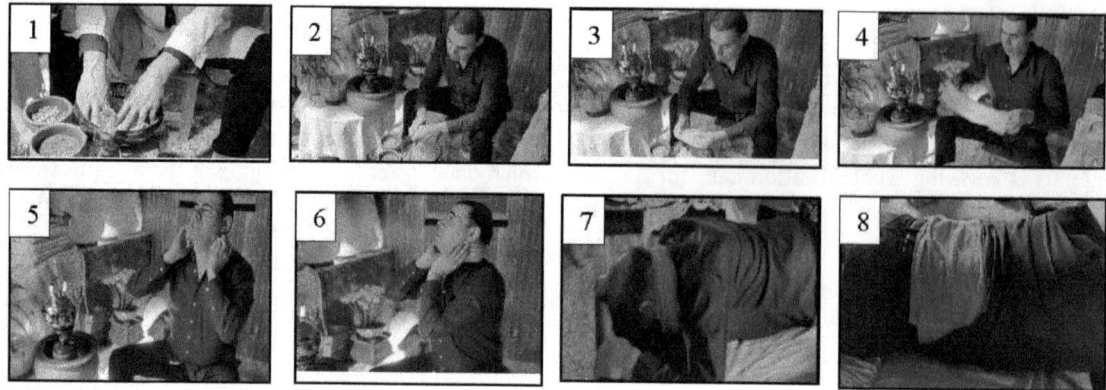

When not to use ice?
- If there is an open wound or blistered skin
- If you have vascular disease or injury
- Hypersensitive to cold
- Should not be applied directly to skin or bones as can lead to frostbite

Heat Therapy

How it works?
"Warm" is the proper temperature. It should be between 76° to 82° Celsius. Improves circulation and blood flow to a particular area due to increased temperature. Relax and soothe muscles and heal damaged tissue. Increases flexibility

Homemade heat packs
- Hot water bottle – tends to stay warm for 20-30 minutes
- Electric heating pad – maintains a constant level of heat if it is plugged in.
- Warming or heated blanket which could be wrapped around.
- Commercial adhesive wrap that sticks to the back and provides several hours of low-level heat.
- Fill a sock with rice and heat it in a microwave.
- Moist hot towel can be used for moist heat.

How can you use heat?
The duration that one needs to apply the heat is based on the type of and or magnitude of injury. For very minor back tension, short amount of heat therapy may be sufficient such as 15-20 minutes. For intense injuries, longer sessions of low-level of heat may be more beneficial such as 30 minutes to 2 hours or more. Applied to head and forehead which reduces spasms and relieves headache. If you are diabetic or having any underlying skin conditions, always check after every 5 minutes for burns.

How to prepare hot pack with a towel:
1. Fill the bowl with water that feels hot, but not scalding, to the touch.
2. You can put some herbs like oregano, mint, 2 teaspoons of salt, freshly squeezed lemon and 2 teaspoons of vinegar.
3. Soak the towel in the hot water, wringing out the excess.
4. Fold the towel into a square and apply it to the area that's in pain.
5. Hold the towel to your skin for up to 20 minutes at a time.

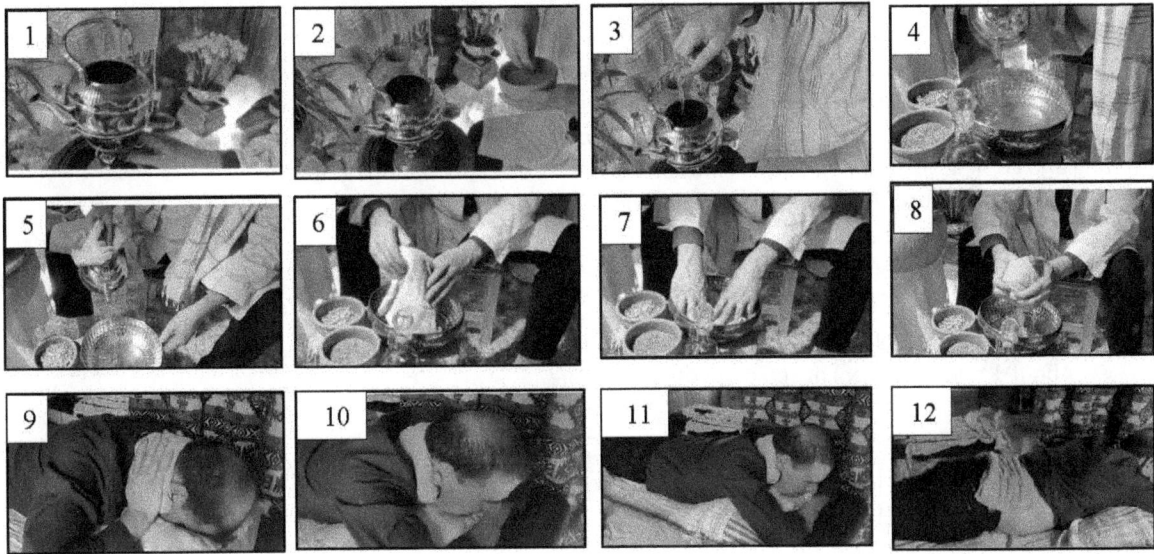

When not to use heat:
- If you have swelling or bruises on the area to the applied
- Diabetes as the skin becomes more sensitive and there is chance of getting burns. Check at regular interval for burns in this case.
- Open wound
- Vascular conditions

Contrast Bath:
Contrast bath therapy is a physical therapy treatment in which all or part of the body is immersed first in hot water, then in ice water, and then the procedure of alternating hot and cold is repeated several times. The contrast bath can help improve circulation around your injured tissue. This is one of many whirlpool treatments physical therapists use to help decrease pain and muscle spasm, increase range of motion and strength, and improve functional mobility.

Goals of Treatment
The goals of treatment will most likely include:
- Decreased pain
- Decreased swelling
- Controlled inflammation
- Improved mobility

How does contrast bath therapy work?
The key to contrast bath therapy is in the rapid changes produced in your circulatory system when you go from very warm water to very cold water. When you submerge part or all of your body in cold water, small blood vessels called capillaries respond to the cold by getting smaller. This is known as vasoconstriction. When you immerse yourself in warm water, the opposite happens. Your blood vessels open up. This is known as vasodilation. This rapid opening and closing of blood vessels near the site of your injury creates a pumping action that's thought to help decrease swelling and inflammation around injuries. Decreasing the swelling and inflammation helps alleviate pain and improve mobility.

How Contrast Bath Therapy Is Administered?
To perform a contrast bath, you need two tubs. One tub should be filled with warm water, and one tub with cold. The warm tub should be between 98-110 degrees Fahrenheit, and the cold tub should be 50-60 degrees Fahrenheit. Once both tubs are the correct temperature, you have to place your injured body part

in the warm tub first, where it should stay for 3-4 minutes. You can do gentle motion exercises during that time. You'll then quickly move the part being treated to the cold tub or bucket. Typically, you'll stay in the cold water for about one minute. This sequence of moving from warm to cold and back again is generally repeated for 20-30 minutes. Contrasting should follow the following basic pattern: three to six alternations between heating and cooling.

- About 2 minutes of heating: comfortably hot
- About 1 minute of cooling: cool, not cold
- About 2 minutes of heating: hotter!
- About 1 minute of cooling: colder!
- About 2 minutes of heating: hot as you can handle
- About 1 minute of cooling: cold as you can handle

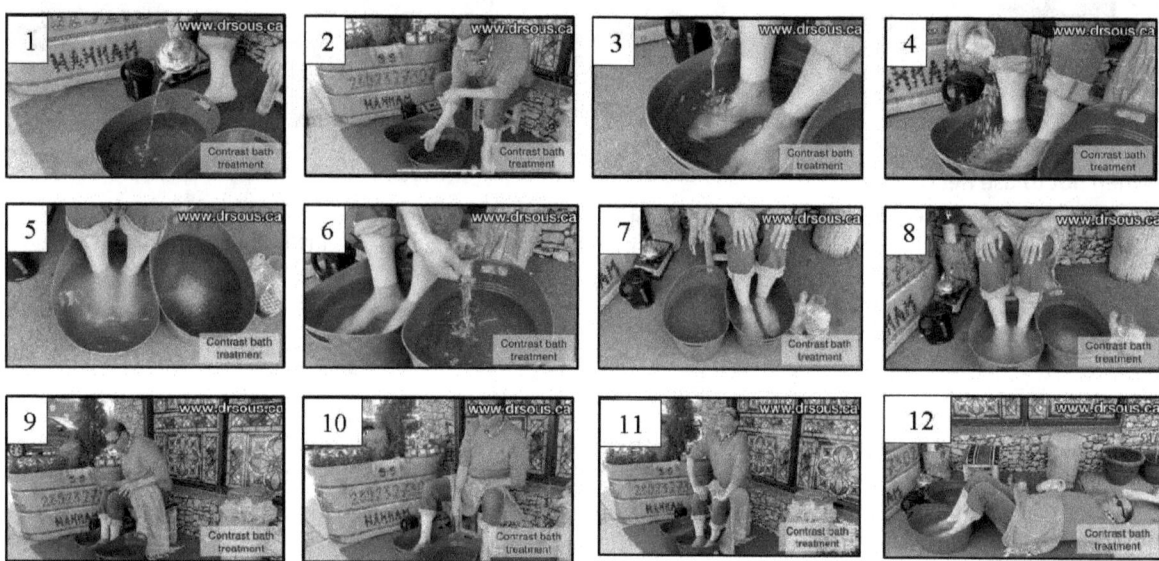

A few tips and rules of thumb for contrast bathing
- Stay warm. You generally want to be more thorough with your heat: at least a minute, but if five minutes depending on how efficient your heating method is. Heat is more comforting and relaxing than cooling, obviously, and inadequate heating is the most common thing people do wrong with contrasting.
- Finish with cold. You should usually finish a contrast session with cold, particularly if you suspect that you might be a little inflamed. Never finish with heat if you're concerned about aggravating inflammation. You might choose to finish with heat if your priority is to have a more relaxing experience.
- Stretch when hot. If you choose to stretch, do it after or even during the heating.

Tips to combine heat and cold therapy in daily routine:
- Keep a heat patch near your bed and use it first thing in the morning to warm up your muscles if you wake up with an achy or stiff back.
- Apply a cold patch before bed if you have exerted your back.
- Use heat therapy after and before sleep if suffering from chronic pain.
- Carry a couple of self-activating heat patches and ice packs in your bag or car while driving or at work.

CHAPTER 5: GENERAL STRETCHING TECHNIQUES

Why stretching is important?

Stretching keeps the muscles flexible, strong, and healthy, and we need that flexibility to maintain a range of motion in the joints. Without it, the muscles shorten and become tight. Then, when you call on the muscles for activity, they are weak and unable to extend all the way. That puts you at risk for joint pain, strains, and muscle damage.

Which muscles should you stretch?
As a rule, if it's not tight and it's not causing you any problems, you don't need to stretch it.

When to Stretch?

Most people understand the importance of stretching as part of a warm-up or cool-down, but when else should you stretch? Stretch periodically throughout the entire day. It is a great way to stay loose and to help ease the stress of everyday life. If you want to improve your range of motion, when is the best time to stretch? One of the best times to stretch is after your exercises, as part of your cool-down. Another great time to stretch is just before going to bed. This works at a neuromuscular level, as the increased muscle length is the last thing your nervous system remembers before going to sleep. Sleep is also the time when your muscles and soft tissues heal, which means your muscles are healing in an elongated, or stretched position.

Stretches for neck and upper back

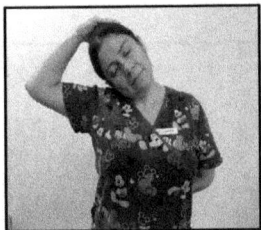 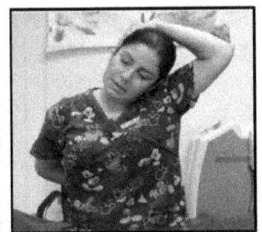

Sides of neck stretch – Put your hand overhead and bend your head to the side. Hold the position for 10 seconds and repeat it for 3-4 times on both the sides.

Posterior neck stretches – Clasp your hands and put it behind your head. Pull your head down gently, keeping your back straight. Hold the position for 10 seconds and repeat it for 3-4 times.

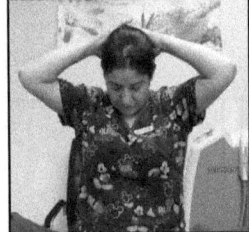 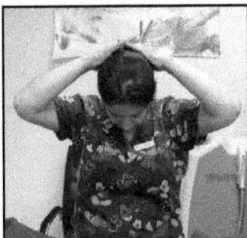

Rotation stretches – Look at an ankle of 45 degrees, put your hand on the head. Pull your head down diagonally and hold for 10 seconds. Repeat for 3-4 times.

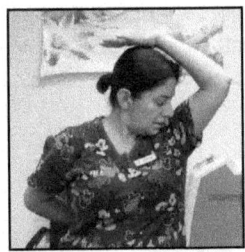 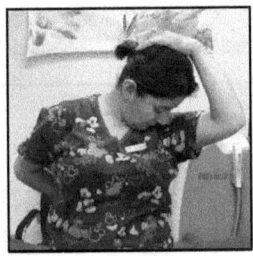 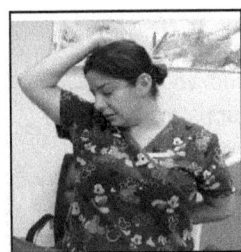 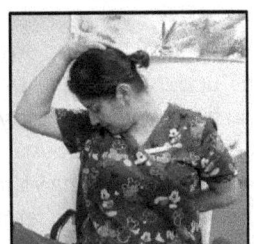

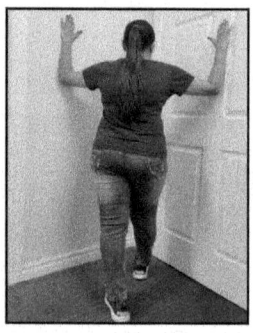 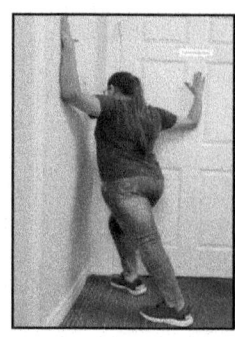

Upper chests stretch – Take a corner of the wall. Stand with your elbows rested on the wall with one leg forwards as a stance position. You need to open your chest while moving forward and close to the wall. Hold the position for 10 seconds and repeat it for 3-4 times

Stretches to relieve your nerve compression: To stretch the median nerve, place open palm on wall with fingertips pointing away from trunk and parallel to the floor. Rotate trunk away from wall keeping the elbow straight and feel the stretch in arm and forearm. Return to the starting position and repeat on the other side.

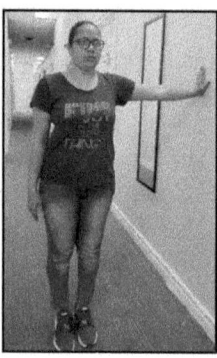 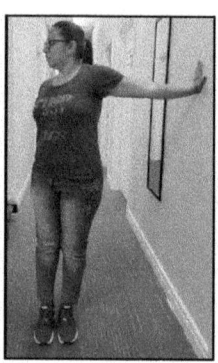 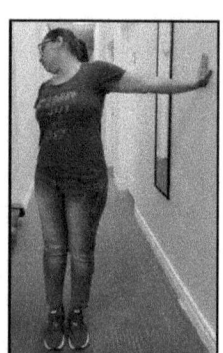

Straighten your arm with your palm facing down and bend your wrist so that your fingers point down. Gently pull your hand toward your body until you feel a stretch on the outside of your forearm. Hold the stretch for 15 seconds. Repeat 5 times, then perform this stretch on the other arm.

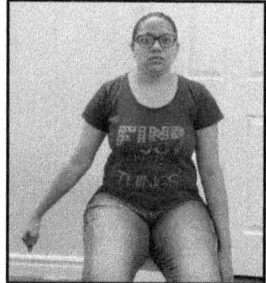 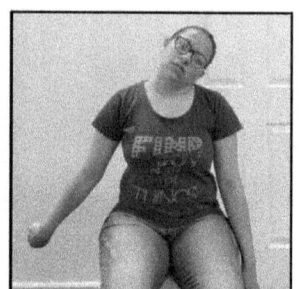

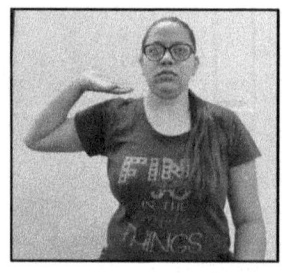 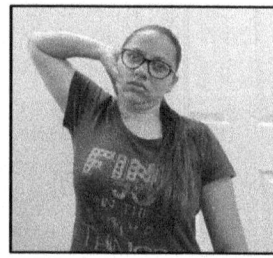

While keeping your head in a neutral position begin with your arm out, palm side of the hand facing up. Bend the elbow toward you, palm side facing you. Rotate the palm of your hand outward and bend your wrist so that the fingers are pointing towards you. Hold the stretch for 15 seconds. Repeat 5 times, then perform this stretch on the other arm.

Child pose - Begin in tabletop position on your hands and knees, with your hands directly under your shoulders and knees under your hips. Extend your arms out in front of you, placing your palms flat on the floor. Slowly sit your hips back toward your heels, dropping your head and chest downward as your arms extend further and reach for the wall in front of you. If this stretch is too much, place a

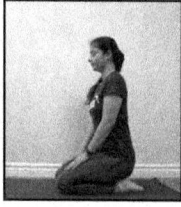 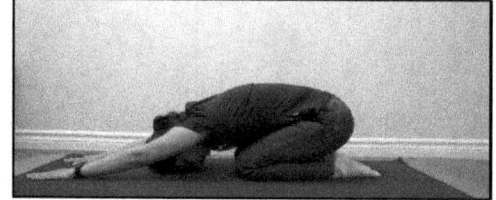

pillow under your belly to prop yourself up a bit and lessen the stretch of the low-back muscles. Hold this pose for 20 to 30 seconds or even longer.

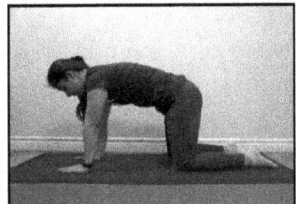 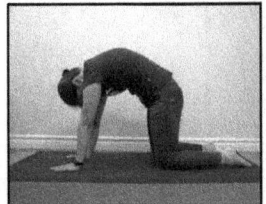 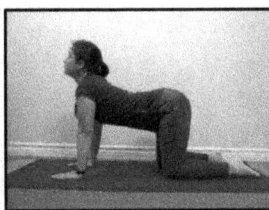

Cat and cow stretch - Begin in tabletop position on your hands and knees, with your hands directly under your shoulders and knees under your hips. Your spine should be parallel to the ground in this position. Then, round your back, stretching your mid-back between your shoulder blades—like how a cat stretches by rounding its back. Hold for five seconds, then relax and let your stomach fall downward as you gently arch your low back and hold here for another five seconds. Repeat these movements for 30 seconds or longer.

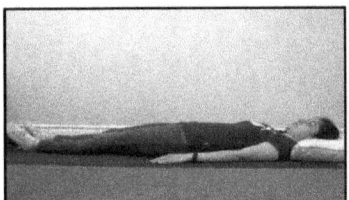 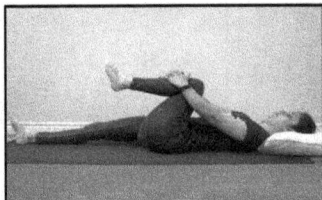

Knee to chest stretch - Begin by lying on your back with your knees bent and feet flat on the floor. Bring your hands to rest either behind your knees or right below your kneecaps. Slowly bring both knees toward your chest, using your hands to gently pull your knees. Hold here 20 to 30 seconds and try rocking your hips side to side and up and down to help massage your low back, then return to starting position.

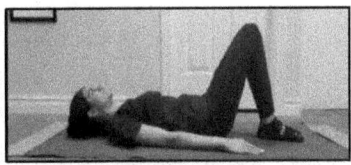

Supine figure of 4 stretch - Lie on your back on a yoga mat with both knees bent and feet planted on the floor. Lift your right leg, flex your right foot, and cross your right ankle over your left thigh. If this is enough stay here or draw your left knee in and hold behind your left thigh to increase the intensity. Hold for 10 to 15 breaths and then switch to the other side.

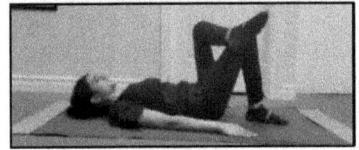 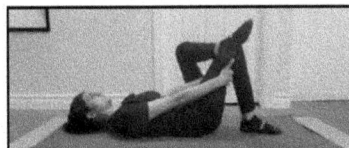 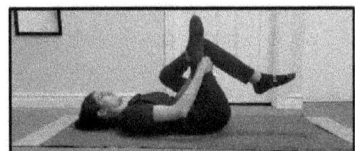

Hamstrings stretch lying down- Lie on your back and lift your right leg up towards your face. Interlace a towel behind your thigh or calf, depending on how tight your hamstrings feel. Keep your opposite leg active and your opposite hip grounded. Your head and shoulders should stay on 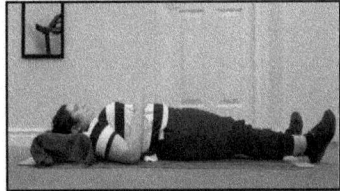 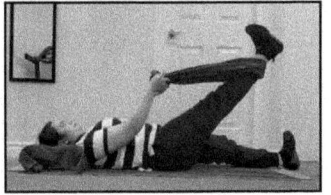 the ground. Hold for 10 breaths. Now, keeping your opposite hip grounded, let your right leg lower out to the right. Only lower the right leg out to the side so far as you can without the opposite hip lifting.

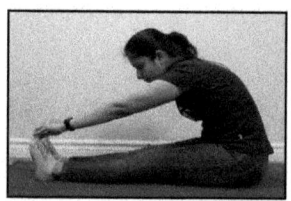 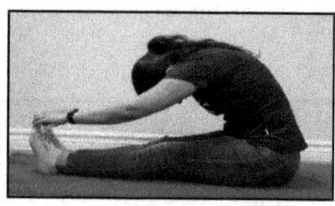

Hamstring stretch in sitting – Sit with your legs extended in front of you. Lean forward with your hands extended and try reaching your toes. Hold the position for 30 seconds. Repeat each for 3 times. Make sure you don't raise your knees while touching your toes.

Thoracic stretch (Thread in needle) – Begin in tabletop position on your hands and knees, with your hands directly under your shoulders and knees under your hips. Your spine should be parallel to the ground in this position. Take your hand and put it inside your opposite shoulder as if you are threading the needle. Reach until the end and hold the position for 30 seconds. You will feel a stretch at your mid back as if your spine is getting unlocked. Repeat this for 3 times on each side.

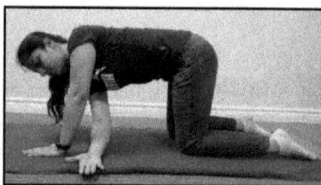 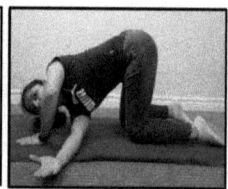 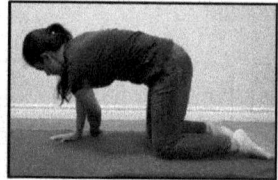 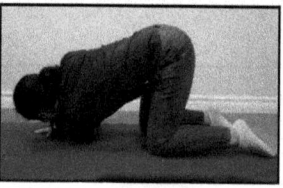

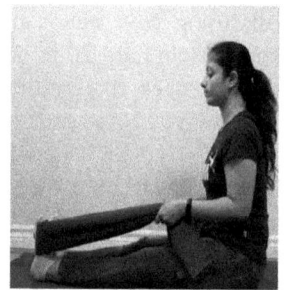

Calf stretches – Sit with your legs extended in front of you. Take a towel and hold it from your foot. Pull your ankle with the towel towards you. Hold the position for 30 seconds and repeat it for 3 times.

Bending Back - Stand pressing hands-on hips to support upper body, elbows lengthened away from armpits. Turn on inner core muscles to support body. Turn on lower buttock muscles to hold pelvis and hips still. Push upper body backwards, feeling breastbone sliding forward and upward. Hold on the position for 10 seconds.

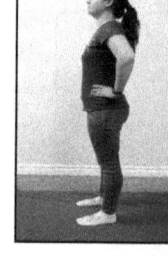 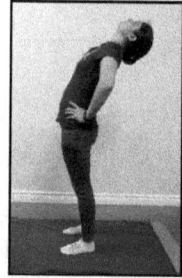

Thoracic stretch on chair – Place your hands on a chair. Walk backward, lowering your chest to the ground. Once your hips are behind your ankles, straighten your legs. Relax the muscles in the fronts of the thighs and gently lift your tailbone. Hold your arms in place and keep pressing your armpits toward the floor. Hold for five to 10 breaths. Take a short break, then repeat two or three times.

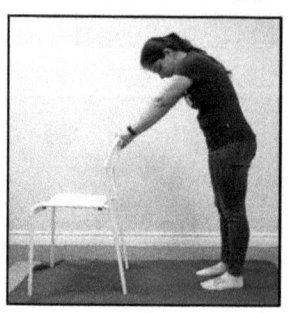 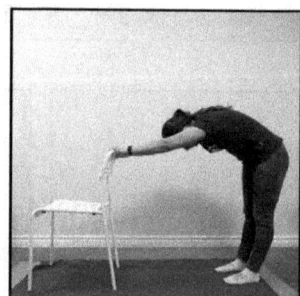

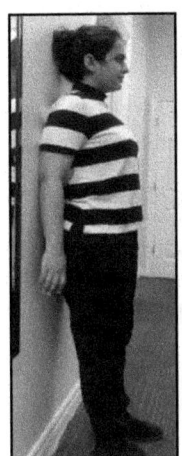 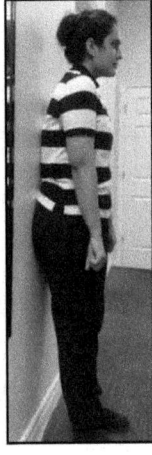

Back extension against wall - Stand against a wall, with your heels and buttocks touching the wall. Squeeze your shoulder blades together. Hold for 5 seconds, then relax. Repeat.

Prone extensions - Lie on your stomach. Slowly prop yourself up on your elbows so your chest is off the ground. If you're able, straighten your arms. Hold for 10 to 20 seconds, then return to start position. Repeat.

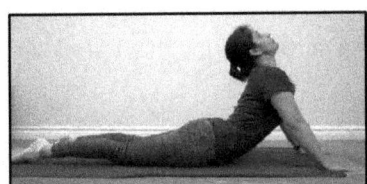 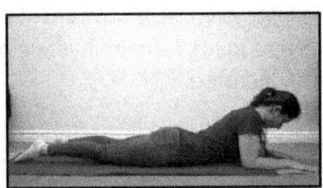

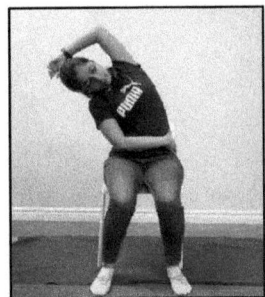 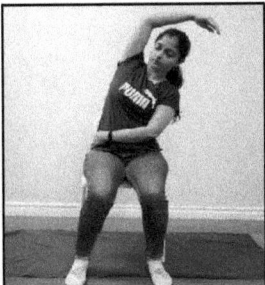

Side stretches in sitting - To start, sit in a chair with your feet flat on the floor. Shift your weight slightly forward to avoid rounding your back. Relax. Keep your ears, shoulders, and hips aligned. Stretch your right arm overhead. Slowly bend to the left. Don't twist your torso. Stay within your pain limits. Hold for 20 seconds. Return to starting position. Repeat 2 to 5 times. Then, switch to the other side.

Side stretches in standing - To start, stand with your feet flat on the floor. Keep your ears, shoulders, and hips aligned. Stretch your right arm overhead. Slowly bend to the left. Don't twist your torso. Stay within your pain limits. Hold for 20 seconds. Return to starting position. Repeat 2 to 5 times. Then, switch to the other side.

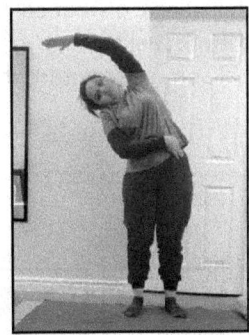 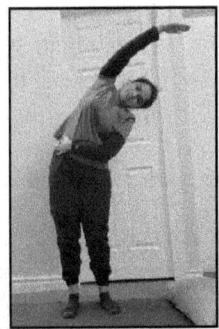

CHAPTER 6: GENERAL MOBILITY EXERCISES

What is mobility / range of motion (ROM) exercises?
Range of motion (ROM) exercises are done to preserve flexibility and mobility of the joints on which they are performed. These exercises reduce stiffness and will prevent or at least slow down the freezing of your joints as the disease progresses and you move
less often.

Why is mobility exercise important?
If muscles and joints remain inactive for a certain period they can deteriorate over time and your range of motion will decrease.

Benefits of mobility exercises
- Improves Circulation
- Improves Muscle Strength
- Maintains Flexibility
- Reduces Pain
- Enhances Physical Performance
- Reduces Stiffness
- Decrease Injury Potential

Tips to follow while doing mobility exercises
- Do the exercises in the same order every time? Go from head to toe, to help you remember the series of moves. Start with neck stretches. Then exercise other body parts in order, moving toward your feet. Do each group of exercises on one side, and then do the same exercises on the other side.
- Move slowly, gently, and smoothly. Avoid fast or jerky motions.
- Try to achieve full range of motion by moving until you feel a slight stretch, but don't force a movement. Stop if you feel pain.
- It is normal to feel some discomfort at first. Regular exercise will help decrease the discomfort over time.

Here are some mobility exercises you can do to for pain relief

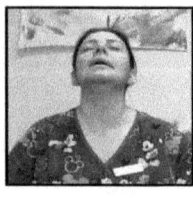 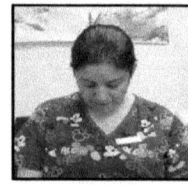 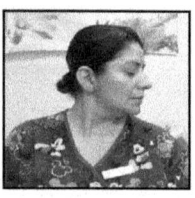
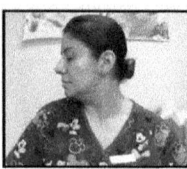 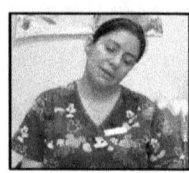 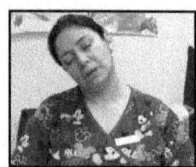

Neck mobility exercises - Do forward, backward, rotations and side bending of your neck. Repeat each movement for 10 times without hold. When you do the movements make sure you don't pull your neck more as it can aggravate the symptom.

Shoulder forward exercises - Raise your arm forward and then up over your head. Try to raise it so that your inner arm touches your ear. Bring your arm back down to your side.

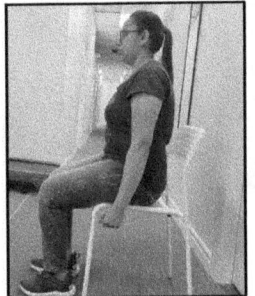 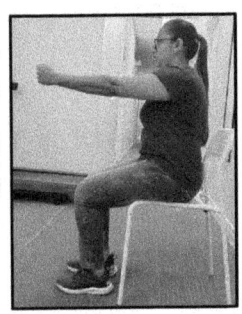

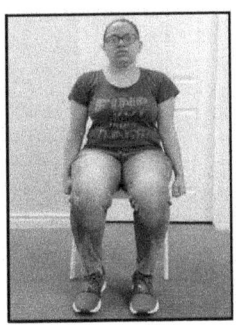 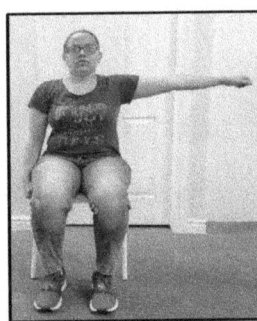

Shoulder side exercises - Raise your arm to the side and then up over your head as far as possible. Return your arm to your side.

Self-neck distraction – Hold on to your hand from the jaw. You need to pull the head upwards and outwards. Feel the stretch on to your neck and hold the position for 30 seconds.

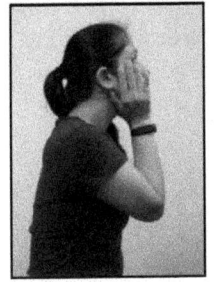

Self-traction for neck - Use the EDGE of a towel. Using the edge, and not the middle of or a folded-up towel is important as you don't want the towel to slip off your skin. Place the edge of the towel on the desired segment. Anchor the towel with the hand on the same side as your troublesome segment as shown. With your opposite hand, reach up and grab the edge of the towel. If you give it a slight tug, you should feel a pulling/stretching sensation behind your neck at the segment. You should not feel any of your symptoms. While pulling the towel (towards your opposite ear), turn your head towards your hand at the same time and hold this position for 3 seconds. Only turn your head in your pain-free range of motion. Your line of pull should be horizontal, to just below the eye. That's 1 rep. Now repeat 10 times.

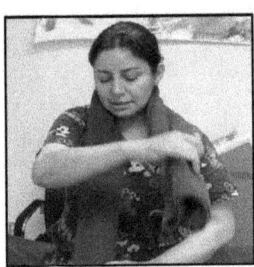 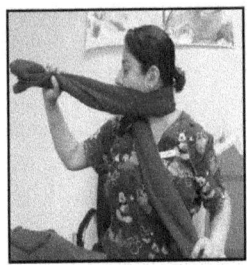 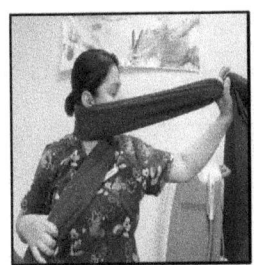 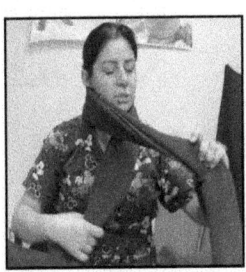

Pelvic tilts - Lie on your back with knees bent and feet flat on floor. Press the small of your back against the floor and tighten your stomach and buttock muscles. Do not push with your feet-all the pull should come from your abdominal muscles. This should cause the lower end of the pelvis to rotate forward and flatten your back against the floor.

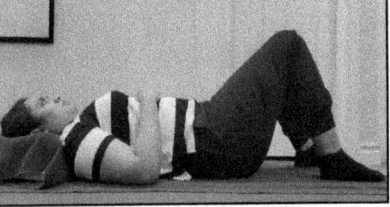

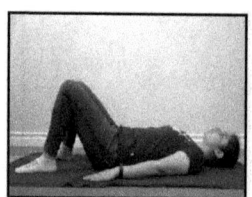 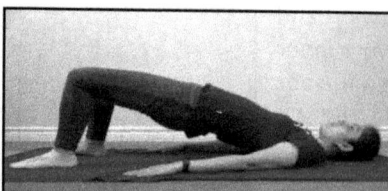

Bridging - Lie on your back with knees bent, shoulder width apart Turn on inner core muscles (press a large, rolled towel between inner thighs to increase and maintain their effort throughout the exercise). Turn on lower buttock muscles to lift hips off the mat, lengthening the thighs away from the belly. Keep inner core muscles on while lowering buttocks back onto mat.

Prone on elbow extensions with neck extension – Lie down on your stomach with weight on your elbow. Lift your upper body with the neck in upwards direction. Hold the position for 5 seconds and repeat it for 10 times

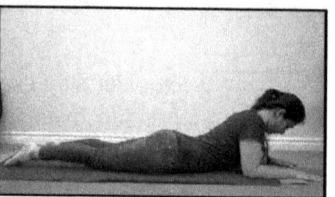 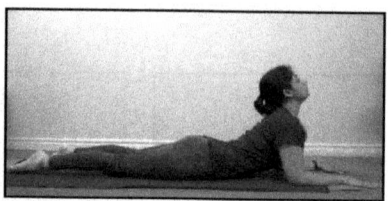

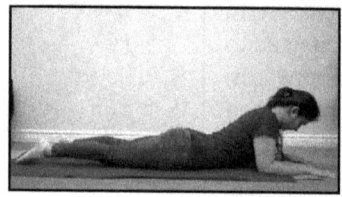 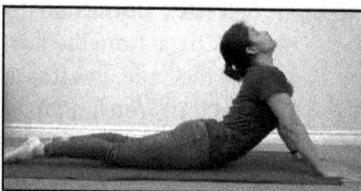

Prone extensions - Lie on your stomach. Slowly prop yourself up on your elbows so your chest is off the ground. If you're able, straighten your arms. Hold for 10 to 20 seconds, then return to start position. Repeat.

Lumbar flexion with rotation - Lie on your back with your hands at your side and your knees bent. Rotate your knees towards the sides.

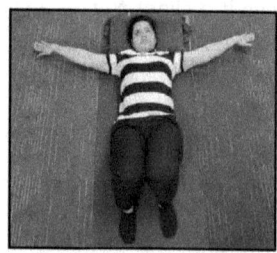 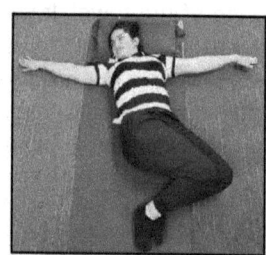 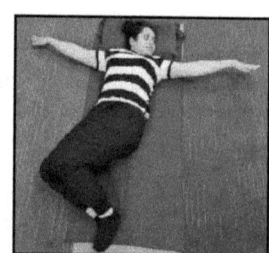

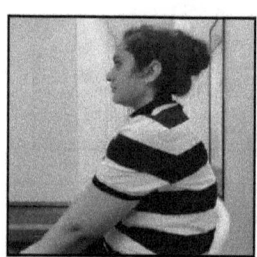 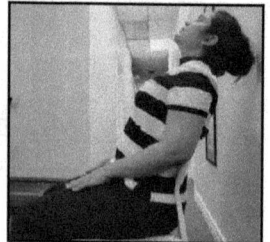

Seated thoracic extension - Sit upright in a chair, with your feet flat on the floor. Place your hands behind your head for support, with your elbows out to the sides. Keeping your head still, slowly roll the top of your spine over the back of the chair. Hold for 5 to 10 seconds, then return to start position. Repeat.

Bending Back - Stand pressing hands-on hips to support upper body, elbows lengthened away from armpits. Turn on inner core muscles to support body. Turn on lower buttock muscles to hold pelvis and hips still. Push upper body backwards, feeling breastbone sliding forward and upward. Hold on the position for 10 seconds.

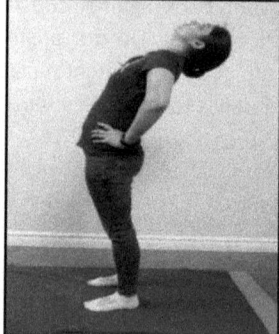 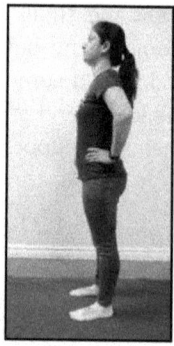

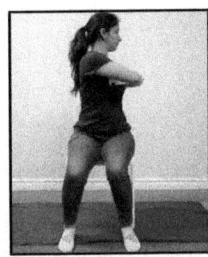 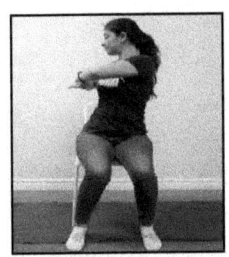

Seated Trunk rotations - Begin the exercise sitting straight on a chair, feet flat on the ground and your head facing forward. Place your left arm behind your left buttocks and your right hand on your left knee. Rotate your trunk looking over your left shoulder – holding when you feel a slight stretch but are still comfortable. Hold position for a few seconds. Swap sides and repeat exercise.

Cat and cow exercise - Begin in tabletop position on your hands and knees, with your hands directly under your shoulders and knees under your hips. Your spine should be parallel to the ground in this position. Then, round your back, stretching your mid-back between your shoulder blades—like how a cat stretches by rounding its back. Hold for five seconds, then relax and let your stomach fall downward as you gently arch your low back and hold here for another five seconds. Repeat these movements for 30 seconds or longer.

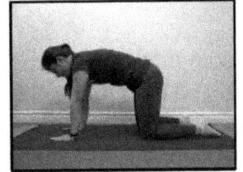 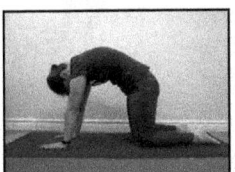

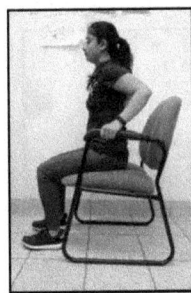 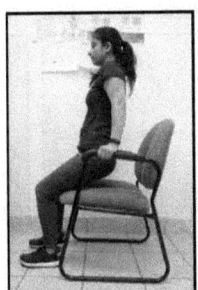

Self-lumbar traction in sitting - Sit in a chair with arm rests. Put your hands on the arm rests. Use your arms to push down until your bottom is slightly lifted from the chair. Hold the position for 30 seconds and repeat it for 3 times.

Self-lumbar traction in standing - Leaning forward over a countertop, support your upper body weight with your arms. Bend your knees and raise your heels. Hold the position for 30 seconds and repeat it for 3 times.

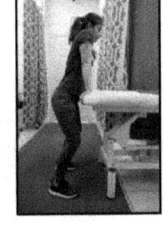

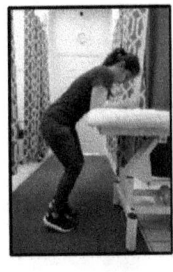 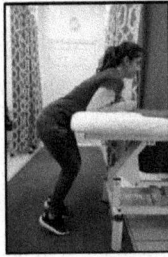

Self-back traction while leaning - Stand facing a sturdy desk, table, or countertop. Reverse your grip on the table and bring your body in contact with the side of the table, keeping your feet right under you. Keep your arms straight, with elbows locked, and sink your body weight, allowing your back to relax. Hold the position for 30 seconds and repeat it for 3 times.

Chair unloading traction for back - Stand between two sturdy chairs, placing your hands on the back of the chair. Keep your arms straight with elbows locked and sink your body weight, allowing your back to relax. Hold the position for 30 seconds and repeat it for 3 times.

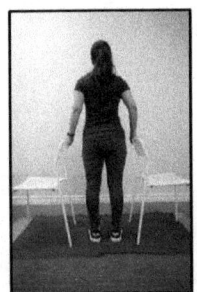 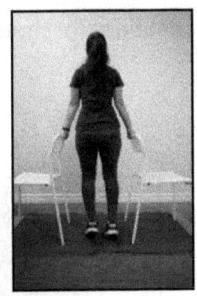

CHAPTER 7: GENERAL STRENGTHENING EXERCISES

What are strengthening exercises?
Strengthening exercises are exercises which are designed to increase the strength of specific or groups of muscles. Strengthening exercises overload the muscle until the point of muscle fatigue. This force and overload of a muscle encourages the growth, increasing the strength.
Here are some strengthening exercises you can follow,

Isometric neck exercises: Tuck your chin in and hold the position for 1o seconds. Repeat it for 10 times.

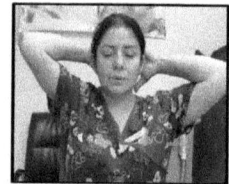 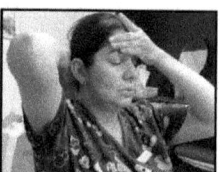
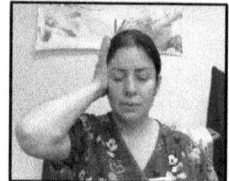 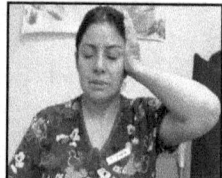

Place your hand on the forehead and tuck your chin in. Give a resistance force with your hand while pushing the head forward at the same time. Make sure there must be no movement, just you need to feel muscle contraction at the lower neck. Details are described in the chapter before. Similarly, put the hand on your side of head and repeat the same process.

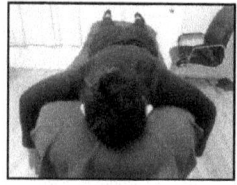 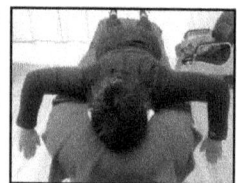

Backward shoulder shrugs - Lift the shoulders up toward the ears and then roll them back, down, and back to the starting position. Repeat this rolling motion for 10 repetitions for three sets.

Standing shoulder crunches - Stand facing the corner of a room. Place your hands on the adjacent surfaces of the wall. Drawing the shoulder blades together, lean forward toward the corner, then push away from the wall back into one's starting posture. Repeat for 10 repetitions for three set.

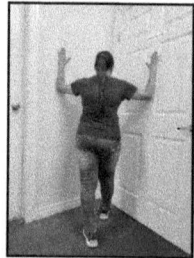 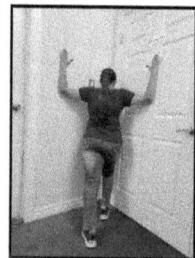

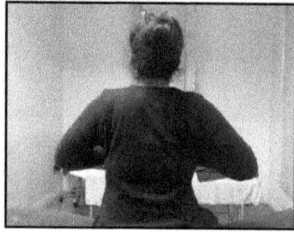 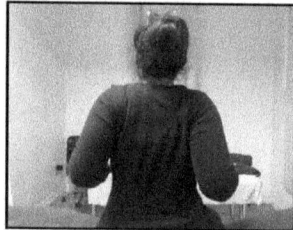 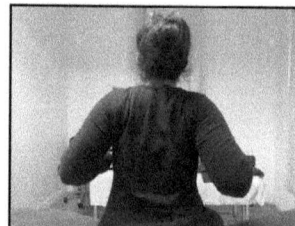

Scapular strengthening – Lie down on your tummy. Abduct your shoulder with elbows bend. Raise your shoulder up and hold the position. Make sure you keep your elbows bent.

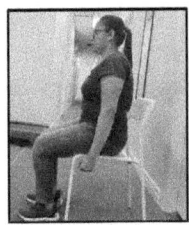 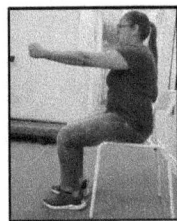

Shoulder flexor strengthening – Sit upright in a chair with your hands relaxed by your sides. Hold a weight in your weaker arm and elbows straight. Keeping your elbow straight, slowly lift your weaker arm up to 90 degrees and hold. Ensure your back and neck muscles remain relaxed as you move your arm. Hold for 10 seconds and repeat it for 10 times on both sides.

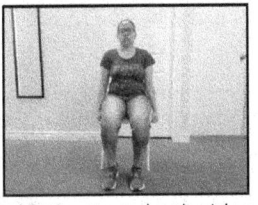 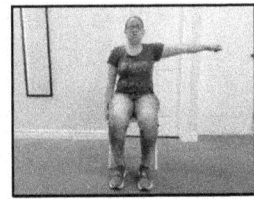

Shoulder abductor strengthening – Sit upright in a chair with your hands relaxed by your sides. Hold a weight in your weaker arm and keep your elbows straight. Keeping your elbow straight, slowly lift your weaker arm up to the side, away from your body up to 90 degrees. Hold for 10 seconds and repeat it for 10 times on both sides.

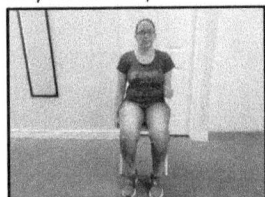 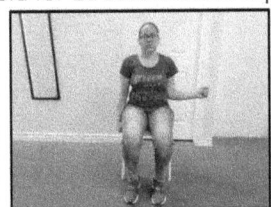

Shoulder rotator strengthening – In sitting position with weight in your hand and forearm supported, rotate arm towards stomach. support or weight in hand) and the elbow held at 90° make a fist and rotate the arm down towards the table in front of you. Try to keep shoulders and back straight.

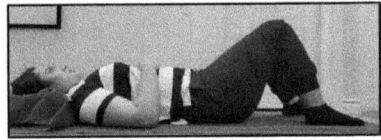

Buttock Squeeze – Lie on your back or your front with legs straight. Squeeze lower buttocks together gently, as if holding a pencil between your buttocks. Hold 6 seconds. Repeat 6 – 8 times.

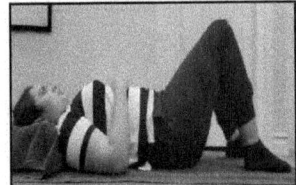 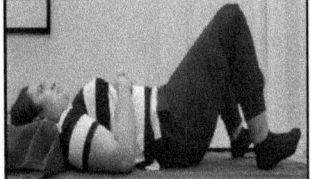

Heel Squeeze - Lie with pillow under belly button, legs apart. Bend knees and put heels together. Turn on core muscles. Keep core muscles engaged and heels pressed firmly together, slowly relax the lower buttock muscles. You would feel the muscles along the front thighs and hips release. Hold 6 seconds. Repeat 6 – 8 times.

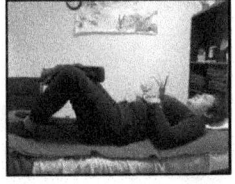

Adductor squeeze - Lean back with your weight on your elbows with your knees bent to about 90 degrees. Put a soft ball or similar-sized object between your knees. Squeeze the ball as hard as you comfortably can and hold for about 3 seconds. Relax and repeat for 10 repetitions.

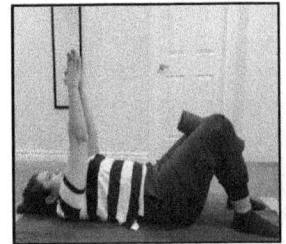 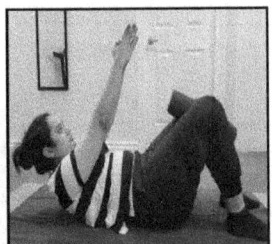

Partial sit ups - Lie on your back with your hands at your side and your knees bent. Use your abdominal muscles to raise your upper back off the floor, while exhaling. Rise up only enough to get your shoulder blades off the floor. Do not thrust yourself off the floor or lift your head with your arms. Keep your knees bent and your feet

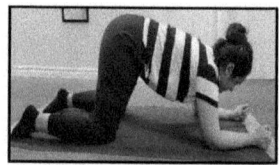 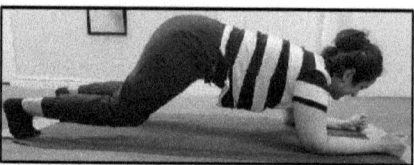

flat on the floor. You should feel the contraction only in your abdominal muscles. Gently lower your upper body down. Make the motions smooth and relaxed.

Short lever modified plank - Lie on belly, legs slightly apart Interlock fingers, place bent elbows behind shoulders. Bend knees and press heels firmly together using your lower buttock muscles. Turn on inner core muscles and hold chin in. Push through forearms and elbows to lift body off the floor, lengthening thighs away from hips. Hold the position for 20 seconds.

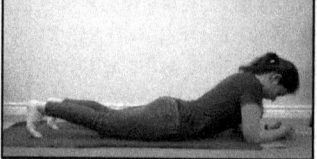 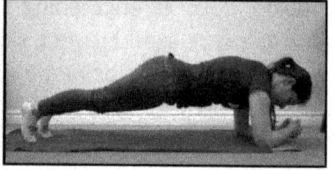

Straight leg plank - Straighten legs, press heels firmly together using lower buttock muscles, toes tugged under. Turn on inner core muscles and hold head in neutral (imagine holding peach under chin). Push through forearms and elbows to lift body off the floor. Lengthen thighs away from lower belly by pressing heels firmly together using lower buttock muscles.

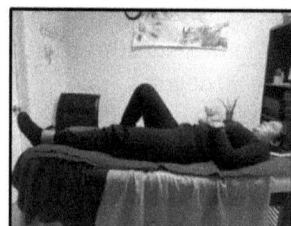 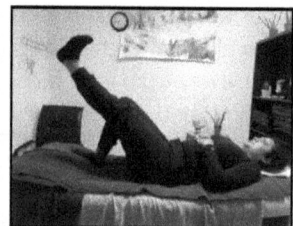

Straight leg raises – Lie on your back with your hips square and your legs laid out comfortably on the floor. Bend the knee of your other leg at a 90-degree angle, planting the foot flatly on the floor. Stabilize the muscles on your straight leg by contracting your quadriceps. Lift the straight leg six inches off the ground. Hold the position for 10 seconds and relax.

Side-lying leg raise - Lie on your left side with your shoulders, hips, and ankles in a straight line. Slowly and controlled, raise your right leg to a 45-degree angle (pain-free range of motion), then lower your leg. Perform 10 repetitions with your right leg. Switch to lying on your right side and perform 10 repetitions with your left leg.

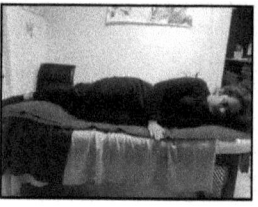 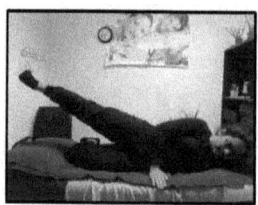

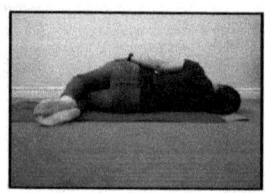 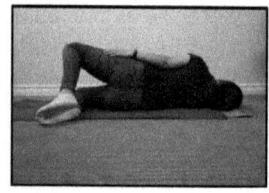

Clam shells - Lay on your side, Place your hand or a pillow under your head. Bend your knees so your heels line up with your hips, keeping your chest open. Pressing your heels together, inhale then exhale opening your top knee away from bottom knee. You should feel your hip and glute working. Try to keep your thighs relaxed. Only go a small way up if your lower back is sore. Do 10 to 20 reps each side.

Arm lifting in four-point kneeling - Float one arm up by pulling shoulder blades down the back, feeling it move along the side of the ribs (palm face in).

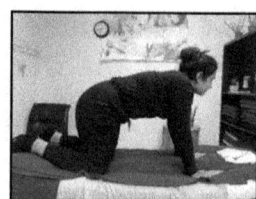 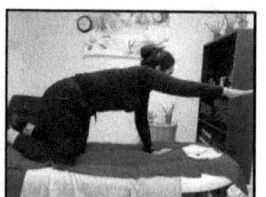

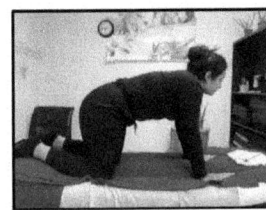 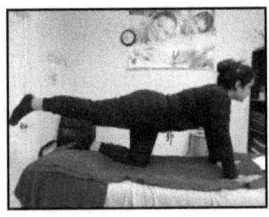

Leg lifting in four-point kneeling. Use lower buttock muscles to slide one leg back on the floor through the toes; lengthening to float leg up until it is straight and level with the hip. Lower leg down, slide back to starting position; ensure your lower belly muscles stay scooped in to prevent pelvis hitch, tip up or drop sideways on the return.

Alternate arm and leg raise - Alternate arm and leg exercise - Start on the floor, on your hands and knees. Tighten your belly muscles. Raise one leg off the floor and hold it straight out behind you. Be careful not to let your hip drop down, because that will twist your trunk. Hold for about 6 seconds, then lower your leg and switch to the other leg. Repeat 8 to 12 times on each leg. Over time, work up to holding for 10 to 30 seconds each time. If you feel stable and secure with your leg raised, try raising the opposite arm straight out in front of you at the same time.

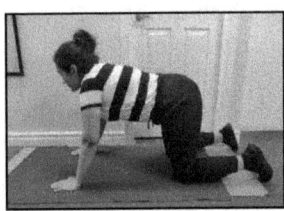 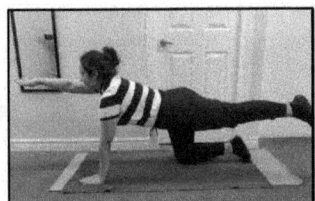

CHAPTER 8: MASSAGE TECHNIQUES FOR PAIN RELIEF

Massage therapy is one of the oldest, safest, effective and the best natural methods which relieve various types of pain. Experts also say that it reduces local inflammation and diminishes the level of depression which results in relaxation.

How massage therapy works in pain?
There are different types of massage techniques performed depending on the area and extent of pain. When performed, it relaxes the muscle which washes out the toxins and waste material in the form of lactic acid and promotes increased blood supply and oxygen to that area.

According to American massage therapy association, there are studies done which proves that massage have several health benefits which includes,
- Increase blood circulation
- Improve range of motion
- Increasing the endorphin level in the body – it is considered the greatest benefit as these substances are responsible for making us feel good and relaxed.

Besides the basic muscular benefits, massage also recovers the entire body. By improving circulation, it encourages nutrients, oxygen, and arterial blood components to visit the area being manipulated. To achieve the maximum benefits of massage, herbs incorporated into the oil during massage are useful in relieving the aches and pains due to inflammation. It is thus created using raw and dried herbs to mix in the carrier oil. By doing this, the infused oil formed has doubled the effects from the carrier oil as well as the herb infused.

How to prepare yourself for massage?
- Set the atmosphere by turning on your favorite relaxing music, lighting a few candles, or plugging in your essential oil diffuser.
- Choose a calming lotion or massage oil or make your own by herbal infused oil.
- Aim to massage each area for 30 seconds to a minute, which will reduce the odds of feeling sore later. And don't massage the area hard. "You can dig too hard in a pain spot and make it more inflamed."
- Keep your fingers and tools away from bony prominences and areas of acute pain, especially in swelling and redness. This can worsen the condition.
- Try pressing your fingers and palms as if you are kneading dough or doing so as you move your hands back and forth in a single long glide. You can also use tips of your fingers to release the pressure.
- Once you are done with massage, clean the area with hot towels (drains off extra oil). You can also use hot packs for 5-10 minutes which will help reduce your stiffness.

Here are some self-massage techniques,

Neck

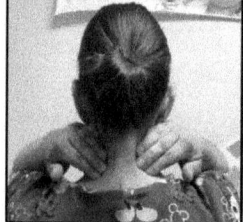 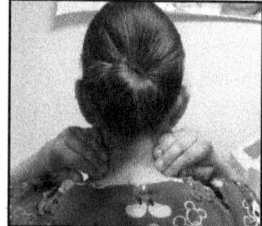 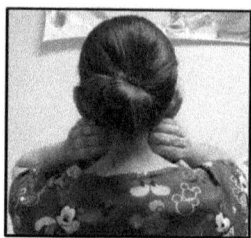 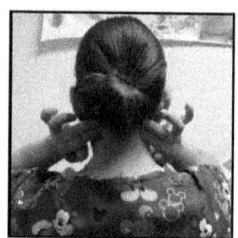

A 24-HOUR HOME REMEDY GUIDE TO YOUR BACK PAIN

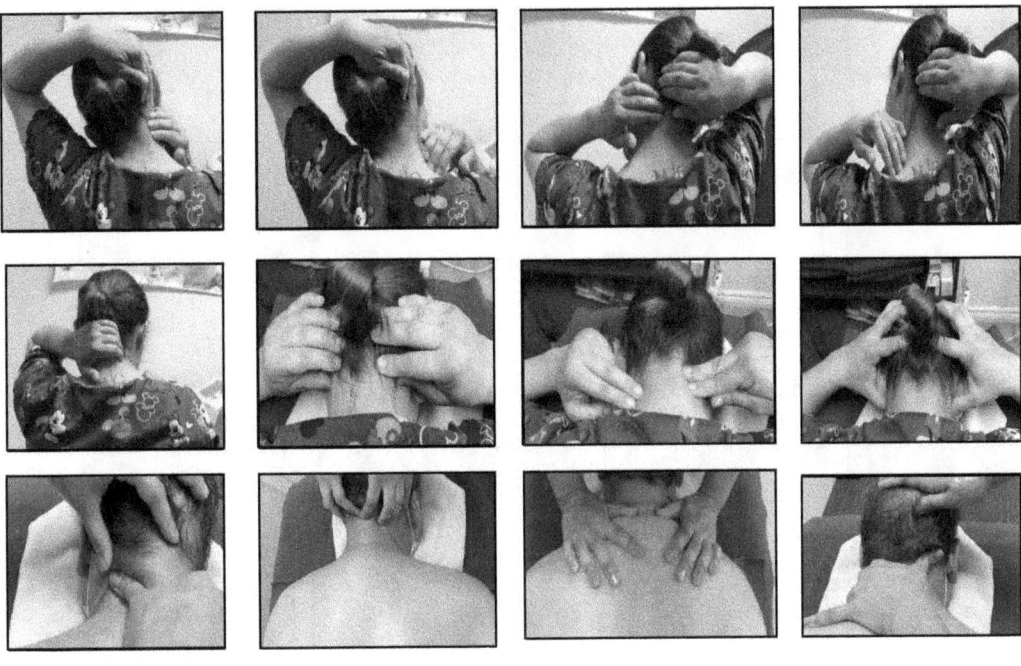

Shoulder and upper back in sitting

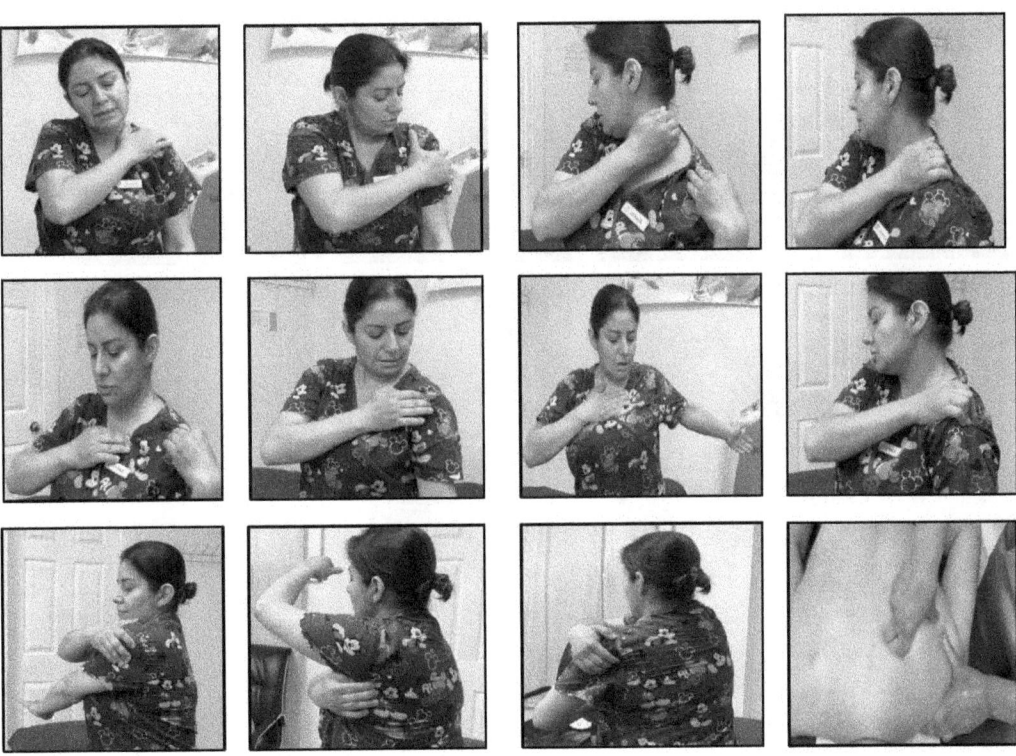

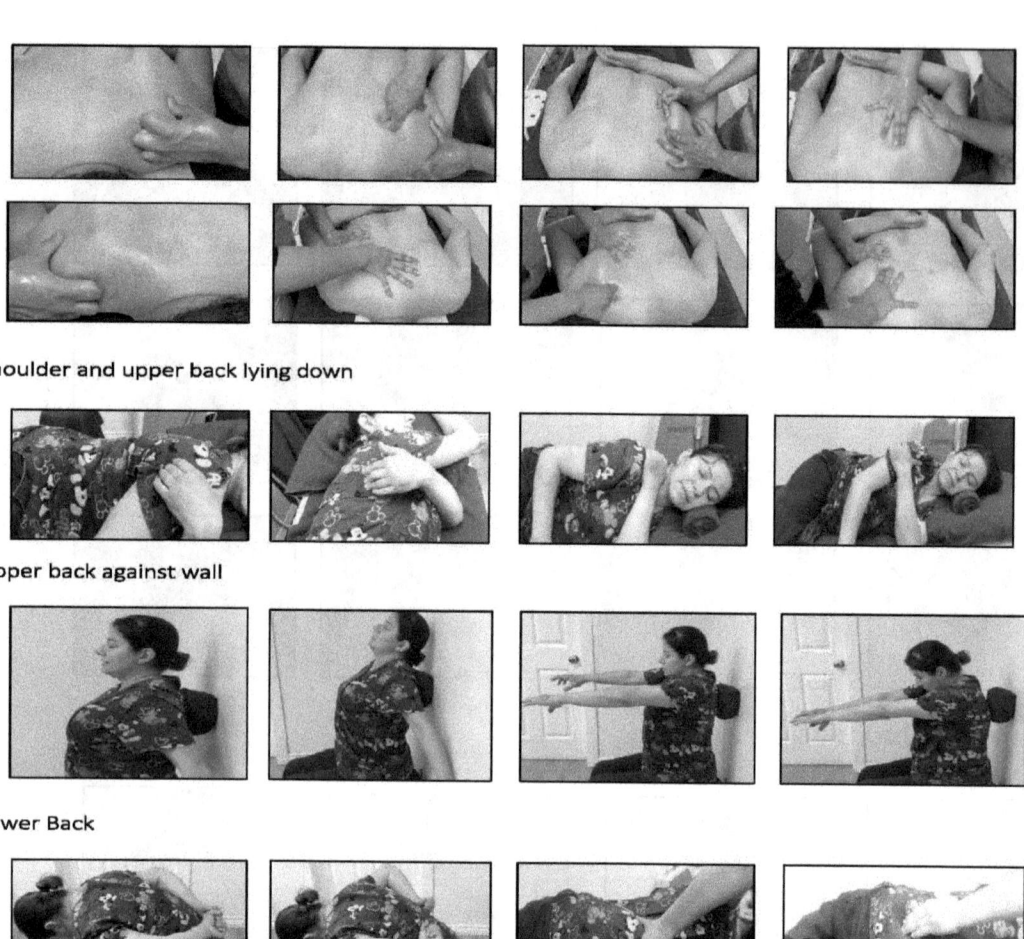

Shoulder and upper back lying down

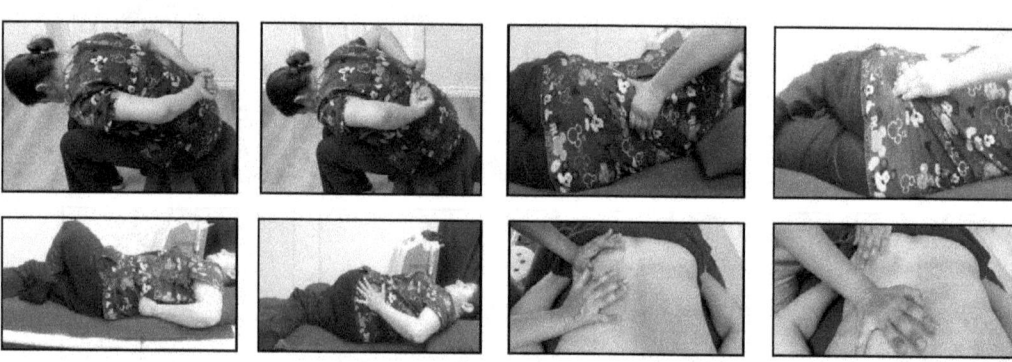

Upper back against wall

Lower Back

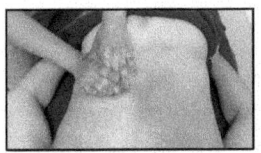 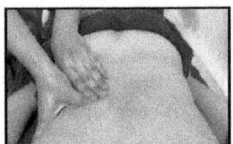 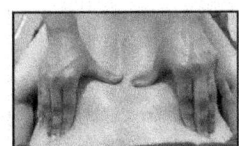 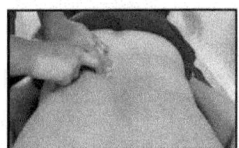

Massage for legs

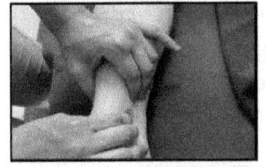 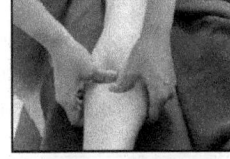 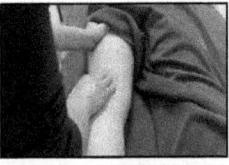 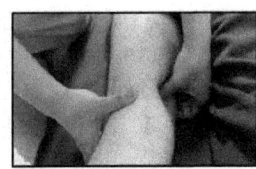

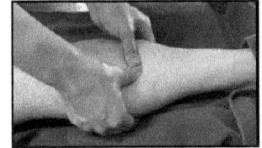 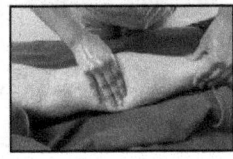 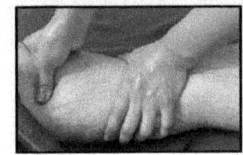 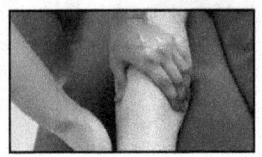

CHAPTER 9: TREATMENT OPTIONS FOR BACK PAIN

Physiotherapy:

It is one of the most widely used forms of treatment adopted for gaining relief from low back pain. It is used in both modes, as a single line of treatment as well as in combination with other treatments such as heat, TENS (Transcutaneous electrical nerve stimulation), ultrasound, infrared therapy or short-wave diathermy.

Ultrasound: One of the therapeutic effects for which ultrasound has been used is in relation to tissue healing. It is suggested that the application of US to injured tissues will, amongst other things, speed the rate of healing & enhance the quality of the repair. 1 MHz frequency is used for deeper penetration. The waves are transmitted through gel and the head is moved in a circular pattern with gentle pressure.

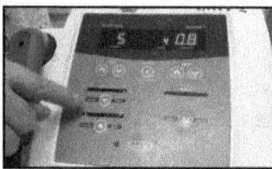 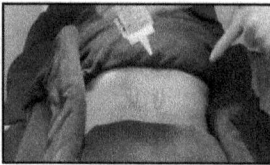 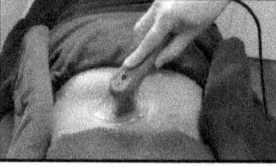 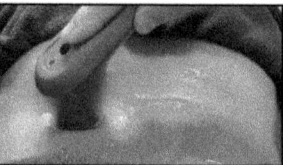

Infrared Therapy: Infrared (IR) or thermal radiation is a band of energy in the complete electromagnetic spectrum. Infrared radiations cause local cutaneous vasodilation due to the release of chemical vasodilator (histamine) as well as possible effect on the blood vessels, occurs after 1-2 mins evident erythema. The rate and intensity of erythema depends on rate and degree of heating. reflex dilation of other cutaneous vessels occurs to maintain normal heat balance prolonged heating leads to sweating and eventually to cooling.

Patient is placed in a comfortable position and the area to be treated is exposed. Nature and effects of treatment are explained. Skin is examined and thermal sensations are tested. Eyes are shielded in case they are irradiated. To achieve maximum penetration, the lamp is placed at right angles to area to be treated. Distance from the lamp can be about 60-75 cm for large lamp (750-1000W) and 45-50cm for smaller ones. Intensity of heat is controlled by altering the position of the lamp or in some lamps by altering the resistance thereby the current to the element. Non-luminous lamp has to be switched on up to 15 mins before application to allow maximum emission

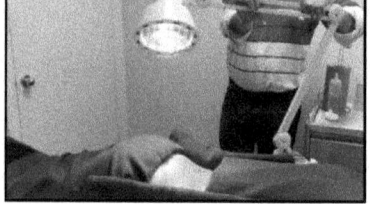

The human back is basically a highly complex system of series of interlocking elements including the vertebrae, discs, facet joints, ligaments, and muscles. Owing to such a complex structure, an episode of back pain needs a strong physiotherapy-based rehabilitation program once the basic medication course has been undertaken.

Chiropractor:

A chiropractor first takes a medical history, performs a physical examination, and may use lab tests or diagnostic imaging to determine if treatment is appropriate for your back pain.

The treatment plan may involve one or more manual adjustments in which the doctor manipulates the joints, using a controlled, sudden force to improve range and quality of motion. Many chiropractors also incorporate nutritional counseling and exercise/rehabilitation into the treatment plan. The goals of chiropractic care include the restoration of function and prevention of injury in addition to back pain relief.

What Are the Benefits and Risks of Chiropractic Care?

Spinal manipulation and chiropractic care are generally considered safe, effective treatments for acute low back pain, the type of sudden injury that results from moving furniture or getting tackled. Acute back pain, which is more common than chronic pain, lasts no more than six weeks and typically gets better on its own.

Naturopathy:

Naturopathic Doctors are qualified to administer acupuncture which has been shown to be a beneficial treatment for low back pain. A Naturopath practitioner applies treatment modalities based on the principles of Naturopathic medicine, which emphasize some of the following beliefs:

- **The Healing Power of Nature:** Nature has healing powers, it is the nature of all things to return to balance; plants, animals and people heal. Naturopathic medicine refers to the inner wisdom that guides internal physical processes that lead to health or disease as 'the healing power of nature,' also called vis medicatrix naturae in Latin.
- **The Triad of Health:** The interaction between the structural, biochemical and mental components of all living beings. The belief that dysfunction in one area leads to disruption elsewhere.

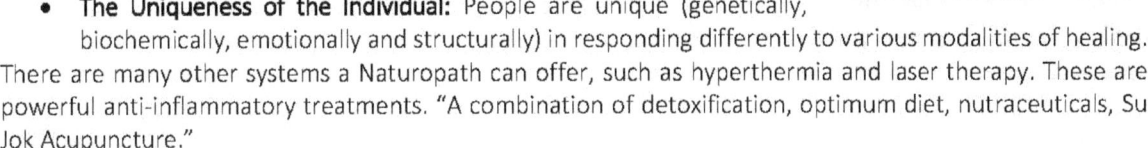

- **The Uniqueness of the Individual:** People are unique (genetically, biochemically, emotionally and structurally) in responding differently to various modalities of healing.

There are many other systems a Naturopath can offer, such as hyperthermia and laser therapy. These are powerful anti-inflammatory treatments. "A combination of detoxification, optimum diet, nutraceuticals, Su Jok Acupuncture."

Acupuncture:

It involves inserting thin needles at certain points on the body. According to traditional Chinese medicine, the body has more than 2,000 of these points. They are connected by pathways or meridians, which create a flow of energy called Qi (pronounced "chee"). Stimulating these points is said to correct the imbalance of qi and improve the flow of energy. Practitioners believe that this helps relieve pain and improve health. It's thought the effects come from stimulating the central nervous system. This may trigger the release of chemicals into the muscles, spinal cord, and brain. These chemicals either alter the experience of pain or produce bodily changes that promote a sense of well-being.

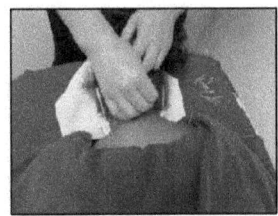 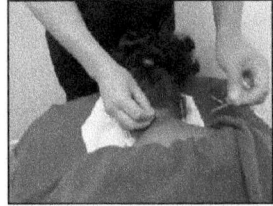 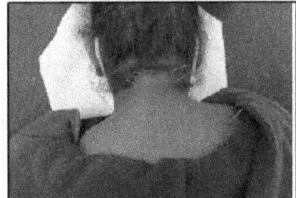 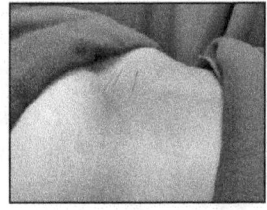

Acupressure:

Acupressure is similar to acupuncture, and both works to stimulate the nervous system to unblock Qi, the body's life force or vital energy. Qi (pronounced chee) flows through channels in the body called meridians. Within meridian channels are hundreds of points or acupoints on the body that correspond to specific body systems. A basic principle of TCM is when Qi is disrupted or blocked, symptoms of physical illness and/or mental distress can develop.

How to Perform Acupressure?
Acupressure may be performed by a qualified acupressure practitioner (see below for information), or you may experience similar benefits by administering it to yourself. Below are some tips on how to perform acupressure on yourself:

- Relax. Take a few deep breaths, relax your jaw and shoulders, find a comfortable position, and close your eyes.

- Firmly press on a point (see below for a list of common acupoints) in a circular or up-and-down motion for about 3 minutes at a time.
- Repeat the motion as often as you like (there's no risk in over-activating an acupoint)

Below are common acupressure points that may help ease back and neck pain:

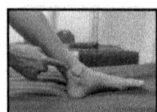
Spleen 6: Located inside your leg above your ankle, this point may be targeted if you have pelvic pain, fatigue, or sleep problems.

Stomach 36: Situated four-fingers-width down from the bottom of your kneecap, this point may help reduce stress and fatigue.

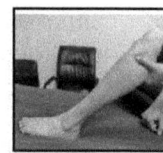

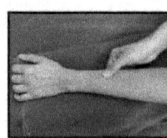
Large Intestine 6: Located at the top of the muscle where the thumb and index fingers are joined, this point may help reduce headaches, neck pain, and stress.

Pericardium 6: Located three-fingers-width down on the inside of the wrist, putting pressure on this point may ease headaches.

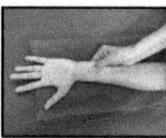

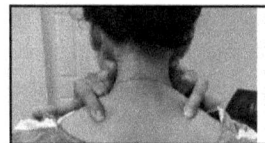
Gallbladder 21: Situated halfway between the top of the neck and shoulder, this acupoint may ease neck and shoulder stiffness and pain, and headaches.

Triple Energizer 3: Stimulated to help ease upper back pain, headaches, neck stiffness, and shoulder pain, this acupoint is located in the groove between the fourth finger and pinky.

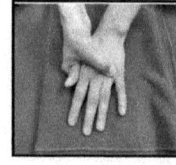

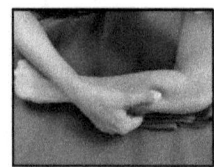
Large Intestine 10: Located on the front side of the elbow, this point may be pressed to relieve shoulder pain and neck tightness.

Cupping therapy:

Cupping therapy is a form of alternative medicine where glass, silicone or plastic cups are placed on the skin to create vacuum suction in order to promote health and healing. Cupping therapy promotes the loosening of soft tissue and connective tissue, scarring and adhesions, moving stagnation and increasing lymphatic flow and circulation. The simple, traditional therapy method shares the benefits of deep tissue massage and muscle relaxation, without lofty fees or a commitment to hours of therapy time.

How is cupping performed?

There are different ways to perform cupping. The steps vary slightly depending on the chosen method. Your provider will leave the cups in place for several minutes. Some treatments involve briefly moving the cups to stretch and massage the area. Depending on the treatment, your provider may place multiple cups on your skin. Cupping methods include Dry: Your provider heats the inside of each cup — typically with an alcohol-soaked cotton ball that is set aflame. The heat sends oxygen out of the cup, creating a vacuum. Some providers use a suction device to remove air from cups. Once placed on your skin, the vacuum force pulls skin up into the cup. Wet: Your provider uses a needle to lightly puncture your skin before, and sometimes after, cupping. Toxins leave the body through the puncture wounds during the cupping procedure.

Does cupping hurt?

No, normally all you feel is a slight pressure from the suction. Pain tolerance varies, but most people who've experienced cupping don't report any pain associated with it. If you've ever held a vacuum cleaner hose over your arm, you know about what it feels like. It might be somewhat uncomfortable for you, but it usually isn't painful. After treatment, you might find that the skin on and around the cupping points is tender, like it would feel if you had a bruise. The nature of cupping makes double-blind studies difficult—unlike simply taking a pill that could be an active medication or a placebo, a patient would certainly know if they'd received a cupping treatment.

What are the side-effects of cupping?

Expect round, bruise-like marks on the cupping points. These marks are the same size as the cups your

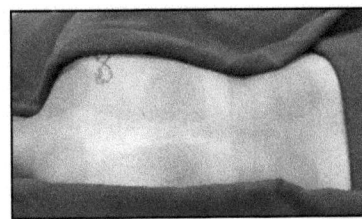

practitioner used and usually disappear on their own in a week or two. During that time, they might change color, just like a bruise would. If you get heated cupping, you might experience some minor burns on your skin from the cups. Your practitioner may give you an ointment to rub into your skin until it heals. Some people report fatigue, headaches, muscle soreness, and nausea after cupping. As the skin heals, you might find that it itches. Avoid scratching, which could lead to infection.

Benefits of cupping?
People mostly use cupping to relieve conditions that cause pain. Some people say it also helps with chronic (ongoing) health issues. Cupping may ease symptoms of:
- Arthritis, including rheumatoid arthritis.
- Back pain, neck pain, knee pain and shoulder pain.
- Breathing problems, such as asthma.
- Carpal tunnel syndrome.
- Gastrointestinal disorders, such as irritable bowel disease (IBD).
- Headaches and migraines.
- High blood pressure (hypertension).

How to do cupping at home?
- Before starting, you have to cleanse, exfoliate, and moisturize the area where you want to do cupping.
- You start by grabbing one of the silicon cups between your thumb and forefinger and squeezing tight.
- While still pinching it closed, you press it to your skin, creating a seal—then let go. This creates a vacuum that sticks the cup to your skin, picking up the skin underneath.
- You drag the cup along your skin in a particular pattern, changing the position of the cup after each stroke.
- During cupping, it's important to always keep the cups moving. That's how you get the massaging action and prevent bruising.

Upper back and neck

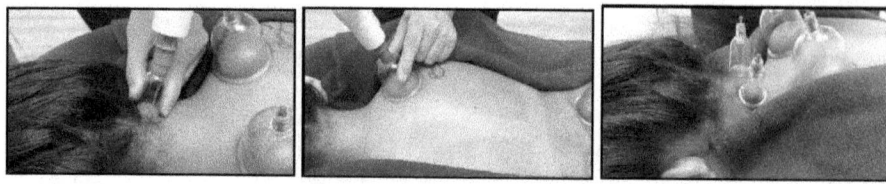

Mid back and lower back:

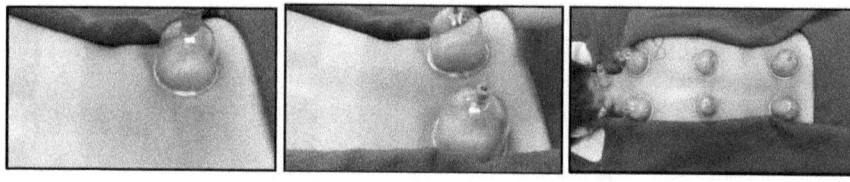

Taking off the cups:

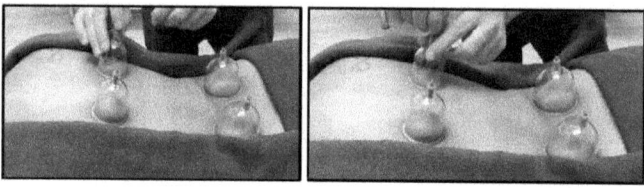

CHAPTER 10: HERBS AND HERB INFUSED OILS

Pain and inflammation are closely related, so reducing inflammation is important. Several herbs have excellent anti-inflammatory properties and following an anti-inflammatory diet will enhance the herbs effects. Herbal medicine has an important role in treating persistent or chronic pain. There are many ways of using herbs from which few are listed below,

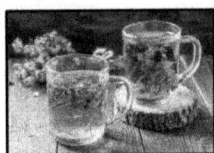
Teas - There are several types of "teas," or herbal beverages. An infusion is made by steeping hot stems, leaves, and flowers of herbs to extract their benefits. Hard materials, like roots, woods, barks, and seeds, need to be boiled, then steeped, for best results. (This is called a decoction.) And a cold extract, which is recommended for the most delicate plants, is made by soaking the herbs in cold water.

Baths - By adding herbs to your tub, you can customize and boost the effectiveness of bath time. A good soak can cleanse, soften, and nourish the skin, rejuvenate a tired body and spirit, and address sore and aching muscles.
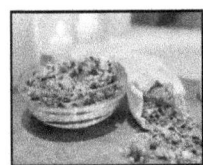

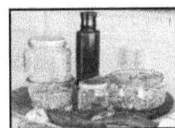
Oils - Infused herbal oils are easy to make and are most effective with massage. It is made simply by soaking dried or fresh herbs in high-quality vegetable, seed, or nut oils.

Poultices (PASTE) – Herbs are crushed or bruised to release their potency, then applied topically, often over a warm or cool piece of cheesecloth or other light fabric.
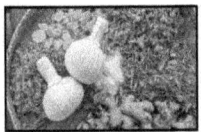

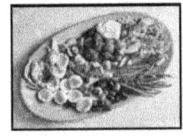
Food ingredient as salad or soups – Herbs are more beneficial when incorporated into your salads and soups. It helps you improve your functions of organ and make the body work effectively.

From ancient time, one of the more versatile use of herbs is mixing it to make infused oil. These oils work in two ways – causes emotional and physical response and penetrates the skin to underlying tissue and distributes their therapeutic properties. There are many herbs found locally who has amazing therapeutic properties and are used to make infused oil. Knowing some of the differences can be helpful to choose the best herb for the situation.

We have conducted a research study with back pain participants. Total 42 participants were involved in the study. They were screened with non-specific low back pain by filling out a questionnaire. Herb infused oil was used for treatment of pain here. It included garden cress seeds, oregano, sesame, Himalayan salt and olive oil. All the herbs had specific properties in relieving pain, inflammation and improving flexibility. The application of oil was explained to the participants. This included first cleaning of the area with lukewarm water and applying the oil directly (3 times a day and keep it on for 5 minutes) with firm pressure. The participants were asked to continue the application regularly, with other back pain preventive measures to be taken. After one week, the participants were assessed again by filling the same back pain questionnaire and results were compared. None of the participants received any kind of treatment during the one-week time which could affect the effectiveness of oil. There was significant decrease of pain at the end of one week for each participant. Thus, herb infused oil was effective in treatment.

We will share you the recipes for the above-mentioned ways. But, first let talk about the important herbs which will help reduce pain, inflammation and promote flexibility. There are few herbs which you will get in your kitchen who has amazing healing properties. Let's see their benefits,

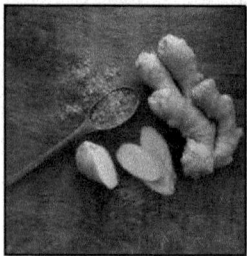

Ginger – It has phytochemicals with excellent anti-inflammatory properties, which relieve pain in joints and muscles. It promotes the circulation of blood and acts as a cure for nausea, headache, and cramps. The easiest way to incorporate ginger in your diet is to have ginger tea. You can also grate the root, wrap cheesecloth around it, soak it in hot water for 30 seconds, and place it on your back for 20 minutes. It also reduces muscle pain and soreness. A topical application of the paste of ginger, cinnamon, sesame oil, and mastic can reduce pain and stiffness in muscles. Ginger also dramatically lowers blood sugar levels.

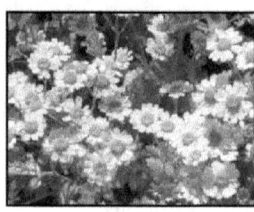

Feverfew - This plant grows throughout the year and belongs to the daisy family. It has an acrid smell, and it is used to treat rheumatoid arthritis, migraines, toothaches, stomach-ache, and headaches. It is available as tinctures, extracts, and capsules. Standardized products have at least 0.2% of parthenopid. There is not much information available about exactly why it works, but it has been a popular remedy for centuries. People report feeling much better after taking the herb. Besides, it doesn't have any significant side effects. These herbs are not ideal for consumption during pregnancy.

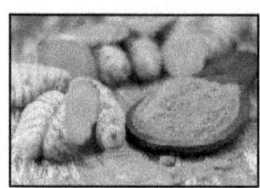

Turmeric - Turmeric has a chemical called curcumin, which helps fight pain because of its antioxidant and anti-inflammatory properties. However, turmeric contains only 3% of curcumin, which is quickly gets eliminated from the body. The liver processes curcumin in two hours and removes it. There is not much absorption that takes place. According to observations, the incorporation of curcumin increases by 2000% when you consume it with black pepper. Turmeric supplements contain not only higher percentages of curcumin but also black pepper to enhance their effectiveness.

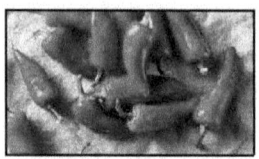

Capsaicin - Found in plants belonging to the Capsicum genus like Chili Pepper, Capsaicin, has medicinal value. It comes in various forms such as ointments, gels, lotions, films, sticks, or creams. These products are basically for the skin. Leaving the lotion on the surface for a few hours offers a tremendous amount of pain relief. Substance P transmits the signals of pain from the peripheral nervous system to the central nervous system, making you aware of the pain. Capsaicin depletes substance P in two days after application. You will feel relatively that the pain has reduced tremendously.

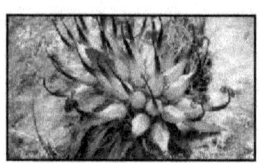

Devil's Claw - A suitable alternative or even addition to turmeric would be Devil's claw. It belongs to the sesame family, and the seeds appear in a flowering plant. It has been used in Sub Saharan Africa for thousands of years as a painkiller. Devil's claw is also known to contain anti-inflammatory properties which relieve back pain. It also eases symptoms of gout, promotes weight loss, improves osteoarthritis, and reduces inflammation in all parts of the body.

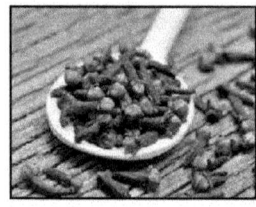

Clove - Clove is a perfect home remedy for toothache since ages. Not many people know that it can also be a cure for back pain. It can be more effective when you consume it in your diet. It can also be used on your back, applied in the form of clove oil. Clove, which forms on the Eugenia Caryophyllids plant, has been shown to possess anti-inflammatory properties that relieve pain. This spice also kills bacteria, fungi, and viruses. These are the functions of the chemical called eugenol. Clove essential oil is quite inexpensive and very beneficial.

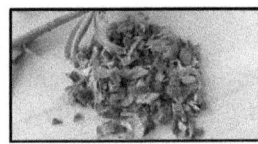

Willow Bark - The White willow bark has been a remedy for centuries to relieve fever, inflammation, and back pain. Nowadays, it is available as a dried herb which can be used to make tea. It is also sold as capsules and in liquid form as extracts. Avoid excess of willow bark. It can be poisonous for children. Salicin that comes in the willow bark is the same compound found in aspirin, and this explains why it works so well.

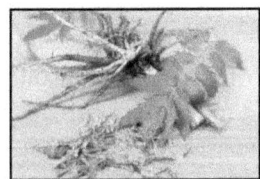

Valerian Root - Muscle spasms are associated with back pain and problems, which is where valerian root excels. This herb is a natural muscle relaxer that also reduces nerve sensitivity. Therefore, if you suffer with back pain that includes muscle spasms, this is one of the best herbs for back pain. Since it can make you drowsy, it is advised that you take it at night and only as directed to avoid overdose.

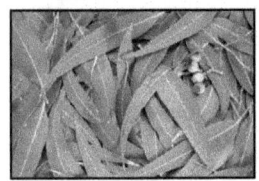

Eucalyptus - You might relate the eucalyptus herb as a remedy for the flu or for colds. While it does help with these conditions, it is also an effective herb for back pain relief due to its ice, cooling effect. The leaf contains tannins which are known to reduce swelling and inflammation, resulting in pain relief. The common use is as a topical pain relief treatment.

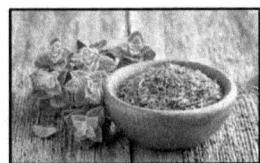

Oregano - Oregano is the herb found locally and widely used in the culinary arts. Besides from its taste this herb also serves in various ailments due to its anti-inflammatory and antioxidant properties. Oregano leaves are high in phenols, which are natural phytochemical compounds with beneficial antioxidant effects. The two most abundant phenols in it are thymol and carvacrol. Among these, Carvacrol — has antimicrobial, antitumor, ant mutagenic, analgesic, anti-inflammatory and antiparasitic properties, making it one of the most active components of oregano when infused in carrier oil.

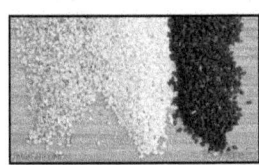

Sesame - Sesame seeds are used for traditional remedy against various ailments for centuries. It has high antibacterial and antioxidant properties. Sesamol, Sesamolin and Sesamin are the antioxidant components present in its seeds. Among these, Sesamin is a lignin with anti-inflammatory properties which helps in pain relief, reduce spasm, and increase range of motion when applied to the affected area. Many studies have proved its therapeutic and healing properties that sesame seeds when infused in oil, applied to the painful area stimulate the blood flow due to its excellent emollient properties.

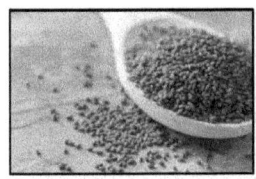

Garden cress seeds - also known as Lepidium Sativum is an edible fast-growing herb which has been used in ancient medicines for a long time. It seeds contains significant amount of plant sterols which are antioxidant and anti-inflammatory compounds. It also contains phenolic compounds which fights at molecular level and inhibits the substance involved in inflammation. The seed when infused in the carrier oil and applied to joints or muscle pain helps recover from muscle weakness, reduce muscle tension, and promotes pain relief.

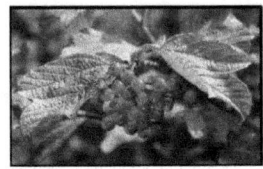

Cramp Bark - Cramp Bark is also known as cranberry bush; this herb is popular due to its ability to treat spasms in the back and uterine pain. It comes in the form of liquid extracts, tinctures and capsules. Native Americans consume cramp bark since ancient time. Most people find it challenging to identify Cramp bark and Black Haw, which is also sometimes referred to by the same name. As the name suggests, it is used to relieve pain from all sorts of cramps. For acute pain, 30 drops of the tincture can be taken every hour until the pain subsides. Cramp bark contains chemicals that significantly reduce muscle spasms. They also decrease heart rate and lower blood pressure. The bioactive compounds are extracted from dried bark and made into tinctures.

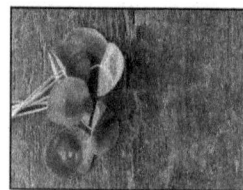

Gotu Kola - Gotu kola is an herb known to boost brain function and is an anti-inflammatory used to treat arthritis pain. While it is used to treat a variety of conditions, it is an effective treatment for back pain.

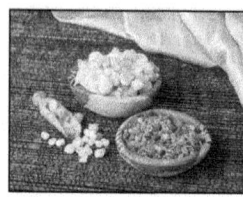

Boswellia - This herb is an extract taken from the gum resin of the Boswellia plant. Due to its anti-inflammatory properties, it is frequently used to treat arthritis and back pain.

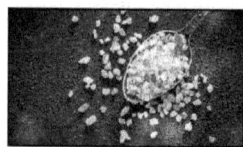

Himalayan Salt - Himalayan Salt is the world's purest and richest, boasting 84 minerals and trace minerals. It's become increasingly popular nowadays, as many have attributed numerous health benefits to it. The healing properties of pink Himalayan salt are believed to restore restful sleep, relieve muscle aches, and increase energy in body. Other than being beneficial for muscle aches and pains, it can also be used to relieve muscle spasms. When infused the salt in carrier oil and applied to the surface, the natural antioxidants present can help to prevent free radical damage and thus reducing the possibility of future muscle pain.

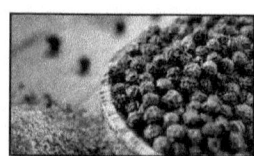

Pepper - Black pepper contains essential oils like piperine, a naturally occurring alkaloid, which is the source of its bold character and heat,15 as well as the monoterpenes sabinene, pinene, terpenene, limonene, and mercene, which give this spice its aromatic qualities. All combined, these oils, when used in aromatherapy, can help ease aching muscles, chilblains, and arthritis, and have curative properties for constipation and sluggish digestion.

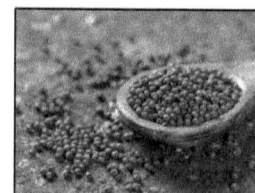

Mustard Seeds - Mustard seeds contain vitamins A, B6 and C (and other vitamins), dietary folate, omega-3 fatty acids, and minerals like magnesium, potassium, selenium, manganese, phosphorus, and copper.11 The seeds also have the following health-promoting plant compounds, which include Glycosylates and isothiocyanates: The former is a compound broken down by myrosinase enzymes to produce isothiocyanates. Sinigrin is also a precursor of a compound called allyl isothiocyanate (AITC), which is produced by the myrosinase enzyme when sinigrin mixes with water.

Using essential oils for back pain:
Apart from the list of herbs mentioned above, you can also use rosemary essential oil, eucalyptus peppermint essential oil, and lavender essential oil. These essential oils treat the back when gently massaged. Directly inhaling these oils also brings some amount of pain relief. Research suggests that these oils can be used in the body as the pain-relieving anti-inflammatory and antioxidant properties. With all the essential oil choices available, it can be confusing to know which ones can help with your back pain. The following oils could help.

Herbs	Benefits
Peppermint oil	Perhaps best-known for its menthol undertones, peppermint oil is one of nature's most potent analgesics. Pure peppermint oil has at least 44 % pure menthol content, which has been widely used for pain of a variety sources.
Wintergreen oil	A close relative to peppermint, wintergreen oil carries similar analgesic properties. Specifically, wintergreen contains methyl salicylate, which is like aspirin. Talk to a doctor if you're taking blood thinners or other medications, as wintergreen can increase the risk of bleeding.
Lemongrass oil	Lemongrass oil has been widely studied for its antifungal properties. One study in mice also evaluated its notable anti-inflammatory properties. Reduction of inflammation may lead to reduced pain, but studies are needed in humans.
Ginger oil	Often used in cooking, ginger has other effects outside of the spice cabinet. Its most notable benefits are anti-inflammatory properties, such as a 2016 study on rheumatoid arthritis showed.
Lavender oil	As one of the most widely studied and popular essential oils, lavender acts as a multipurpose oil for a variety of ailments. According to one clinical review, lavender oil can help alleviate headaches and muscle pain. Such benefits may transfer to back pain as well.
Eucalyptus oil	Known for both its anti-inflammatory and antibacterial properties, eucalyptus oil can have analgesic effects in muscles and joints. A 2015 clinical review found that the oil has promise in treating ailments like arthritis, the flu, and wounds.
Roman and German chamomile oils	While chamomile is best known for its soothing and calming properties (the reason why many people drink chamomile tea when sick), the essential oil has other noted benefits. These include reduced muscle spasms and overall inflammation. Take care when using chamomile if you have a ragweed allergy, as the plants come from the same family
Rosemary oil	Rosemary is more than just a cooking herb. Rosemary essential oil has clinically proven benefits. These include reduced pain from rheumatic disorders and menstrual cramps. Such anti-inflammatory and analgesic effects may also be helpful for back pain.
Sandalwood oil	Sandalwood oil contains anti-inflammatory properties. Such effects have been studied for their similar effects to over-the-counter medications. Reducing inflammation in the back with sandalwood oil could possibly decrease pain, too.
Olive oil	Olive oil is valued not only for its flavor, but also for its range of wellness benefits. Olive oil is rich in oleic acid, a type of monounsaturated fat. Studies have shown that oleic acid is linked to reduced biomarkers of inflammation17 such as C-reactive protein. This oil when infused with herbs, doubles the benefits with its rich properties and gives the best results. Extra virgin olive oil is considered the highest-quality olive oil to be used as carrier oil with herbs. It is unrefined and contains more nutrients compared to other processed varieties.

RECIPES FOR NECK AND UPPER BACK PAIN

The first recipe:

Ingredients are,

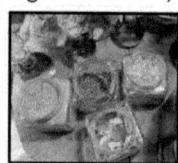

3 teaspoons of turmeric powder,
Half a teaspoon of black pepper
A teaspoon of lemon peel
A teaspoon of Himalayan salt
¾ cup of regular drinking cups of olive oil

Method:

- Take all the ingredients and coarse grind in the mixture. Take the powder and add olive oil into it and stir it up. You can store this in a dark color bottle to prevent it from direct sunlight.
- Also, it can be placed in a refrigerator to ensure its protection.
- Take small amount of oil, massage on your upper back with gentle pressure, try working on the areas which are stiff.
- After massage, you can take a hot compress and gently wipe off your skin.
- Massage can be done once in a day.

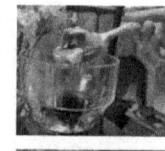
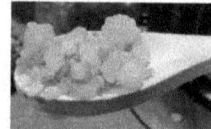
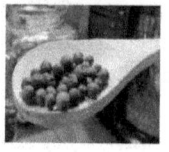
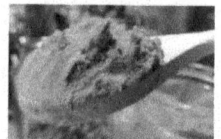
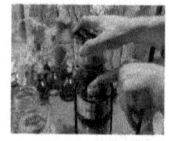
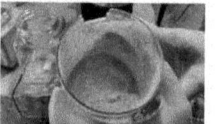
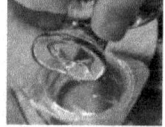
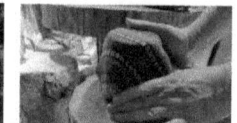

Benefits:

- Relieves acute pain
- Stimulates blood circulation
- Stimulates and revitalizes nerves
- Reduces inflammation
- Moisturizes the skin and nourishes the muscle

The second recipe:

Ingredients are,

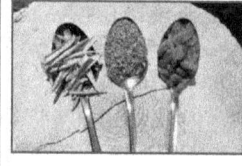

3 teaspoons ground dry olive leaves
6 teaspoons of dried sour grapes
3 teaspoons of dried wild thyme
Half a cup of drinking cups of extra-virgin olive oil

Method:

- Take the amount of dried olive leaves, thyme, and dried sour grapes, grind the dry ingredient until it becomes like powder.
- Then, add virgin olive oil and mix it well.
- And put in an airtight container, away from heat and sun or in the fridge
- Take small amount of oil, massage on your upper back with gentle pressure, try working on the areas which are stiff.
- Use it 3 to four times a day with gentle pressure on back.
- After massage, you can take a hot compress and gently wipe off your skin.

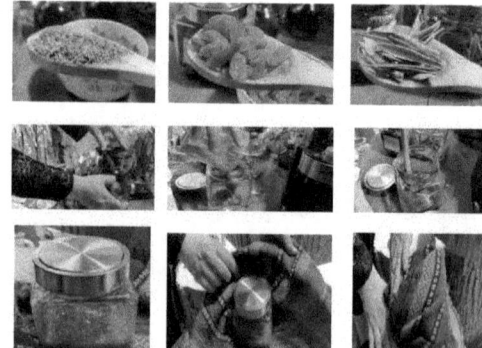

The third recipe:
Ingredients are,
A teaspoon of hot pepper
5 spoons of green tea
3 teaspoons of sesame seeds
2 teaspoons of salt
A full cup of extra-virgin olive oil

Method:
- Take all the dry ingredients and grind it in a coffee grinder until it becomes a fine powder.
- Add virgin olive oil to it and mix well.
- Place it in an airtight container, away from heat and sun and in the fridge
- Use 3 times a day (morning, noon, and evening) with gentle pressure on the back.
- After massage, you can take a hot compress and gently wipe off your skin.
- Make sure you stir the mixture before using.

Benefits:
- Eliminates pain directly
- Stimulates blood circulation
- It stimulates and revitalizes the nerves and aids in healing
- Eliminates inflammation
- Nourishes muscle and moisturizes the skin

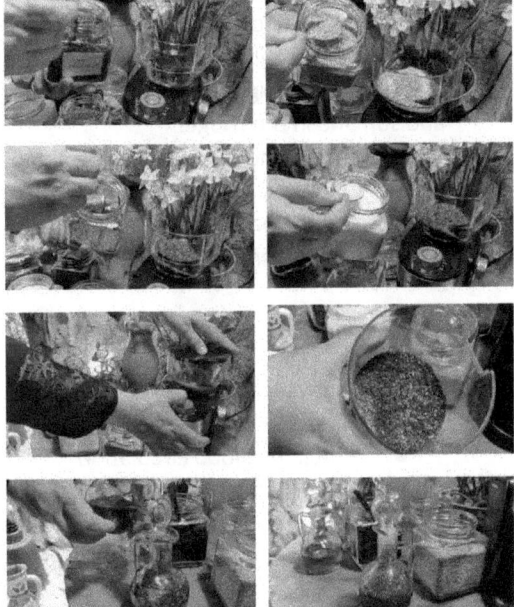

The fourth recipe:
Ingredients are,
3 teaspoons of fine turmeric powder
3 teaspoons of sage powder
A teaspoon of cinnamon powder
A cup of regular cups olive oil

Method:
- Take all the dry ingredients and grind it in a coffee grinder until it becomes a fine powder
- Add virgin olive oil to it and mix well.
- Place it in an airtight container, away from heat and sun and in the fridge
- Use 3 times a day (morning, noon, and evening) with gentle pressure on the back.
- Make sure you stir the mixture before using.
- After massage, you can take a hot compress and gently wipe off your skin.

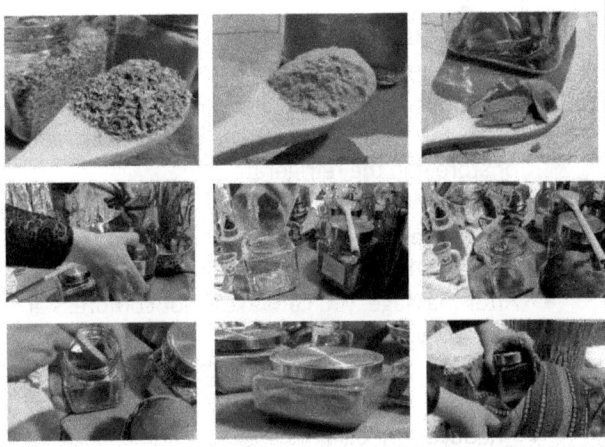

The fifth recipe:
Ingredients are,

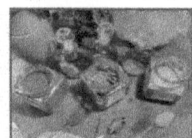

3 teaspoons of sesame seeds
2 teaspoons of cinnamon bark
4 teaspoons of Cress seeds
Half a large cup of olive oil

Method:
- Take all the dry ingredients and grind it in a coffee grinder until it becomes a fine powder
- Add virgin olive oil to it and mix well.
- Place it in an airtight container, away from heat and sun and in the fridge.
- Take a small amount and Use 3 times a day (morning, noon, and evening) with gentle pressure on the back.
- Make sure you stir the mixture before using.

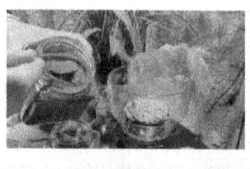 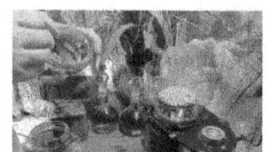
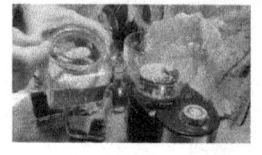 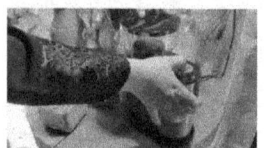
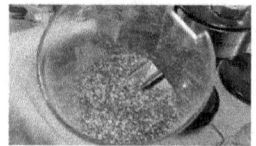 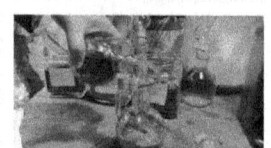
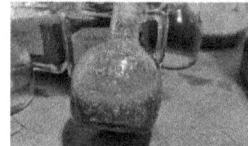 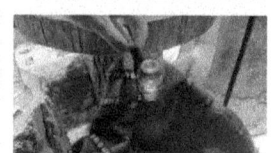

Benefits:
- Reduces the pain
- It activates the free nerve endings and blocks the pain receptors.
- Stimulates blood circulation
- Reduces inflammation and swelling

The sixth recipe:
Ingredients are,

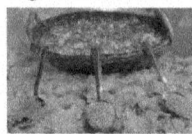

A teaspoon of black mustard
A teaspoon of sesame
3 teaspoons of ground bay leaves
Half a large cup of drinking glasses of olive oil

Method:
- Take all the dry ingredients and grind it in a coffee grinder until it becomes a coarse powder.
- Add virgin olive oil to it and mix well
- Place it in an airtight container, away from heat and sun or store it in the refrigerator.
- Use 3 times a day (morning, noon, and evening) with gentle pressure on the back.
- Make sure you stir the mixture before using.
- After massage, you can take a hot compress and gently wipe off your skin.

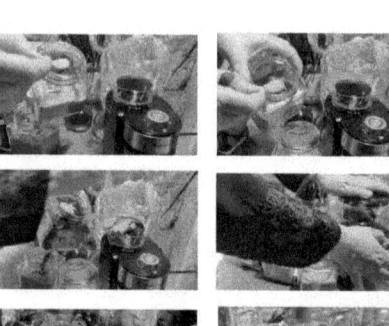
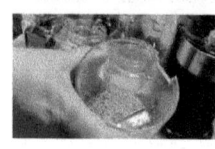 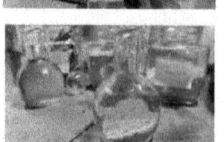

Benefits:
- Reduces the pain

- It activates the free nerve endings and blocks the pain receptors.
- Stimulates blood circulation
- Reduces inflammation and swelling

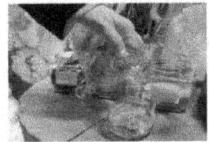 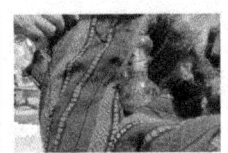

The seventh recipe:
Ingredients are,

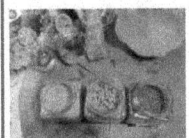

A teaspoon of chili powder
5 teaspoons of chamomile powder
3 teaspoons of turmeric
Half a large cup of extra-virgin olive oil

Method:
- Do not but any powders from the store. Instead use whole herbs to enhance more benefits.
- Take all the dry ingredients and grind it in a coffee grinder until it becomes a coarse powder.
- Add virgin olive oil to it and mix well.
- Place it in an airtight container, away from heat and sun or store it in the refrigerator.
- Use 2 times a day (morning, evening) with good pressure on the back.
- Make sure you stir the mixture before using.
- After massage, you can take a hot compress and gently wipe off your skin.

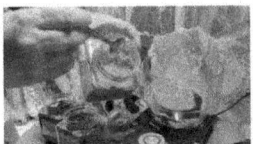 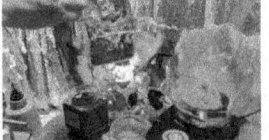
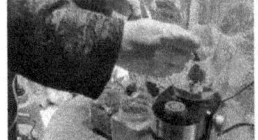 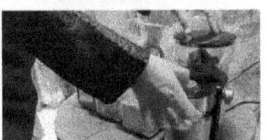
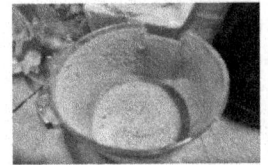 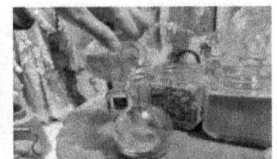
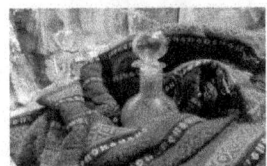

Benefits:
- Relieving acute pain
- Relaxes the muscle and calms the nerves, in addition to softening and lightening the skin
- Stimulates nerves
- Reduces inflammation

The eighth recipe:
Ingredients are,

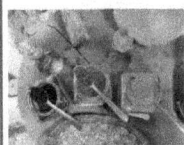

5 teaspoons of mustard
5 teaspoons of black seeds
5 teaspoons of chia seeds
1 cup of olive oil

Method:
- Take all the dry ingredients and grind it in a coffee grinder until it becomes a coarse powder.
- Add virgin olive oil to it and mix well.

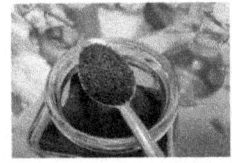 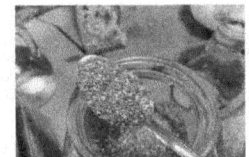

- Place it in an airtight container, away from heat and sun or store it in the refrigerator.
- Use 4 times a day with gentle pressure on the back.
- Make sure you stir the mixture before using.
- After massage, you can take a hot compress and gently wipe off your skin.

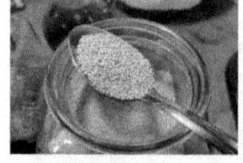
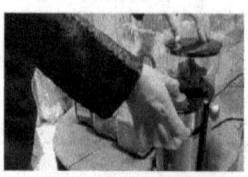
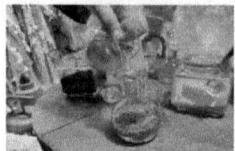
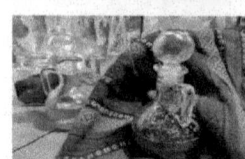

Benefits:
- Relieving acute pain
- Relaxes the muscle and calms the nerves, in addition to softening and lightening the skin
- Stimulates nerves
- Reduces inflammation

The ninth recipe:
Ingredients are,
5 teaspoons of ground ginger
2 teaspoons of fenugreek
3 teaspoons of bay leaf powder
2 teaspoons of wild thyme powder
Half cup of olive oil

Method:
- Take all the dry ingredients and grind it in a coffee grinder until it becomes a coarse powder.
- Add virgin olive oil to it and mix well.
- Place it in an airtight container, away from heat and sun or store it in the refrigerator.
- Use 3 times a day with gentle pressure on the back.
- Make sure you stir the mixture before using.
- After massage, you can take a hot compress and gently wipe off your skin.

Benefits:
- Relieving acute pain
- Relaxes the muscle and calms the nerves, in addition to softening and lightening the skin
- Stimulates nerves
- Reduces inflammation

The tenth recipe:
Ingredients are,
Half a cup of apple cider vinegar
5 teaspoons of table salt
A teaspoon of turmeric
2 teaspoons garlic powder
A cup of olive oil
Method:
- Take all the dry ingredients and grind it in a coffee grinder until it becomes a coarse powder.
- Add virgin olive oil to it and mix well.
- Place it in an airtight container, away from heat and sun or store it in the refrigerator.
- Use 3 times a day with gentle pressure on the back.
- Make sure you stir the mixture before using.

- After massage, you can take a hot compress and gently wipe off your skin.

Benefits:
- Relieving acute pain
- Relaxes the muscle and calms the nerves, in addition to softening and lightening the skin
- Stimulates nerves
- Reduces inflammation

The eleventh recipe:
Ingredients are,

>7 teaspoons of bran
>4 teaspoons cinnamon powder
>3 teaspoons of wild thyme
>2 teaspoons of laurel powder
>Half a large cup of olive oil

Method:
- Take all the dry ingredients and grind it in a coffee grinder until it becomes a coarse powder.
- Add virgin olive oil to it and mix well.
- Place it in an airtight container, away from heat and sun or store it in the refrigerator.
- Use 3 times a day with gentle pressure on the back.
- Make sure you stir the mixture before using.
- After massage, you can take a hot compress and gently wipe off your skin.

Benefits:
- Relieving acute pain
- Relaxes the muscle and calms the nerves, in addition to softening and lightening the skin
- Stimulates nerves
- Reduces inflammation

RECIPES FOR ACUTE LOWER BACK PAIN

The first recipe:
Ingredients are,
A teaspoon of basil
4 teaspoons of green thyme
1 teaspoon of cumin
A teaspoon of garlic powder

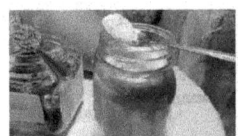 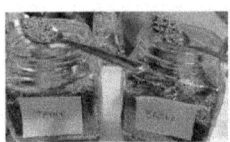 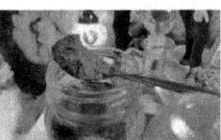

Method:
- Take all the dry ingredients in a bowl and mix well.
- Add virgin olive oil to it and mix well.
- Place it in an airtight container, away from heat and sun or store it in the refrigerator.
- Use 3 times a day with gentle pressure on the back.
- Make sure you stir the mixture before using.
- After massage, you can take a hot compress and gently wipe off your skin.

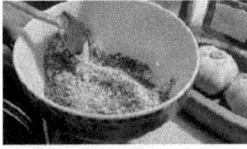 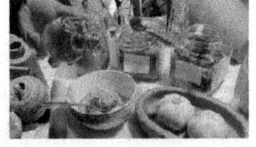
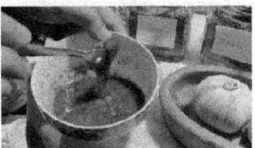 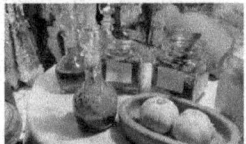

The second recipe:

Ingredients are,
5 teaspoons of parsley
3 teaspoons of fennel
5 teaspoons bay leaf powder
2 teaspoons of moringa seeds
A large cup of olive oil

Method:
- Take all the dry ingredients and grind it in a coffee grinder until it becomes a coarse powder.
- Add virgin olive oil to it and mix well.
- Place it in an airtight container, away from heat and sun or store it in the refrigerator.
- Use 3 times a day with gentle pressure on the back.
- Make sure you stir the mixture before using.
- After massage, you can take a hot compress and gently wipe off your skin.

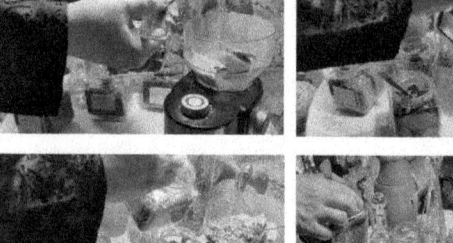
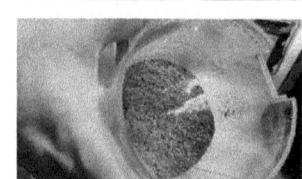
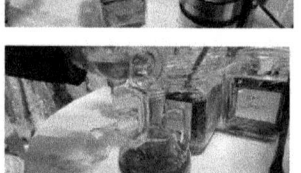

Benefits:
- Relieving acute pain
- Relaxes the muscle and calms the nerves, in addition to softening and lightening the skin
- Stimulates nerves
- Reduces inflammation

The third recipe:

Ingredients are,
2 teaspoons of cloves
3 teaspoons of sage powder
3 teaspoons of coriander powder
A teaspoon of honey

Method:
- Take all the dry ingredients and grind it in a coffee grinder until it becomes a coarse powder.
- Add honey to it and mix well.
- Add olive oil to it and mix well.
- Place it in an airtight container, away from heat and sun or store it in the refrigerator.
- Use 3 times a day with gentle pressure on the back.

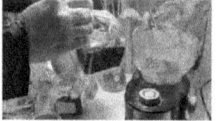
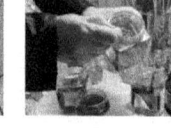
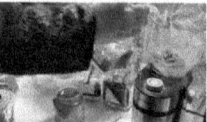
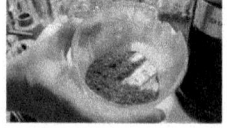

Benefits:
- Relieving acute pain
- Relaxes the muscle and calms the nerves, in addition to softening and lightening the skin
- Stimulates nerves

The fourth recipe:

Ingredients are,
3 teaspoons of fenugreek
3 teaspoons of mustard
3 teaspoons of mint
A large cup of olive oil

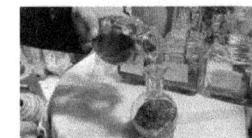 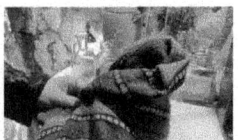

Method:
- Take all the dry ingredients and grind it in a coffee grinder until it becomes a coarse powder.
- Add virgin olive oil to it and mix well.
- Place it in an airtight container, away from heat and sun or store it in the refrigerator.
- Use 2-3 times a day with gentle pressure on the back.
- Make sure you stir the mixture before using.

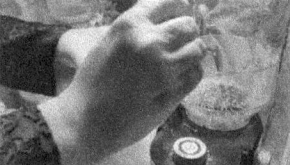 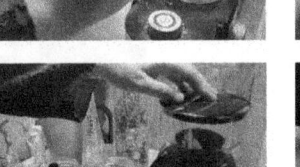 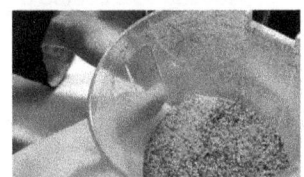 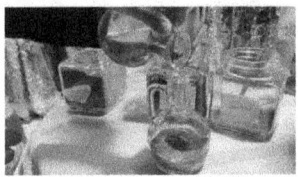 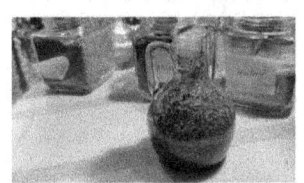

Benefits:
- Relieving acute pain
- Relaxes the muscle and calms the nerves, in addition to softening and lightening the skin
- Stimulates nerves

The fifth recipe:

Ingredients are,

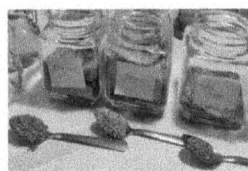

6 teaspoons of chia seeds
3 tablespoons of flaxseed
2 tablespoons of green thyme
A large cup of olive oil

Method:
- Take all the dry ingredients and grind it in a coffee grinder until it becomes a coarse powder
- Add virgin olive oil to it and mix well
- Place it in an airtight container, away from heat and sun or store it in the refrigerator.
- Use 3 times a day with gentle pressure on the back.
- Make sure you stir the mixture before using.

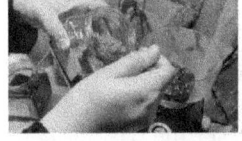 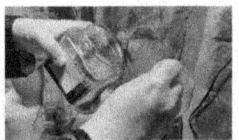 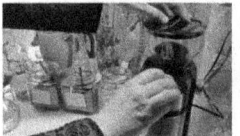 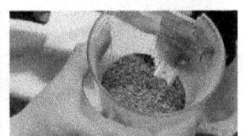

RECIPES FOR CHRONIC LOWER BACK PAIN

The first recipe:

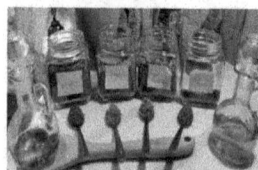

Ingredients are,
3 teaspoon mints
2 teaspoons of sage
3 teaspoons of green thyme powder
3 tablespoons of chia seeds
Half a large cup of olive oil

Method:
- Take all the dry ingredients and grind it in a coffee grinder until it becomes a coarse powder.
- Add virgin olive oil to it and mix well.
- Place it in an airtight container, away from heat and sun or store it in the refrigerator.
- Use 2-3 times a day with gentle pressure on the back.
- Make sure you stir the mixture before using.

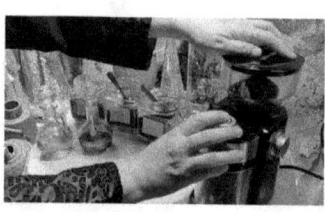 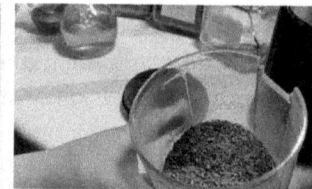
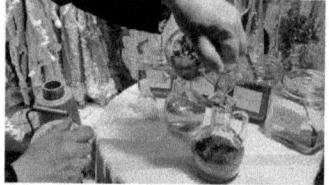 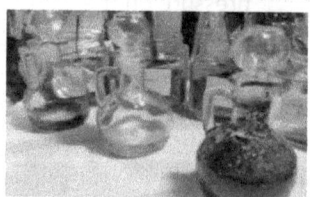

The second recipe:
Ingredients are,

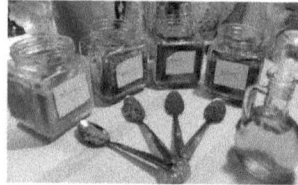

5 teaspoon turmeric
4 teaspoons of basil powder
4 teaspoons of cress seeds
6 teaspoons of mint
Half cup of olive oil

Method:
- Take all the dry ingredients and grind it in a coffee grinder until it becomes a coarse powder.
- Add virgin olive oil to it and mix well.
- Place it in an airtight container, away from heat and sun or store it in the refrigerator.
- Use 2-3 times a day with gentle pressure on the back.
- Make sure you stir the mixture before using

Benefits:
- Relieving acute pain
- Relaxes the muscle and calms the nerves, in addition to softening and lightening the skin

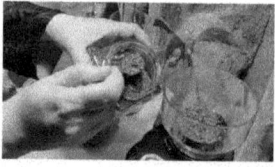 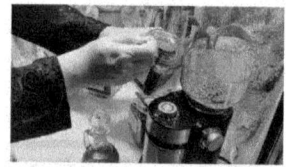
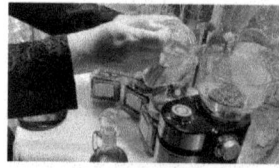 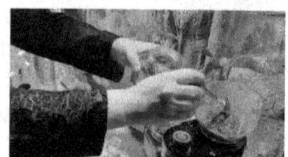
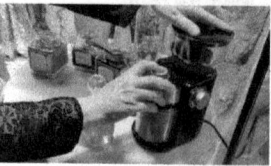 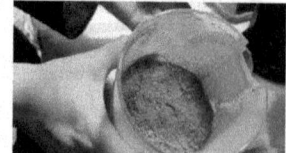

- Stimulates nerves
- Reduces inflammation

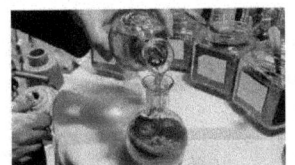 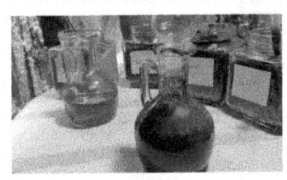

The third recipe:
Ingredients are,

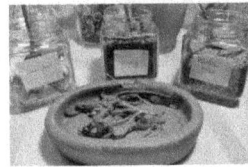

3 teaspoons of fennel
5 teaspoons of chicory
10 teaspoons lemon peel and dry orange peel
Half cup of olive oil

Method:
- Take all the dry ingredients and grind it in a coffee grinder until it becomes a coarse powder.
- Add virgin olive oil to it and mix well.
- Place it in an airtight container, away from heat and sun or store it in the refrigerator.
- Use 2-3 times a day with gentle pressure on the back.
- Make sure you stir the mixture before using.

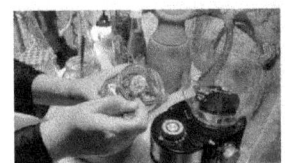 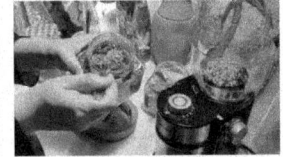
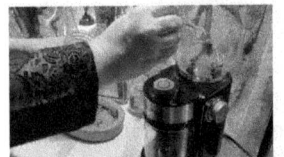 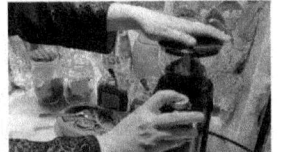
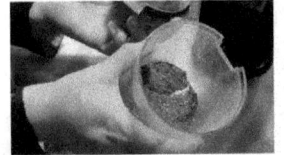 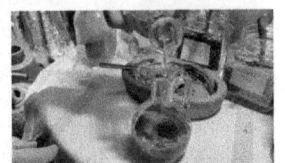
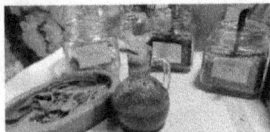 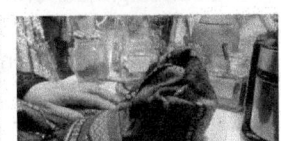

Benefits:
- Relieving acute pain
- Relaxes the muscle and calms the nerves, in addition to softening and lightening the skin
- Stimulates nerves
- Reduces inflammation

The fourth recipe:
Ingredients are,

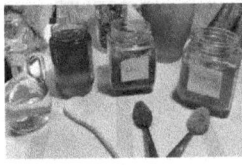

3 teaspoons of honey
5 teaspoons of basil
4 teaspoons of turmeric
Half cup of olive oil

Method:
- Take all the dry ingredients and grind it in a coffee grinder until it becomes a coarse powder.
- Add virgin olive oil and honey to it and mix well.
- Place it in an airtight container, away from heat and sun or store it in the refrigerator.
- Use 2-3 times a day with gentle pressure on the back.
- Make sure you stir the mixture before using.

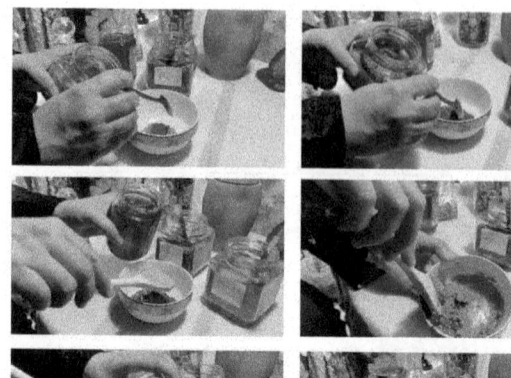

Benefits:
- Relieving acute pain
- Relaxes the muscle and calms the nerves, in addition to softening and lightening the skin
- Stimulates nerves
- Reduces inflammation

The fifth recipe:
Ingredients are,

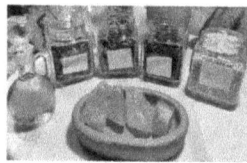

3 teaspoons of bran
5 teaspoons of linden
3 tablespoons of juniper
5 tablespoons of violets
A cup of olive oil

Method:
- Take all the dry ingredients and grind it in a coffee grinder until it becomes a coarse powder.
- Add virgin olive oil and honey to it and mix well.
- Place it in an airtight container, away from heat and sun or store it in the refrigerator.
- Use 2-3 times a day with gentle pressure on the back.
- Make sure you stir the mixture before using.

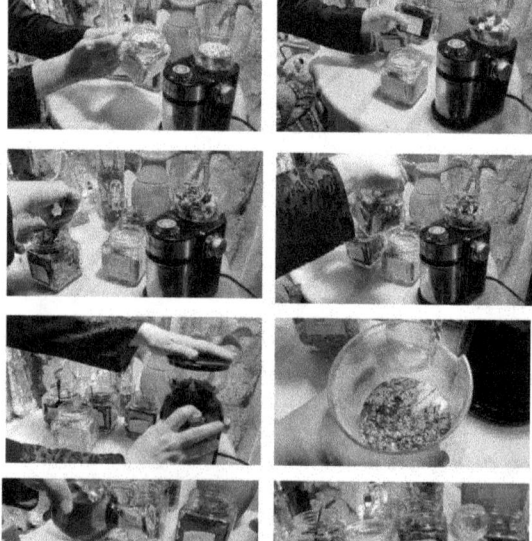

Benefits:
- Relieving acute pain
- Relaxes the muscle and calms the nerves, in addition to softening and lightening the skin
- Stimulates nerves
- Reduces inflammation

The sixth recipe:
Ingredients are,

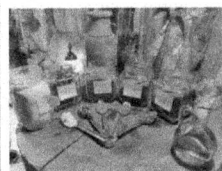

5 spoons of ginger
2 tablespoons of powdered milk
5 tablespoons of Moringa
3 teaspoons of wild thyme
A cup of olive oil

Method:
- Take all the dry ingredients and grind it in a coffee grinder until it becomes a coarse powder.
- Add virgin olive oil and honey to it and mix well.
- Place it in an airtight container, away from heat and sun or store it in the refrigerator.
- Use 2-3 times a day with gentle pressure on the back.
- Make sure you stir the mixture before using.

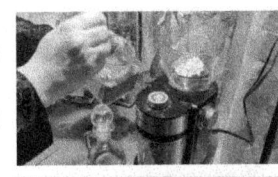 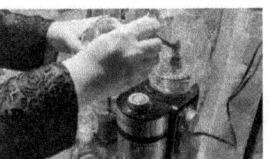
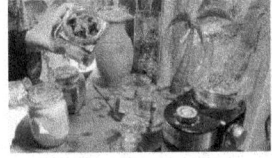 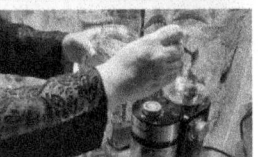
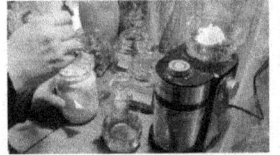 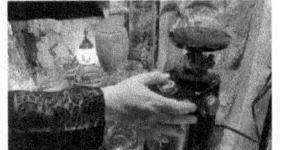
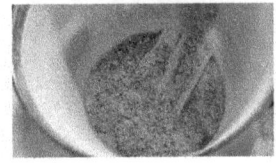 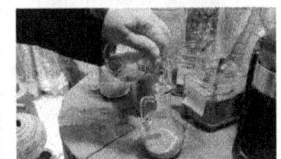

Benefits:
- Relieving acute pain
- Relaxes the muscle and calms the nerves, in addition to softening and lightening the skin
- Stimulates nerves
- Reduces inflammation

The seventh recipe:
Ingredients are,

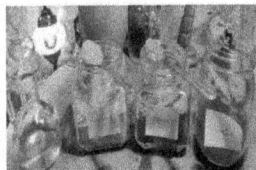

3 teaspoons of cumin
6 teaspoons of turmeric
5 teaspoons of green thyme
A cup of olive oil

Method:
- Take all the dry ingredients and grind it in a coffee grinder until it becomes a coarse powder.
- Add virgin olive oil and honey to it and mix well.
- Place it in an airtight container, away from heat and sun or store it in the refrigerator.

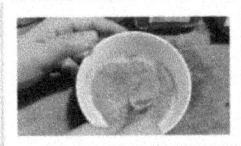 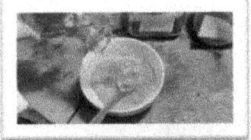
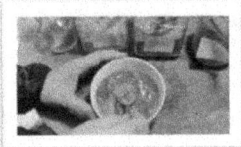 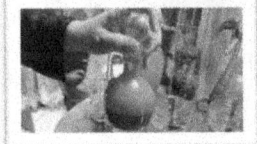

- Use 2-3 times a day with gentle pressure on the back.
- Make sure you stir the mixture before using.

Benefits:
- Relieving acute pain
- Relaxes the muscle and calms the nerves, in addition to softening and lightening the skin
- Stimulates nerves
- Reduces inflammation

The eighth recipe:
Ingredients are,

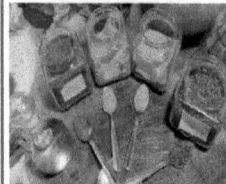

6 teaspoons of cress seeds
5 teaspoons of turmeric
5 spoons of pepper
5 spoons of sesame
A cup of olive oil

Method:
- Take all the dry ingredients and grind it in a coffee grinder until it becomes a coarse powder.
- Add virgin olive oil to it and mix well.
- Place it in an airtight container, away from heat and sun or store it in the refrigerator.
- Use 2-3 times a day with gentle pressure on the back.
- Make sure you stir the mixture before using.

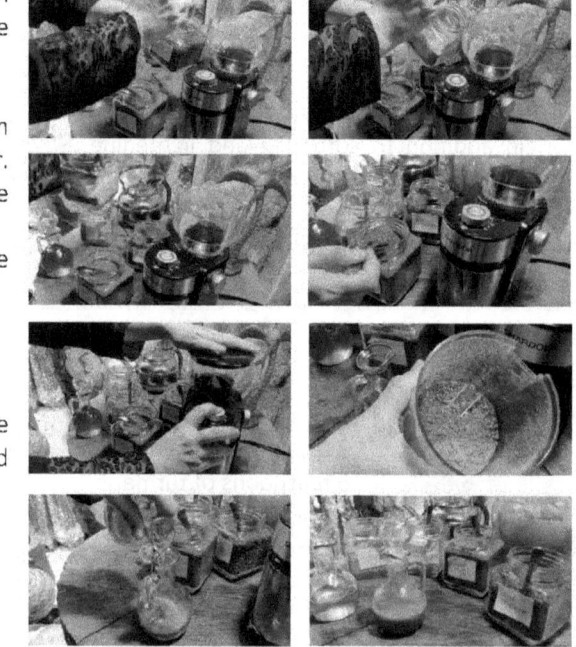

Benefits:
- Relieving acute pain
- Relaxes the muscle and calms the nerves, in addition to softening and lightening the skin
- Stimulates nerves
- Reduces inflammation

The ninth recipe:
Ingredients are,

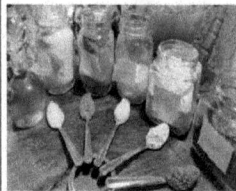

5 spoons of camphor
3 tablespoons of cumin
6 tablespoons of mango
3 tablespoons of powdered milk
2 teaspoons of flour
Half cup of olive oil

Method:
- Take all the dry ingredients and grind it in a coffee grinder until it becomes a coarse powder.
- Add virgin olive oil and honey to it and mix well.
- Place it in an airtight container, away from heat and sun or store it in the refrigerator.
- Use 2-3 times a day with gentle pressure on the back. Put a hot towel after massaging.
- Make sure you stir the mixture before using.

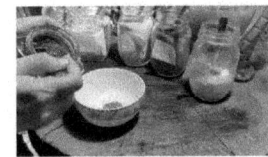
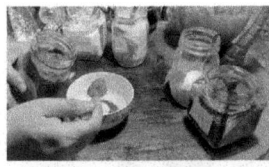
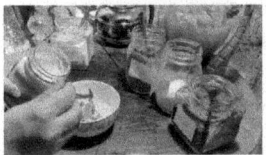
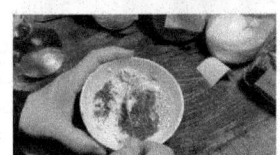
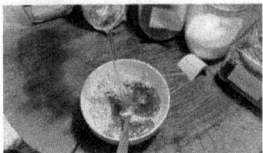
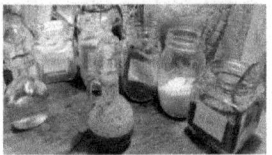

Benefits:
- Relieving acute pain
- Relaxes the muscle and calms the nerves, in addition to softening and lightening the skin
- Stimulates nerves
- Reduces inflammation

The tenth recipe:
Ingredients are,

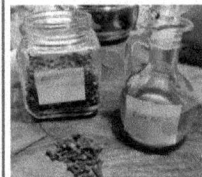

6 spoons of cloves
A normal cup of olive oil

Method:
- Add virgin olive oil to the clove and mix well.
- Let it cool down before using.
- Place it in an airtight container, away from heat and sun or store it in the refrigerator.
- Use 2-3 times a day with gentle pressure on the back. Put a hot towel after massaging.
- Make sure you stir the mixture before using.

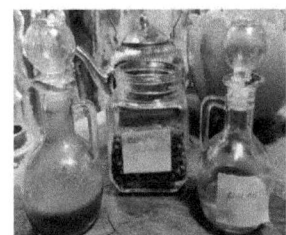

Benefits:
- Relieving acute pain
- Relaxes the muscle and calms the nerves, in addition to softening and lightening the skin
- Stimulates nerves
- Reduces inflammation

The eleventh recipe:
Ingredients are,

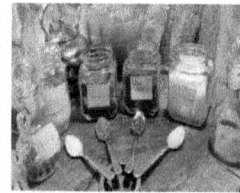

3 teaspoons of lavender oil
3 teaspoons of coconut powder
3 teaspoons of pepper cone
3 teaspoons of mint
3 teaspoons of camphor
1 cup of olive oil

Method:
- Mix all the ingredients together and coarse grind it.
- Add lavender oil and olive oil to the mixture and mix well
- Place it in an airtight container, away from heat and sun or store it in the refrigerator.
- Use 2-3 times a day with gentle pressure on the back. Put a hot towel after massaging.
- Make sure you stir the mixture before using.

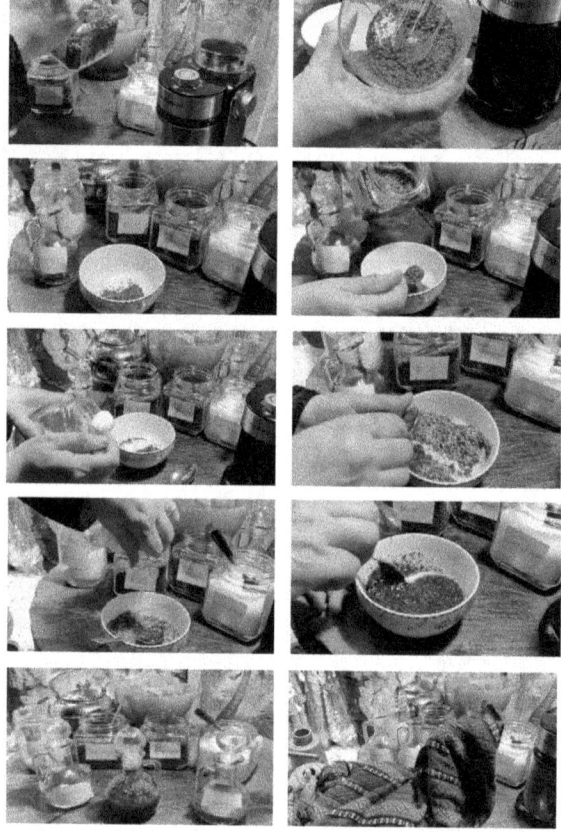

Benefits:
- Relieving acute pain
- Relaxes the muscle and calms the nerves, in addition to softening and lightening the skin
- Stimulates nerves
- Reduces inflammation

The twelfth recipe:
Ingredients are,

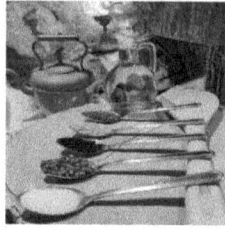

5 teaspoons lavender
3 teaspoons of sesame seeds
2 teaspoons of black seeds
2 teaspoons of pepper cone
2 teaspoons of salt
A full cup of extra-virgin olive oil

Method:
- Take all the dry ingredients and grind it in a coffee grinder until it becomes a coarse powder.
- Add virgin olive oil and mix well.
- Place it in an airtight container, away from heat and sun or store it in the refrigerator.
- Use 2-3 times a day with gentle pressure on the back. Put a hot towel after massaging.
- Make sure you stir the mixture before using.

Benefits:
- Relieving acute pain
- Relaxes the muscle and calms the nerves, in addition to softening and lightening the skin

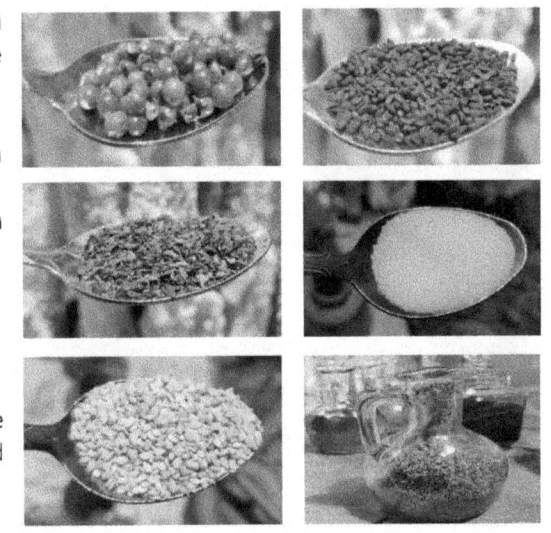

CHAPTER 11: HERBAL TEAS FOR RELAXATION AND PAIN RELIEF

Herbal teas have been used for centuries, both for their health benefits and for pleasure. Some people claim that certain herbal teas have properties that can help reduce symptoms of stress, anxiety, and other mental health concerns. Some herbal teas may help take the edge off occasional stress and anxiety, while others may be better used as a routine complementary therapy for an underlying condition.

Herbal Teas	Benefits
Ashwagandha tea	<ul><li>Reducing stress</li><li>Reducing anxiety and depression</li><li>Reducing fatigue and increasing physical endurance</li><li>Boosting immune system</li><li>Improving fertility</li><li>Promote longevity</li><li>Protecting the brain</li><li>Protecting digestive system</li></ul>
Barley Tea	<ul><li>Boosts Your Immune System</li><li>Improves Blood Flow and Circulation</li><li>Prevents Tooth Decay</li><li>It Can Help You Unwind</li><li>Can Increase Weight Loss</li><li>May Boost Fertility in Men</li></ul>
Chamomile tea	<ul><li>Slowing or preventing osteoporosis</li><li>Treating diabetes and lowering blood sugar</li><li>Reducing inflammation</li><li>Cancer treatment and prevention</li><li>Helping with sleep and relaxation</li><li>Treating cold symptoms</li><li>Treatment for mild skin conditions</li><li>Reducing menstrual pain</li></ul>
Cinnamon Tea	<ul><li>Loaded with antioxidants</li><li>Lowers inflammation and may improve heart health</li><li>May help reduce blood sugar</li><li>May promote weight loss</li><li>Fights off bacteria and fungi</li><li>May reduce menstrual cramps and other PMS symptoms</li></ul>
Cranberry Tea	<ul><li>Antioxidants</li><li>Urinary tract infection</li><li>Oral Hygiene's</li><li>Boost immune system and fights infection</li><li>Vitamin packed</li><li>Stress relief</li></ul>

	- Eye Health - Kidney health - Fat burning
Hibiscus Tea	- Packed With Antioxidants - May Help Lower Blood Pressure - May Help Lower Blood Fat Levels - May Boost Liver Health
Ginger Tea	- 1Blood pressure and heart health - Pain relief - Immune support and cancer prevention - Weight and blood sugar control
Rosehip Tea	- Rich in antioxidants - May have antidiabetic properties - May improve bone health - May have cancer-fighting properties
Lemon tea	- Natural antibacterial - Treats insomnia - Treats diabetes - Natural antibacterial - Lavender Tea Health Benefits - Improves Sleep
Lemongrass tea	- Relieving anxiety. Many people find sipping hot tea to be relaxing, but lemongrass tea may offer further anxiety-reducing properties. - Lowering cholesterol. - Preventing infection. - Boosting oral health. - Relieving pain. - Boosting red blood cell levels.
Valerian Root	- Insomnia - Menopausal Symptoms - Anxiety - Stress Management
Turmeric tea	- Eases arthritis symptoms. ... - Helps prevent Alzheimer's disease. ... - Helps prevent cancer. ... - Maintains ulcerative colitis remission. ... - Boosts the immune system. ... - Lowers cholesterol. ... - Can help treat uveitis.
TULSI	- High Cholesterol - Metabolic Syndrome - Anxiety
Sage tea	- Rich in anti-inflammatory and antioxidant compounds

	- May promote healthy skin and wound healing
- Promotes oral health
- May have anticancer properties
- Improves blood sugar control
Rosemary Tea	- High in antioxidant, antimicrobial, and anti-inflammatory compounds
- May help lower your blood sugar
- May improve your mood and memory
- May support brain health
Rose tea	- Naturally caffeine-free
- Hydration and weight loss benefits
- Rich in antioxidants
- May alleviate menstrual pain
Honey bush	- Rich in antioxidants
- May support a healthy immune system
- May aid weight loss
- May protect against heart disease
Rooibos Tea	- Low in Tannins and Free from
- Caffeine and Oxalic Acid
- Packed With Antioxidants
- May Boost Heart Health
- May Reduce Cancer Risk
Peppermint Tea	- May Ease Digestive Upsets
- May Help Relieve Tension Headaches and Migraines
- May Freshen Your Breath
- May Relieve Clogged Sinuses
Olive leaves tea	- relax and ease arthritic pain
- reduce bad cholesterol
- lower glucose levels
- lower blood pressure
- strengthen the cardiovascular system – a heart tonic
- stimulate the immune system
- help fight infections

CHAPTER 12: HERBAL POULTICE (PASTE) RECIPES FOR PAIN RELIEF

What is herbal poultice (paste)?

A poultice is simply a way to apply herbal matter directly to the skin. Typically, the herbs are mixed with water or oil and applied much like a paste. If the herb is particularly potent, such as with onion, mustard, garlic, or ginger, the skin may be protected by a thin cloth, or the herbs might be placed in a cloth bag or a clean sock. Herbal poultices may be hot, which increases circulation in the area, or cold, which can quickly relieve the pain of a sunburn or the sting of an insect bite. Certain herbs can fight infection, reduce inflammation, draw poison from the skin, relieve aches and pains, or soothe chest congestion.

Precautions for using herbal poultice
- An allergic reaction is possible when applying any substance directly on your skin. Test a small area on your forearm before applying the poultice to the affected area.
- Do not apply any type of paste or cloth poultice to a wound that appears to be seriously infected.
- If you're making a heated poultice, it should be warm — not hot — to avoid burning your skin.
- Ten to fifteen minutes is the usual time for this poultice to be applied to the skin, and when it is removed a little olive oil should be applied.

Here are some recipes for herbal poultice for pain relief,

Neck and shoulder pain

Recipe 1: Figs with oats and turmeric

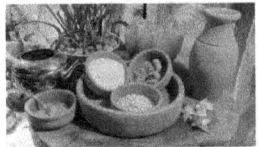

Ingredients
5 dried figs
1 cup of milk
3 tablespoons oatmeal
4 teaspoons turmeric

Method:
- Boil the oats with milk, add turmeric, and then mix well.

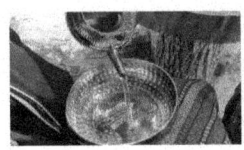 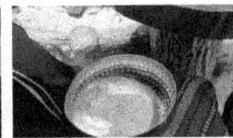 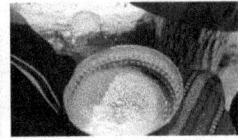 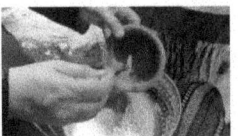

- Add figs in the mixture and blend it well until it becomes paste.

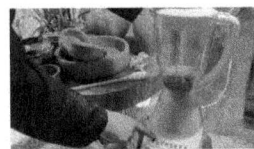 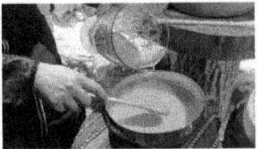 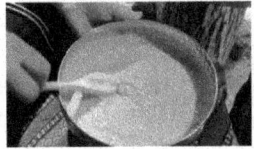

- Apply the paste directly to the neck without any barrier such as gauze or cloth three to four times a day.
- Keep the paste for 10-15 minutes. It can also be stored in container to be used several times later.

Benefits:
- Reduces pain

- Activates circulation
- Nourishes the muscle
- Relaxes the nerves and muscles
- Reduces inflammation.

Recipe 2: Banana and avocado with cinnamon

Ingredients:

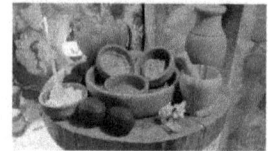

1 banana
1 medium-sized avocado
1 teaspoon cinnamon
1/4 cup yogurt

Method:
- Mash the banana and avocado in a bowl.

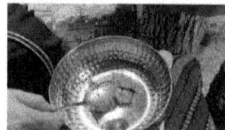 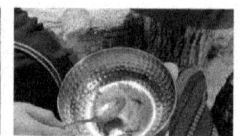

- Add cinnamon to it and then mix everything with yogurt.

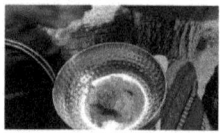 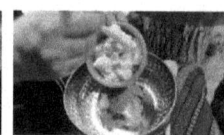 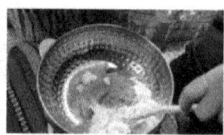 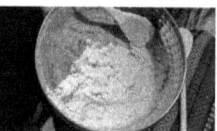

- Put on the gauze and apply 2-3 times a day and the duration of treatment an hour on the back.
- Can be applied for a week or until the pain ends.

Benefits:
- Relieves pain
- It helps the nerves relax.
- Nourishes the muscle
- Reduces inflammation.
- It activates circulation.

Recipe 3

Ingredients:

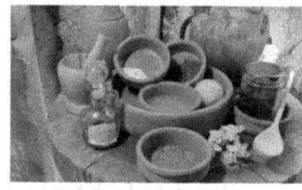

2 Egg outer covering or peel.
1/4 cup lemon juice
3 tablespoons cress seed
3 teaspoons honey
1 teaspoon pepper
3 teaspoons olive oil

Method:
- Grind the egg peel until smooth powder and then add lemon juice and olive oil and mix well.

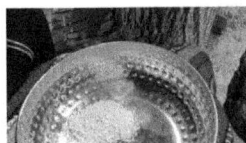 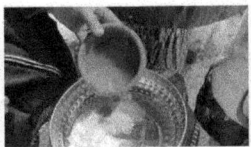 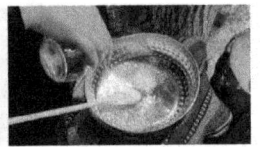

- Add grounded pepper and cress seeds and finally add honey until a sticky paste is formed.

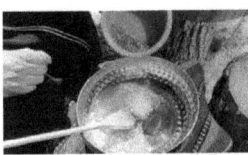 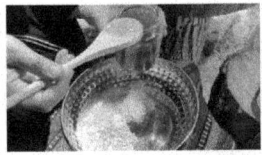 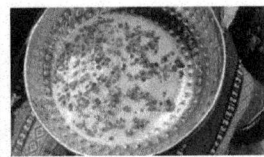

- You can apply it topically and on top of it a hot towel can be placed.

Benefits:
- Relieves pain in the neck and back
- Nourishes the muscle
- Activates circulation
- Stimulates nerves
- Reduces inflammation.

For Back Pain
Recipe 1:
Ingredients:

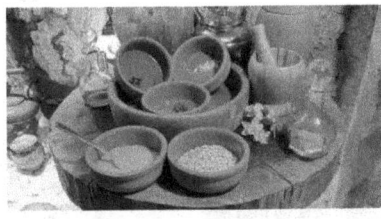

2 teaspoons ginger
1 cup of hot water
1 teaspoon cloves
1 teaspoon cinnamon
1/4 cup vinegar
3 tablespoons tahini
4 tablespoons oatmeal

Method:
- Boil the oats with water and then add cloves, cinnamon, and ginger.

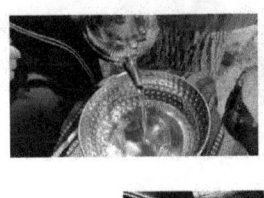 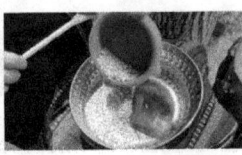 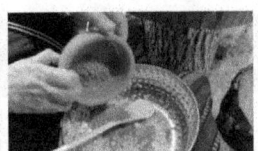 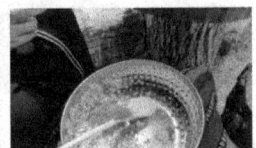

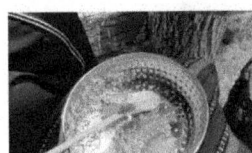 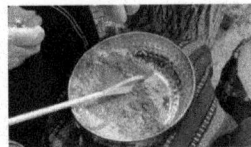 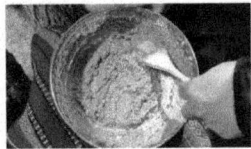

- When it becomes a coherent mixture then add tahini on top of it.

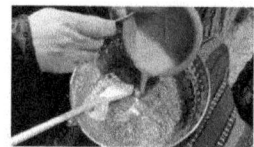
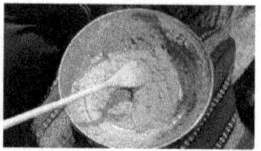

- Apply directly to the area of pain and this is for the sharp back pain which can be in the lower or middle back.

Benefits:
- Relieves pain
- It reduces inflammation and stimulate the nerves.
- Activates circulation, nourishes the muscle.

Recipe 2
Ingredients:

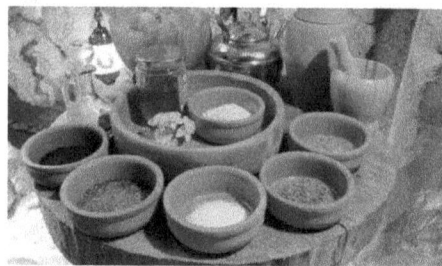

1 teaspoon camphor
2 tablespoons black seed
2 tablespoons thyme
3 teaspoons lavender oil
3 teaspoons mint
3 teaspoons basil
3 teaspoons honey
3 teaspoons flour or oatmeal

Method:
- Grind the materials well and then mix them with honey and flour or oatmeal to make a paste.

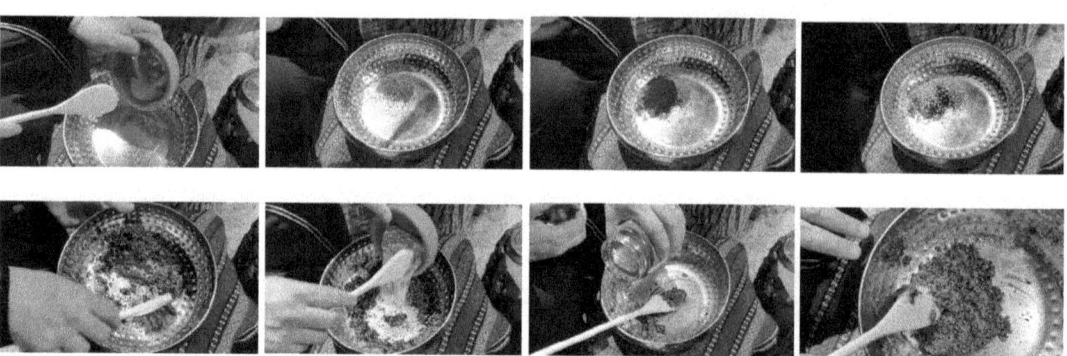

- Apply topically to the place 2-3 times a day for a week. Can be applied to the neck and back, for a month.

Benefits
- Relieve pain
- Activates circulation
- Stimulates nerves
- Reduces flames
- Nourishes the muscle

Recipe 3:
Ingredients:

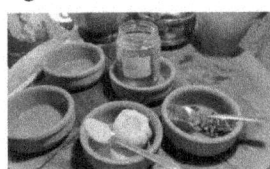

3 tablespoons wheat flour
3 tablespoons ginger powder
3 tablespoons fenugreek
2 tablespoons chia seed
1/4 cup olive oil

Method:
Grind the material in a grinder and then add olive oil gradually until it becomes a paste, apply the paste directly to the area of pain.

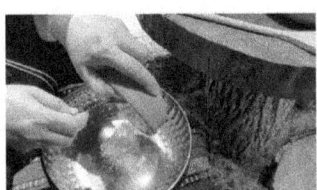 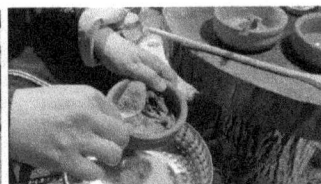 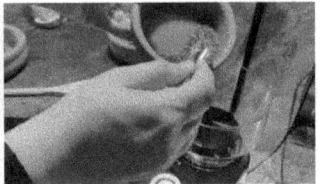

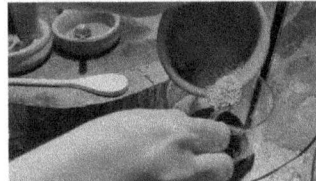 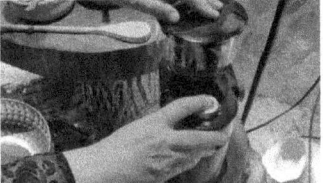

Benefits
- Reduces pain
- Activates circulation
- Reduces inflammation
- Stimulates nerves
- Nourishes the skin and muscle

Recipe 4:

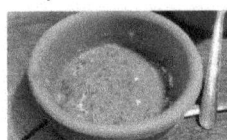

3 cloves garlic
Slice of aloe vera
Spoonful of cloves
1 teaspoon honey

Method:
- Beat garlic in mortar and pastel and mash it until it becomes like paste.

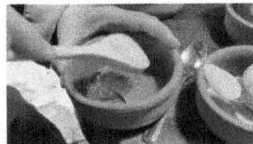 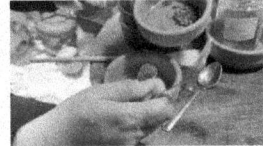 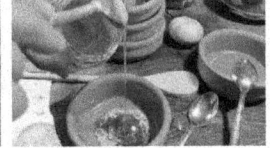 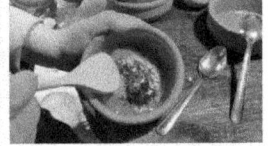

- Always use the paste through a screen may be a cloth, should not put directly on the skin for fear of allergic reactions.
- Can be used 3 times a day for a week until healing in case of severe pain. Should not use on neck.

Benefits:
- Reduces pain
- Stimulates nerves
- Activates circulation
- Nourishes the muscle.
- Reduces inflammation

CHAPTER 13: HERBAL INHALATIONS AND GARGLING FOR RELAXATION

Steam inhalation, also known as steam therapy, has been around since ancient times. The Egyptians were the first known users of inhalation therapy and often included dry plants and minerals in their preparations. Today, steam therapy is still a common non-pharmacologic treatment to help clear mucus and open the nasal passages, throat, and lungs. There are several ways to inhale steam, which is created by boiling water with various herbs and then breathing in the steam it releases.

BENEFITS OF STEAM INHALATION:

A stuffy nose is triggered by inflammation in the blood vessels of the sinuses. The blood vessels can become irritated because of an acute upper respiratory infection, such as a cold or a sinus infection. The main benefit of breathing in moist, warm steam is that may help ease feelings of irritation and swollen blood vessels in the nasal passages. The moisture may also help thin the mucus in your sinuses, which allows them to empty more easily. This can allow your breathing to return to normal, at least for a short period of time.

Steam inhalation may provide some temporary relief from the symptoms of:
- the common cold
- the flu (influenza)
- sinus infections
- bronchitis
- nasal allergies

How to do steam inhalation with herbs?
The most common method of steam inhalation is a do-it-yourself treatment.
- Put two quarts of water in a pot.
- Heat the water until it's not quite boiling, just steamy.
- Put two handfuls of herbs in the water and let steep for 10 minutes.
- Create a tent with a towel over your head to inhale the steam.
- Inhale the steam for no more than 10 minutes.
- Keep the decoction, or extract, of water and herbs on your counter for a few hours after you're finished.

At that point, the herbs have become more concentrated, and the chemicals they release into the air from their essential oils can be left to dissipate in the air, where they can continue to help refresh you and your environment. You can toss the liquid after a few hours. Additional steam therapy methods include inhaling steam from baths, showers, and steam rooms. These methods are the best way to use steam inhalation to relieve symptoms of sore throat and nasal congestion in children. In recent years, portable steam inhalers, also known as vaporizers, have become popular. Herbs most beneficial for steam inhalation: Many herbs can help increase the beneficial effects of steam therapy. Here are five popular choices:

Thyme	This herb is an expectorant (helps loosen mucus) and has antibacterial properties. It's the most used essential oil for steam therapy because it has great benefits, and it's not an irritant like some stronger oils can be
Mint	Mint leaves in steam therapy decoctions is very effective. It has a nice scent, and it helps loosen mucus and is also antibacterial, but cautions against using peppermint essential oil for steam therapy, as it is very strong. Spearmint oil used in vaporizers may be a better choice.
Eucalyptus	It has cooling qualities and is used as a natural decongestant and can help with respiratory ailments. It's great for loosening mucus, but use it in small doses, as it can be overpowering

Basil	It's a decongestant and is naturally antiseptic and antibacterial. It is an essential oil which can be used to sharpen concentration and alleviate some of the symptoms of depression. It may relieve headaches and migraines
Rosemary	This herb has antiviral, anti-inflammatory, and antimicrobial properties. It is a stimulating essential oil that can boost mental activity and sharpen your focus. It can also be used to ease pain and cramping

The best part of using these herbs that they are readily available locally, or even in your own indoor or outdoor herb garden.

Physiology behind inhalation of Essential Oils:

Essential Oils have tiny molecules, which disperse into the air (especially when diffused) and enter through the nose. When inhaled, the scent molecules reach the olfactory epithelium, which consists of millions of receptor cells located at the top of the nostrils, just below and between the eyes. Odors are then converted to messages, which are converted and relayed to the brain for processing. Inhalation provides the most direct route to the brain. With every breath, some scent molecules inescapably travel to the lungs. Some molecules are absorbed by the mucous lining of the respiratory pathway. Other molecules reach the alveoli and are transferred into the bloodstream.

Therefore, inhalation of essential oils not only influences emotions but also has a physical impact. Interaction with the limbic system (emotional brain). During inhalation, odor molecules travel through the nose and affect the brain through a variety of receptor sites, one of which is the limbic system, which is commonly referred to as the "emotional brain." The limbic system is directly connected to those parts of the brain that control heart rate, blood pressure, breathing, memory, stress levels, and hormone balance. This relationship helps explain why smells often trigger emotions. Knowing this, we can hypothesize how inhalation of essential oils can have some very profound physiological and psychological effects.

What do essential oils do?

- Basil essential oil is used to sharpen concentration and alleviate some of the symptoms of depression. It may relieve headaches and migraines. It should be avoided during pregnancy.
- Bergamot essential oil is said to be useful for the urinary tract and digestive tract. When combined with eucalyptus oil it may help relieve skin problems, including those caused by stress and chicken pox.
- Black pepper essential oil is commonly used for stimulating the circulation, muscular aches and pains, and bruises. Combined with ginger essential oil, it is used to reduce arthritis pain and improve flexibility.
- Chamomile essential oil can treat eczema.
- Citronella essential oil is a relative of lemongrass and acts as an insect repellent
- Clove essential oil is a topical analgesic, or painkiller, that is commonly used for toothache. It is also used as an antispasmodic antiemetic, for preventing vomiting and nausea, and as a carminative, preventing gas in the gut. It has antimicrobial, antioxidant, and antifungal properties.
- Eucalyptus essential oil can help relieve the airways during a cold or flu. It is often combined with peppermint. Many people are allergic to eucalyptus, so care should be taken.
- Geranium essential oil can be used for skin problems, to reduce stress, and as a mosquito repellant.
- Jasmine essential oil has been described as an aphrodisiac. While scientific evidence is lacking, research has shown that the odor of jasmine increases beta waves, which are linked to alertness. As a stimulant, it might increase penile blood flow.
- Lavender essential oil is used as an antiseptic for minor cuts and burns and to enhance relaxation and sleep. It is said to relieve headache and migraine symptoms.
- Lemon essential oil is said to improve mood and to help relieve the symptoms of stress and depression.
- Rosemary essential oil may promote hair growth, boost memory, prevent muscle spasms, and support the circulatory and nervous systems.

- Sandalwood essential oil is believed by some to have aphrodisiac qualities.
- Tea tree essential oil is said to have antimicrobial, antiseptic, and disinfectant qualities. It is commonly used in shampoos and skin care products, to treat acne, burns, and bites. It features in mouth rinses, but it should never be swallowed, as it is toxic.
- Thyme essential oil is said to help reduce fatigue, nervousness, and stress.
- Yarrow essential oil is used to treat symptoms of cold and flu, and to help reduce joint inflammation.

Useful oil for Respiratory system

- Thyme oil: can remove excess mucus in the airways, eliminate infection and open airways that can worsen respiratory symptoms. How to use: This essential oil can be added to the vaporizer by 3-6 drops,
- Lavender oil: It has some soothing and anti-inflammatory properties that make it ideal for the respiratory system. It can reduce swelling in the respiratory tract and calm muscle spasms, preventing bronchospasm that can cause wheezing. How to use: You can add lavender oil to a warm bath and inhale the resulting aromatic vapors deeply or mix lavender oil with jojoba oil.
- Eucalyptus oil: It is known to be a demulcent and expectorant that can also break up excess mucus in the respiratory tracts. It is soothing for infections of the throat and breathing passages. How to use: Add 5 drops of camphor oil to the vaporizer or diffusers.
- Tea tree oil: It stimulates an immune system response in the form of excess mucus production in inflamed airways. Tea tree oil can counteract this injury directly by the body. How to use: Add five to six drops to a bowl of hot water. Put a towel on your head and take deep breaths.
- Frankincense oil: It will cut the mucus and relieve tightness in the chest, promoting normal and healthy breathing, even during an asthma attack. How to use: Many people choose to spread frankincense oil in the air for all-day, which gives relief from breathing conditions. A diluted version of this oil (along with coconut oil) can also be applied to your chest at night, as it will help you breathe normally throughout the night without interruption while you sleep.
- Clove oil: It can prevent the respiratory tracts from developing allergies, and this oil relieves muscle tension in the throat as well, so that breathing continues without interruption. How to use: Clove oil has a wonderful scent, which makes it a popular choice for diffusing it in rooms, as well as for steam inhalation treatments. Some people choose to mix it with a carrier oil (such as almond or olive oil) and apply it to the chest. However, sensitivity to this oil is very high, so never apply undiluted oil to the skin.
- Mint leaves oil: Armed with decongestant, antispasmodic, sedative, and anti-inflammatory properties. It can open breathing passages and prevent an asthma attack from becoming more severe.
- Chamomile oil: This legendary anti-inflammatory oil can calm respiratory inflammation and support the immune system, and it does not have any significant catalytic reactions. It can also act as a repellent to get rid of excess mucus from the throat and lungs, making asthma attacks less severe. How to use: You can add a few drops of chamomile oil to a cup of hot chamomile tea during a steam inhalation treatment to help you keep your breathing easy throughout the day.
- Peppermint oil: Peppermint oil is one of the essential oils you always have because it not only smells great, but it also helps relieve pain. You can use peppermint essential oil to treat several health problems. Research has found peppermint oil to be a good natural oil for relieving headaches, improving depression, relieving muscle pain, clearing congestion, and soothing skin ailments.

Antibacterial oils

- Lemon essential oil: Lemon essential oil comes in the top list as one of the best scented essential oils for your home that also have medicinal properties. It removes germs from surfaces and kills bacteria on the skin. Apply 4-6 drops.
- Clove essential oi: Clove is another essential oil that smells good and has many therapeutic uses to help improve your health. Contains antimicrobial and antioxidant properties, only use 2-3 drops.

- Oregano oil: Oregano oil is commonly used with carrier oils to help treat and prevent wound infections. Studies have shown that oregano essential oil is effective against infection with staphylococcus aureus bacteria.
- Sage oil: It works to expel parasites, fungi and bacteria from the house and cleanse the general atmosphere of the house by dropping a few drops of oil in the vaporizer. 2-4 drops
- Ginger oil: It sterilizes the house and has a pleasant smell that helps to expel bacteria from the house and even mosquitoes and bugs can be placed 5 drops.

For anxiety, stress & relaxation.
- Lavender oil: Inhalation of lavender oil has been proven to improve sleep quality. Specialist in complementary and alternative medicine has confirmed the positive effect in combating mild sleep disorders. Use 3 drops into a diffuser
- Thyme essential oil: Thyme essential oil has anti-inflammatory, anti-fungal, and anti-bacterial properties. It has been shown that when used alone or in combination with other natural health-promoting compounds, it reduces snoring. Use 2 drops.
- Peppermint essential oil. Inhaling peppermint essential oil can aid in rest and relaxation due to its aromatic scent. Use 2-5 drops only.
- Lemon oil: Lemon essential oil is extracted from fresh lemon peels by cold pressing method. It is great in cases of anxiety and stress. Use 3 drops.
- Fennel oil: Fennel essential oil is extracted by crushing the seeds of the fennel plant and then extracting the oil through a process of steam distillation. Helps relax because of its fragrant smell.
- Eucalyptus oil: The leaves of eucalyptus trees are dried, crushed, and distilled to extract the essential oil. The scent of eucalyptus oil can help soften mucus in the respiratory tract, which may help reduce snoring by 2-3 drops.
- Vetiver oil: Vetiver essential oil can help you breathe better while you sleep. Use 5 drops.
- Clove oil: Clove oil is made by distilling the dried flower buds of the clove tree. You can use 1-2 drops.
- Sage oil: The use of sage oil before bedtime contributes to improving breathing quality at high rates, using 2-5 drops.

The most important oil to improve blood circulation:
- Camphor essential oil is characterized by stimulating blood vessels and stimulating blood circulation. Use 5-6 drops.
- Cypress oil: is an excellent oil for those who feel tired, weak, and exhausted, and it is a stimulant for blood vessels. Use 4 drops.
- Ginger oil: The refreshing smell helps the body to be active and it is preferable to put this oil in the morning or in the offices. You can use 3 drops.
- Coriander essential oil: This oil is characterized by its direct entry into the nose, cleansing of the urticarial veins, stimulating the blood, and thus stimulating blood circulation.
- Black pepper oil: The pepper plant is characterized by suppressing appetite and stimulating the digestive and respiratory system, due to stimulating and revitalizing the blood. And therefore, the effectiveness is stronger by fumigation than using it as oil. Use 1-2 drops.
- Cumin oil: Cumin is a substance that stimulates blood circulation and relaxes the digestive system. Use 2-4 drops.
- Lavender oil: is characterized by the aromatic substance inside it and its wonderful smell that makes it beneficial wherever and however it is applied. It also helps in stimulating blood circulation. Use 2-3 drops.
- Headache treatment: Camphor oil: is characterized by its strength and aroma that helps relieve pain and stimulates nerves. 2-3 drops

- Citrus oils: These oils are great for applying to headaches, as it helps in relieving it and help sleep. Use 6 drops of it.
- Peppermint oil: It is characterized by its strong smell, which inhaled helps relieve headaches. Use 3 drops.
- Lavender: It is characterized by giving a feeling of comfort and relieving pain. You can use 2-3 drops.
- Rose, violet, and basil oil: Basil helps relieve headaches due to its wonderful aromatic smell. Apply 3-4 drops of basil oil, 2-3 drops of rose and violet oil. The combination of these oils contributes to accelerating the recovery from headaches, especially migraines.
- Nut oil: This fruit has many benefits, not to mention its oil, and it has benefits for hair, cramps, and pain, and when inhaled, it has the ability to relieve headaches, especially migraines. You can use 2-5 drops.
- Jasmine oil: Jasmine is distinguished by its essential oil that is used in perfumes and sometimes in sherbets, and Jasmine tea, which is very comfortable for head problems and headaches, even nervous tension. Use 1-2 drops.

Here are some recipes for inhalation:

Recipe 1:
Ingredients
- 5 cups lukewarm water
- 1 teaspoon vinegar
- 6 teaspoons rosemary
- 2 teaspoons thyme

Method:
Put the water in a bowl and boil and add herbs to it. When the water is boiling, and you see steam coming out of it switch the flame off and add vinegar and cover it. Put a towel on the face with the bowl inside and inhale for half an hour or 20 minutes and then wash face with cold water. Repeat the process daily for a week.

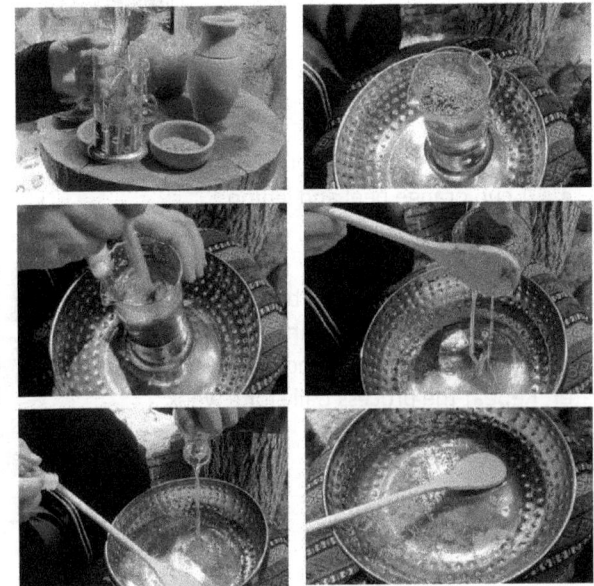

Recipe 2:
Ingredients
- 5 cups lukewarm water
- 5 teaspoons of lavender oil
- 3 teaspoons chamomile
- 3 drops of lemon oil

Put water in a bowl and boil and add herbs to it and then add vinegar and put a towel on the face and inhale for half an hour or 20 minutes and then wash face with water. Repeat the process daily for a week.

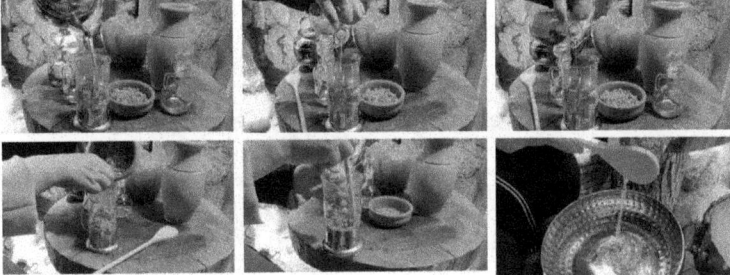

Lavender oil treats dry skin or eczema. It is very useful for relaxing.

Recipe 3:
Ingredients:
- 5 cups lukewarm water
- 1 teaspoon Camphor

Put the water in a bowl and boil then add camphor. Put a towel on your face and inhale from the bowl for half an hour or 20 minutes and then wash face with water repeat the process daily for a week.

Benefits
- Calm the nerves.
- Stimulates the body and vitality.
- Good pain reliever.

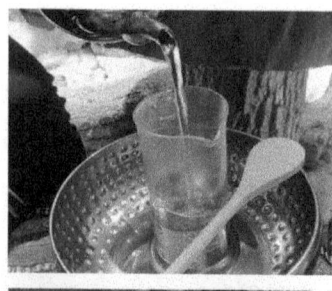
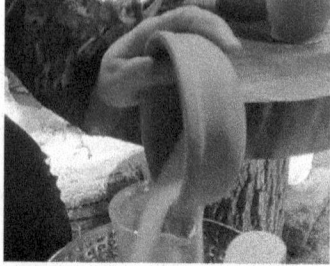
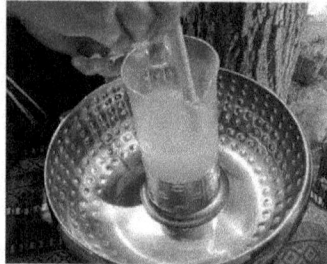
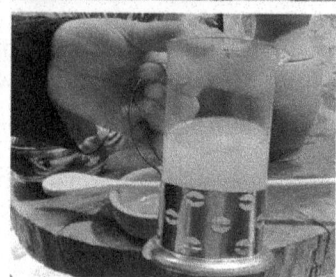

Recipe 4:
Ingredients:
- 5 cups lukewarm water
- 1 cup orange peel and lemon
- 3 teaspoon vinegar

Put the water in a bowl and boil then add vinegar. Put a towel on the face and inhale from the bowl for half an hour or 20 minutes and then wash face with water. Repeat the process daily for a week.

Benefits
- Reduces pain
- Calm the nerves.
- Detox
- It fragments skin pores and stimulates circulation.

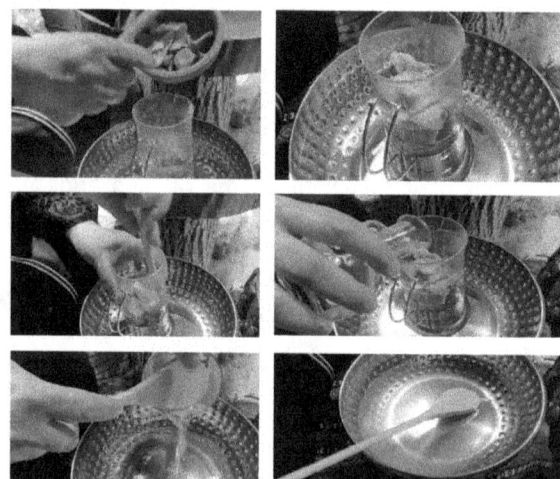

Steps involved to prepare for inhalation:
You'll need the following materials:
- a large bowl
- water
- a pot or kettle and a stove or microwave for heating up water
- towel

Here's the process:
1. Heat up the water to boiling.
2. Put the ingredients in the boiling water as mentioned in the above following recipes. You can choose any recipe according to your condition.
3. Carefully pour the hot water into the bowl.
4. Drape the towel over the back of your head making a tent over your head.

5. Turn on a timer.
6. Shut your eyes and slowly lower your head toward the hot water until you're about 8 to 12 inches away from the water. Be extremely careful to avoid making direct contact with the water.

7. Inhale slowly and deeply through your nose for at least two to five minutes.
Don't steam longer than 10 to 15 minutes for each session. However, you can repeat steam inhalation two or three times per day if you're still having symptoms.

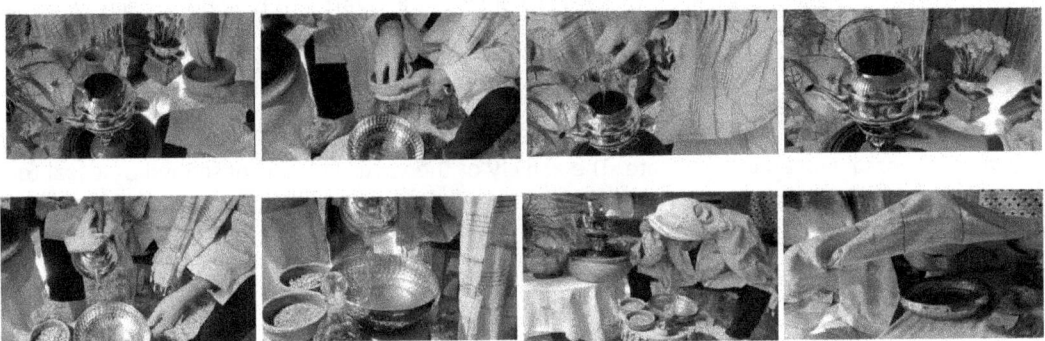

GARGLING

A traditional home remedy of gargling warm saltwater is sometimes recommended to soothe a sore throat. Physiological changes that occur when you do saltwater gargle: Soreness of throat is generally due to the infection of the bacterium called Streptococcus. So, it is called strep throat. A strep throat is usually inflamed due to bacteria making widespread damage on our soft tissues or mucosa. These inflammations (known as edemas) are usually filled with water. When we gargle with warm salt water that is saltier than our body fluids (hypertonic solution), through osmosis the salt draws out the edema fluid.

The principle behind it is that if a porous partition separates dilute and concentrated solutions then the dilute solution permeates through the porous partition into the concentrated solution.
This process does not stop till the concentration of both the solutions is equal. Salt water is more concentrated than the water in bacteria. The membrane of the cell of inflammatory tissue acts as a porous partition. So, the salt draws water from the swollen cells that are causing pain and the inability to swallow foods.
Not only that, it will also draw water from the bacteria. When the bacteria gradually lose their body fluid, they cannot remain active after dehydration. So, they wither and die. This phenomenon is called plasmolysis.

The other benefits are; when the salt water enters the throat, the solution helps to neutralize acids in the throat, restoring the natural pH balance that had been disrupted by the sore throat. By doing this, the burning sensations are relieved, and the mucous membranes become less irritated, which can speed healing.

Benefits of saltwater gargle:
Saltwater gargles can be effective for treating mild pain, discomfort, and tickles in the mouth and throat. Maintains the pH level. The mixture helps to neutralize the acids in the throat that is produced by bacteria. It helps to maintain a healthy pH balance, which prevents the growth of unwanted bacteria in the mouth.
- Sore throats: Saltwater gargles can be an effective way to relieve discomfort from sore throats. Clears nasal congestion Gargling with salt water also helps to remove the mucus build-up in your respiratory tract and nasal cavity. The concoction reduces the inflammation and relieves the pain in the throat. Apart from that, it flushes out the bacteria and virus, which if left unattended can lead to congestion.
- Gives relief from tonsillitis: Tonsils are two lump tissues located at the back of the throat, which gets inflamed due to a bacterial and viral infection. Inflamed tonsillitis might cause pain in swallowing the food. Gargling with salt water can help you get relief from the pain and ease these symptoms.

- Canker sores: Canker sores are painful ulcers that can develop in the mouth. Gargling with salt water may help ease pain and promote healing of the sores.
- Allergies: Some allergies, such as hay fever, can cause a person's nasal passages and throat to swell, which can be uncomfortable. Though gargling with salt water will not prevent the allergy, it may help alleviate some of the throat discomforts.
- Respiratory infections: Gargling with salt water may help relieve the symptoms of the common cold.
- Dental health: Regularly gargling with salt water can assist in removing bacteria from the gums, which helps in cleaning and preventing the buildup of plaque and tartar. A buildup of bacteria in the mouth can lead to gum disease and tooth decay.

How does gargling help in relaxation?

It innervates the heart, lungs, and gut, it can powerfully alter your physical reaction to stress and improve your mental and emotional state. The activity of the vagus nerve is described by Vagal tone— the higher the tone, the better the parasympathetic response and the calmer we feel. Gargling for 10-20 seconds can be a strong stimulus for the vagus nerve.

Here are some recipes for gargling:

Recipe 1
Ingredients:
- Half a teaspoon of salt
- 3 teaspoons chamomile
- 2 tablespoons honey
- 1 cup of water

Method:
Put the chamomile in water and boil then add honey and salt and stir well and gargle with it 3 times a day.

Benefits:
- Pharyngeal cleanses protect against germs and viruses
- Reduces inflammation
- Stimulates nerves
- Activates circulation

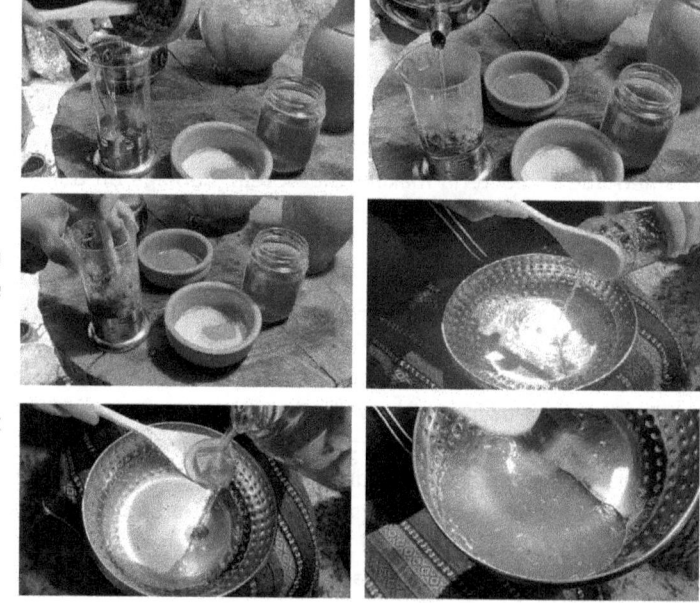

Recipe 2:
Ingredients
- 2 teaspoons mint
- 2 teaspoons green tea
- 2 teaspoons of sage
- ½ a teaspoon of table salt

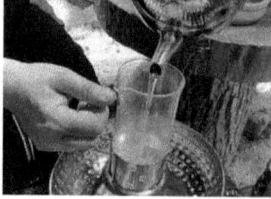
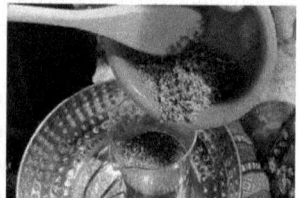

Method:
Boil everything together and drain and then add salt to it and gargle with it 3-4 times a day.

Benefits
- Pharyngeal cleanses protect against germs and viruses.
- Protects against diseases and reduces infections
- Relieves pain and congestion
- Stimulates nerves and tasteful senses
- Activates circulation

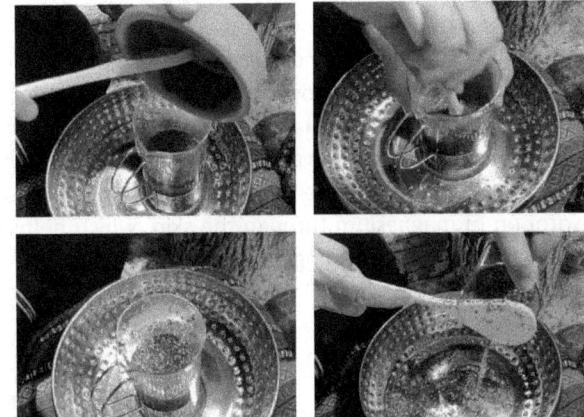

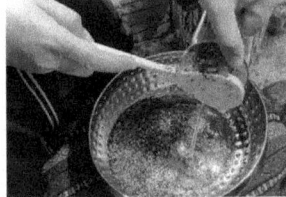 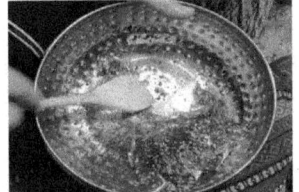

Recipe 3:
Ingredients:
- 2 teaspoons salt
- 2 cups warm water

Method:
This gargle is an inexpensive natural remedy and easily available in every house. Boil water and then add salt to it and gargle 3-4 times a day.

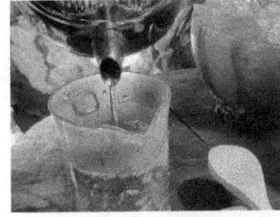 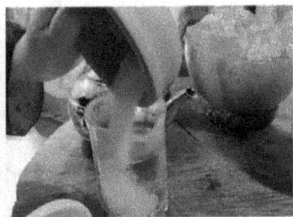
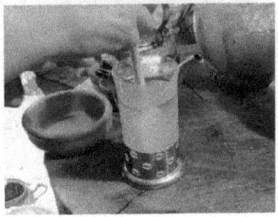 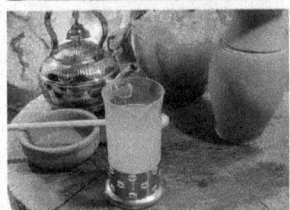

Benefits:
- Protects against diseases and reduces infections
- Relieves pain and congestion
- Stimulates nerves and tasteful senses
- Benefits in light pain relief
- Strengthens gums and reduces infections

CHAPTER 14: BODY AND FOOT SOAK RECIPES FOR RELAXATION

But first let us understand how soaking helps?

Salt is considered a home remedy for generations. Soaking the foot with it relieves aches and pains, reduces inflammation, improves blood circulation, reduces, or removes unpleasant odors from the feet, and has anti-fungal and microbial properties. It helps with skin infections and wounds, including athlete's foot, nail fungus and small wounds. In addition, there is a lot of research indicating that it helps to remove toxins from the body and relieve stress. Skin absorption of minerals relieves cramping and foot pain, enhances the absorption of magnesium through the skin, which helps relax muscles and nerves and relieves foot pain. It has antibacterial and antifungal properties, improving blood flow to the skin, thus enhancing the chances of recovery.

Recipes for body soaking

Recipe 1
Ingredients:

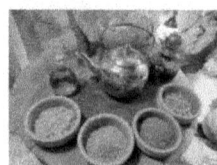

A cup of Epsom salt/Dead Sea or homemade table salt
Half a cup of apple cider vinegar
Dry chamomile, mint, basil, and thyme

Method:
- Mix all the dry herbs and boil it with water until simmers.

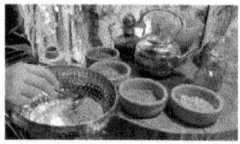 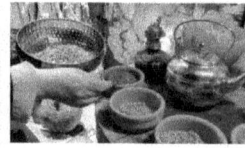 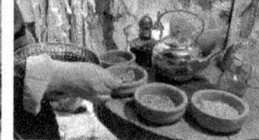

- Add warm water and stir well.

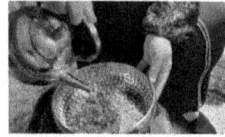 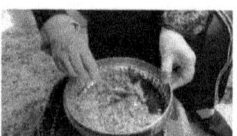

- Add salt, apple cider vinegar and stir well.

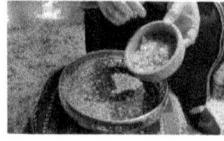 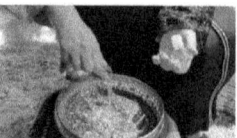

- Soak your body in tub filled with this mixture every evening for 15-20 minutes. (You can be there for longer time if you need).

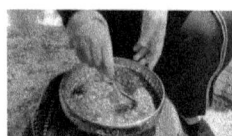 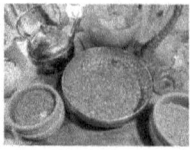

Benefits:
- It reduces toxins present in the body and lessens the pain
- Reduces infections, bacteria, and fungus
- Stimulates blood circulation
- Nourishes the skin and make it smooth.

Recipe 2
Ingredients:
> Half a cup of Dead Sea Salt or Epsom salt
> 10 teaspoons of dry or fresh mint leaves
> 10 teaspoons of dry or fresh mint leaves
> 10 teaspoons of rosemary
> 5 A cup of apple cider vinegar
> teaspoons of chamomile

Method:
- Mix all the dry herbs in a bowl.

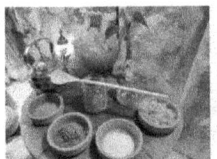 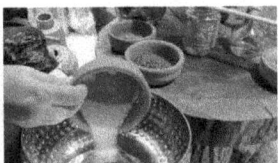 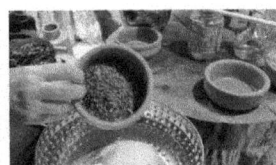 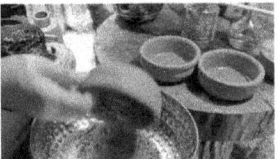

- Add warm water, salt, and apple cider vinegar into it and mix well.

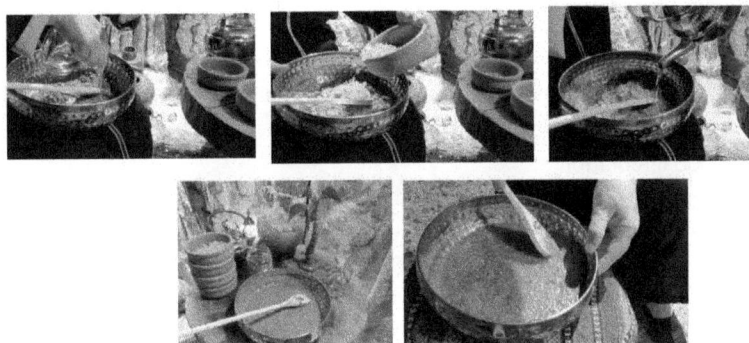

- Soak your body in tub filled with this mixture every evening for 15-20 minutes. (You can be there for longer time if you need).

Benefits:
- It reduces toxins present in the body and lessens the pain
- Reduces infections, bacteria, and fungus
- Stimulates blood circulation
- Nourishes the skin and make it smooth.

Recipe 4
Ingredients:

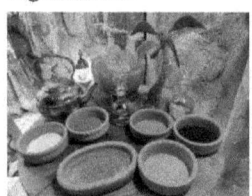

A large cup of dead sea salt, Himalayan salt, or Epsom salt
4 teaspoons of ginger
4 teaspoons basil
5 teaspoons of olive oil
A cup of apple cider vinegar

Method:
- Mix all the dry herbs in a bowl.

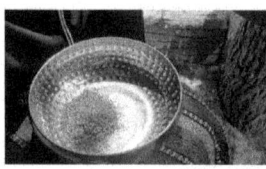 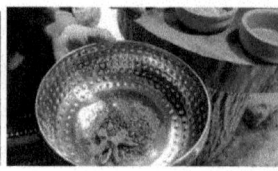 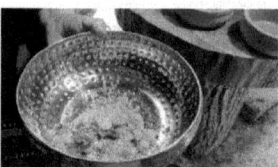

- Add warm water, olive oil, and apple cider vinegar into it and mix well.

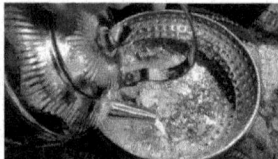 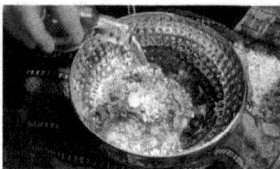 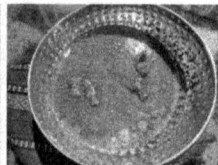

- Then, soak your body in tub filled with this mixture every evening for 15-20 minutes. (You can be there for longer time if you need).

Benefits:
- It reduces toxins present in the body and lessens the pain
- Reduces infections, bacteria, and fungus
- Stimulates blood circulation
- Nourishes the skin and make it smooth.

Recipe 5
Ingredients:
10 teaspoons of table salt
A large cup of apple cider vinegar
3 teaspoons of mint
3 teaspoons of sesame
5 teaspoons of wild thyme
5 teaspoons of black seed powder
5 teaspoons of flaxseed

Method:
- Take flax seeds, black seeds, sesame seeds, and grind it well. Take it in a bowl.

A 24-HOUR HOME REMEDY GUIDE TO YOUR BACK PAIN

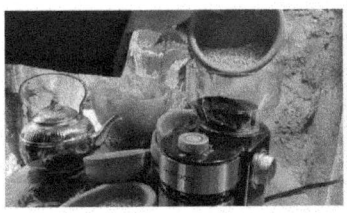 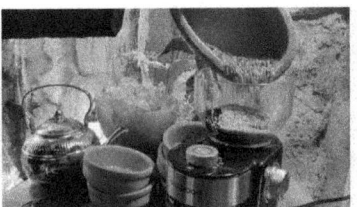 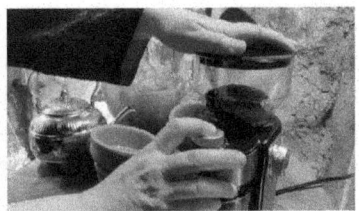

- Mix all the dry herbs (mint, thyme, and salt) in a bowl.

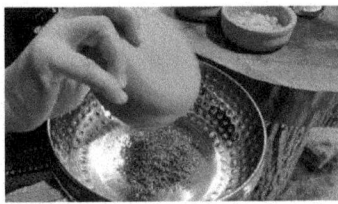 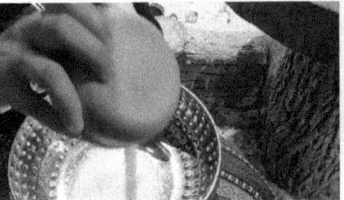 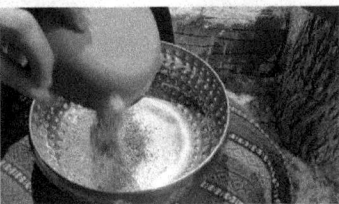

- Add warm water, olive oil, and apple cider vinegar into it and mix well.

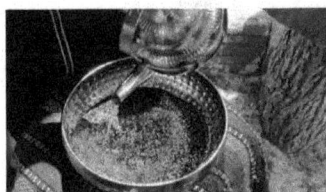 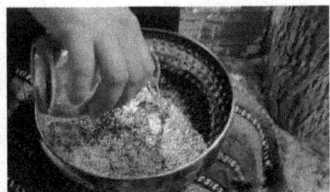 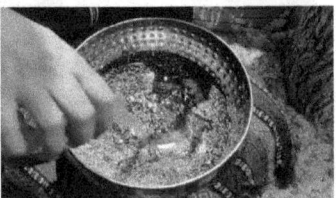

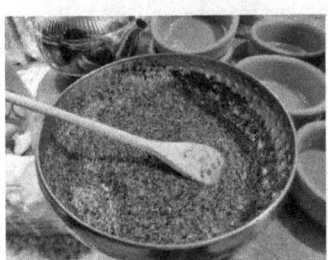

- Then, soak your body in tub filled with this mixture every evening for 15-20 minutes. (You can be there for longer time if you need).

Benefits:
- It reduces toxins present in the body and lessens the pain
- Reduces infections, bacteria, and fungus
- Stimulates blood circulation
- Nourishes the skin and make it smooth.

Recipes especially for foot soaking:

Recipe 1

Ingredients:

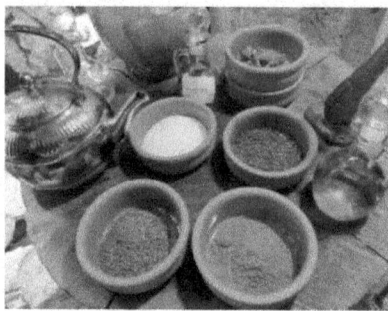

2 teaspoons of fennel

3 tablespoons of mint

5 spoons of ginger

4 tablespoons of sage

4 tablespoons of table salt

A cup of white vinegar

Method:

- Mix all the dry herbs in a bowl.

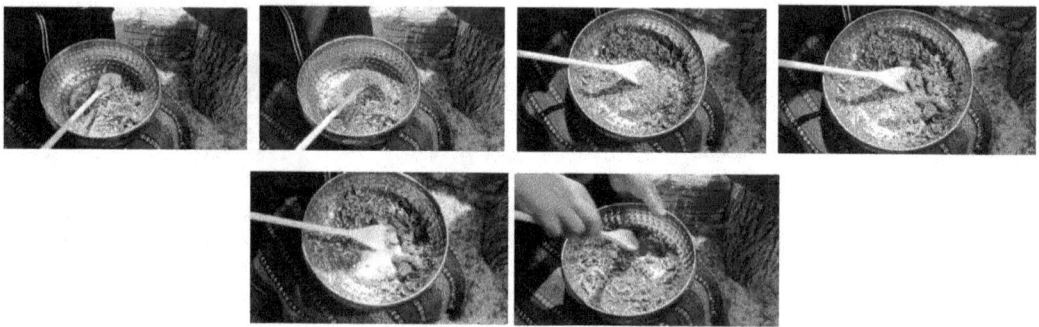

- Add warm water, olive oil into it and mix well.

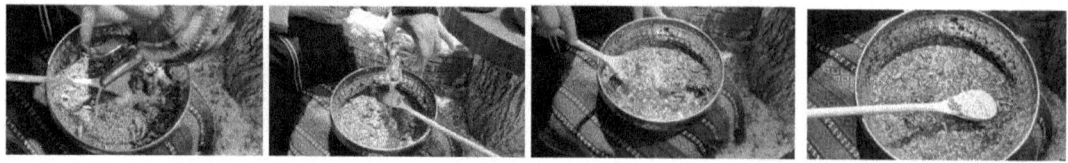

- Then, soak your feet in tub filled with this mixture every evening for 15-20 minutes. (You can be there for longer time if you need).
- Prefer a bowl or tub which is non-metallic.

Recipe 2
Ingredients:
3 tablespoons of ginger

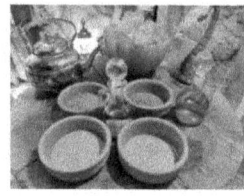

2 tablespoons of lavender

4 tablespoons of mint

3 tablespoons of cumin

2 tablespoons of hot pepper

7 tablespoons of table salt

A cup of food vinegar, preferably white

Method:
- Mix all the dry herbs in a bowl.

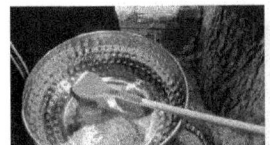 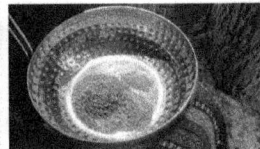 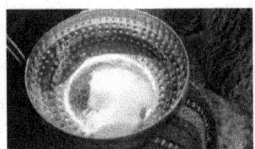 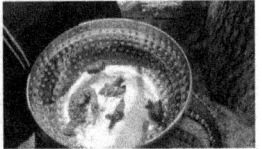

- Take hot pepper and grind it well. Take it in a bowl and mix with the other herbs.

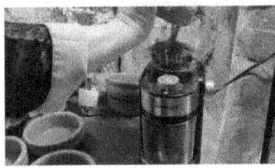 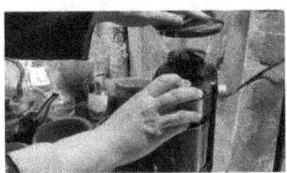 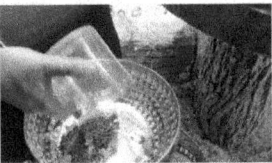

- Add warm water, olive oil, and lavender into it and mix well.

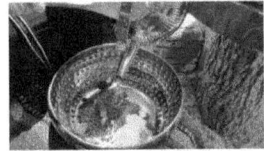 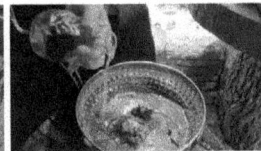 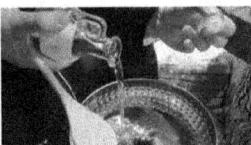 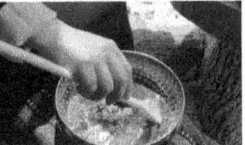

- Then, soak your feet in tub filled with this mixture every evening for 30 minutes. (Repeat it for 2 times a day).
- Prefer a bowl or tub which is non-metallic.

Recipe 3

Ingredients:
- A cup of apple cider vinegar
- 3 teaspoons of Moringa
- 3 teaspoons of sesame seeds
- 5 teaspoons of cinnamon
- A quarter cup of olive oil

Method:
- Mix all the dry herbs (moringa and cinnamon powder) in a bowl.

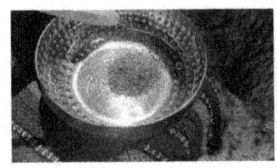 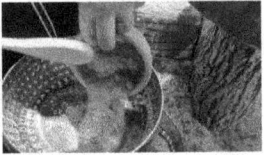

- Take sesame seeds and grind it well. Take it in a bowl and mix with the other herbs.

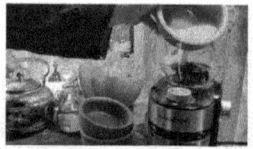 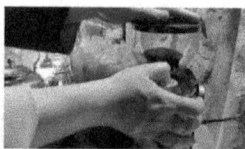 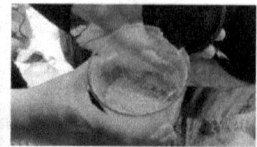 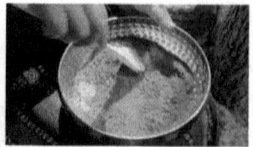

- Add warm water, olive oil into it and mix well.

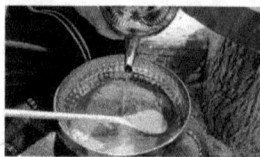 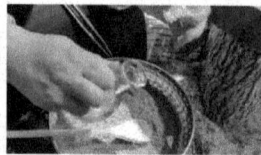 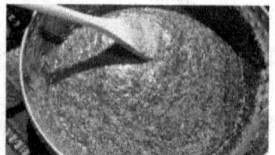 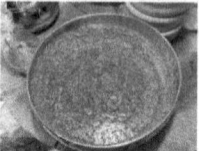

- Then, soak your feet or the whole body in tub filled with this mixture every evening for 15-20 minutes. (You can be there for longer time if you need).

Benefits:
- It reduces toxins present in the body and lessens the pain
- Reduces infections, bacteria, and fungus
- Stimulates blood circulation
- Nourishes the skin and make it smooth.

Recipe 4
Ingredients:

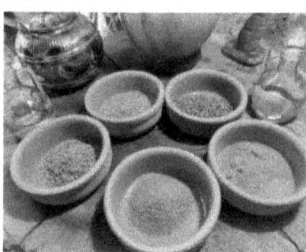

A cup of apple cider vinegar
3 tablespoons of coriander seed
5 spoons of moringa sowing
5 spoons of cinnamon
3 tablespoons of basil
2 tablespoons of thyme
A cup of extra-virgin olive oil

Method:
- Mix all the dry herbs in a bowl.

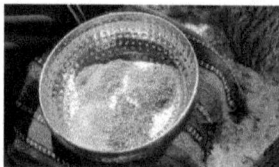 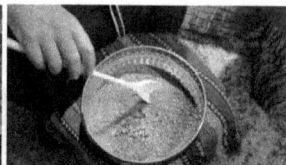

- Add warm water, olive oil into it and mix well.

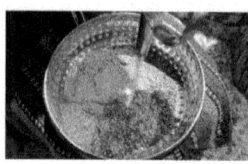 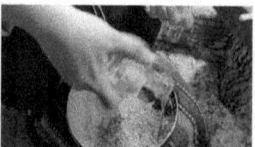 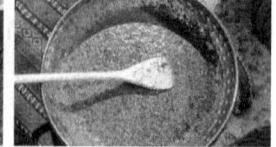

- Then, soak your feet or whole body in tub filled with this mixture every evening for 30 minutes. (Repeat it for 2 times a day).
- Prefer a bowl or tub which is non-metallic for foot.

How to prepare foot soak:

To best ease soreness, a foot soak should be between 92°F and 100°F. foot soak involves immersing the feet in warm water. Follow these steps to perform a foot soak:

1. Fill a basin or foot spa or a bucket with enough warm water to cover the feet up to the ankles.
2. Add any of the following ingredients mentioned above for foot soak, according to your conditions to the water.
3. Place the feet in the soak for about 20 to 30 minutes.
4. Dry thoroughly after the soak and then moisturize the feet.

An Epsom salt foot soak can dry out the feet, so it is best not to do it every night. Try soaking the feet once or twice a week to make sure it does not cause dryness. Always end your foot soak with moisturizer.

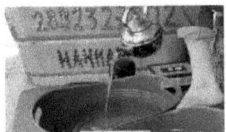 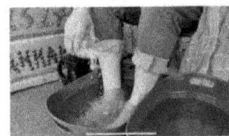 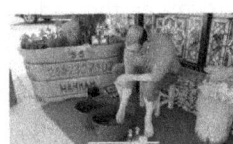 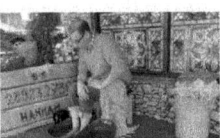

Benefits:

- It reduces toxins present in the body and lessens the pain
- Reduces infections, bacteria, and fungus
- Stimulates blood circulation
- Nourishes the skin and make it smooth.

CHAPTER 15: SCRUBS AND PEELING RECIPES TO REJUVINATE SKIN AND REDUCE PAIN

How peeling relieves pain?
Sugar and ingredients used peels the skin, provides it with different minerals, opens the pores, stimulates the flow of blood circulation, and purifies the body from toxins, as olive oil moisturizes the skin and removes stains. This overall promotes recovery from pain and nourishes the muscles.

For Head and Neck:
Recipe 1:
Ingredients:
- Half a cup of sea salt, Epsom or normal
- Half a cup of virgin olive oil
- 1 teaspoon grated lemon or juice
- 2 tablespoons honey
- 1 teaspoon of Turmeric, mint, green tea and dill.

Method:
- Mix the dry ingredients together, then add honey and mix well.

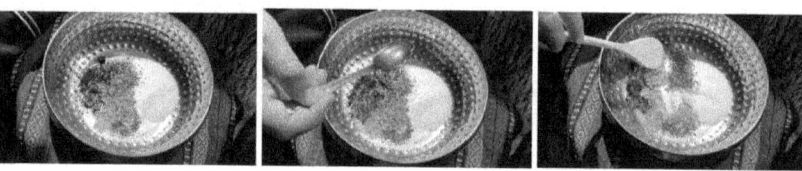

- After that, add lemon juice and mix well.

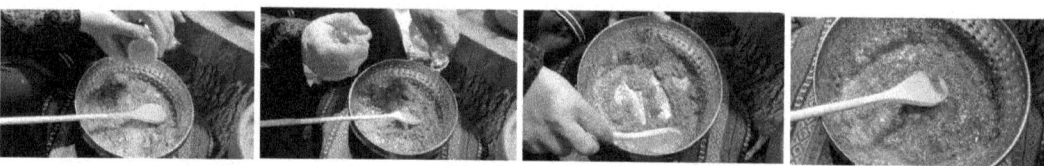

- Massage the body with mixture before bathing, making gentle circular movements.
- Shower with hot water after several minutes without using soap or wipe it with hot towel.
- Dry the skin, then apply a moisturizing cream or lotion

Benefits:
- Relieves pain and stimulates nerves
- Activates blood circulation and nourishes the muscle
- Reduces skin infections and nerve infections

Recipe 2
Ingredients:
- A teaspoon of chamomile.
- A teaspoon of anise.
- Five teaspoons of salt
- Five spoons of caraway.
- A teaspoon of sage.
- Half a cup of white vinegar

- 2 tablespoons honey

Method:
- Mix all the dry ingredients in a bowl and add honey.

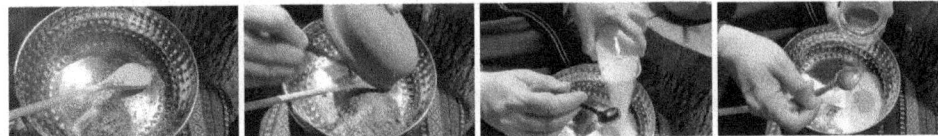

- Add vinegar to the mixture and mix well.

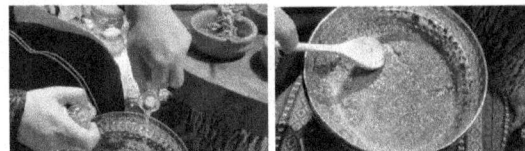

- Massage the body with mixture before bathing, making gentle circular movements.
- Shower with hot water after several minutes without having to use soap.
- Dry the skin, then apply a moisturizing cream or lotion

Benefits:
- Reduces acute pain
- Activates blood circulation and relieves tension from the muscle.
- Stimulates nerve.

Recipe 3
Ingredients:
- 2 tbsp. sugar
- 2 tablespoons honey
- 2 tablespoons coarse salt
- 3 teaspoons oats
- Half a cup of lemon juice
- Half a cup of olive oil
- 1teaspoon of cress seeds, sesame, flaxseed, sage, and mint.

Method:
- Take the grains and grind and mix well.

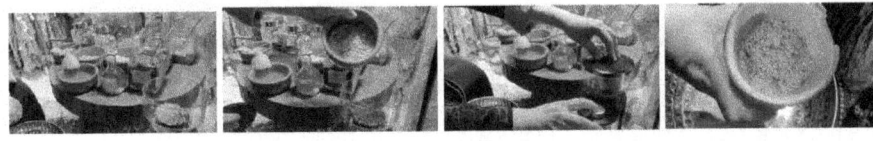

- Add honey, sugar and salt together to lemon juice, mix and add to the dry mixture.

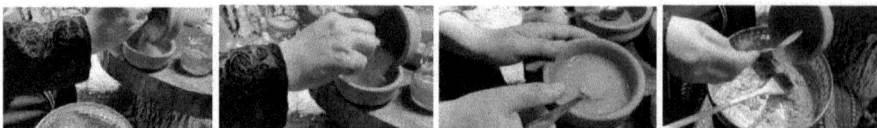

- Add olive oil to the mixture and stir it well.

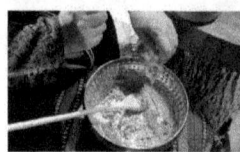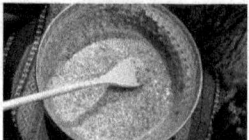

- Massage the body with mixture before bathing, making gentle circular movements.
- Wash the area with lukewarm water or wet towel and then massage in circular movements.
- Shower with hot water after several minutes without having to use soap.
- Dry the skin, then apply a moisturizing cream or lotion

Benefits:
- Relieves pain and stimulates nerves
- Activates blood circulation and nourishes the muscle
- Reduces inflammation.

Recipe 4
Ingredients:
- 1/4 cup olive oil
- Three teaspoons of mint
- ¼ cup of sugar
- Three tablespoons of green tea
- 2 teaspoons turmeric
- Half a cup of table salt or Himalayan salt

Method:
- Mix all ingredients together until a rough paste is formed.

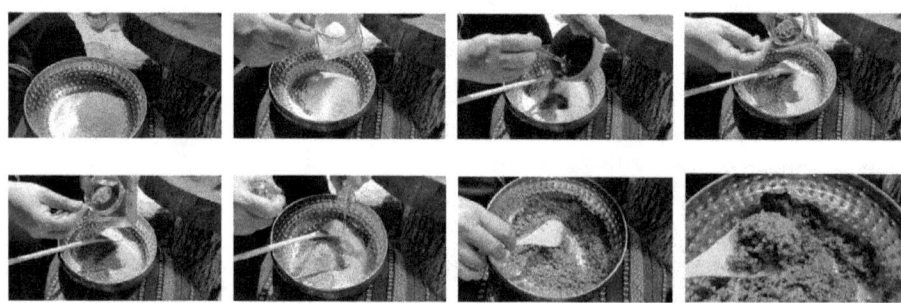

- Clean your skin, then apply the sugar mixture to it.
- Massage the neck and head using your fingers with circular movements on the area.
- For 5-10 minutes, you need one to two minutes on each part of the body.
- Wash your body using a moisturizing peeler with warm water.

Benefits:
- Relieves pain and stimulates nerves
- Activates blood circulation and nourishes the muscle
- Reduces inflammation

Recipe 5
Ingredients:

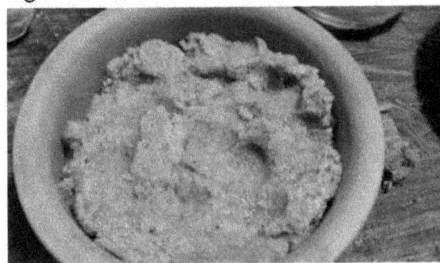

½ a cup of Oatmeal
½ a cup of brown sugar
½ a cup of honey
1 teaspoon of Thyme
1 teaspoon of lavender
2 teaspoon of cloves powder
2 teaspoon of ginger powder
¼ a cup of olive oil

Method:
- Mix all the ingredients together until a smooth mixture and then add the liquid ingredients and mix well until it becomes a dough.

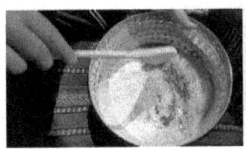 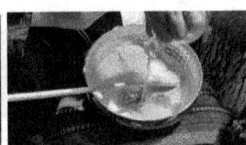 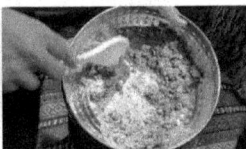 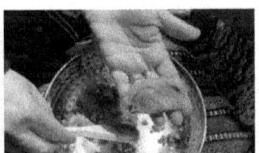

- Clean with lukewarm water or a wet towel and then apply the scrub mixture to the area.
- Massage your skin using your fingers with circular movements for 5-10 minutes.
- Wash your body and apply a moisturizing lotion afterwards.

Benefits
- Activates blood circulation and flush out toxins from your body.
- Reduces inflammation.
- Relieves pain and stimulates nerves.

Recipes for acute back pain

Recipe 1
Peeled sea salt
Salt has antibacterial properties that can help treat certain skin diseases. Salt is also a preservative, so the sea salt peeler can maintain itself naturally. Use ground sea salt because coarse sea salt can be very harsh on your skin. Sea salt peelers may be too abrasive for sensitive skin. Be careful if you have a wound in your skin because salt can hurt it. Because there's no salt smell, you might want to add some of your favorite essential oils to your own salt peeler.

Ingredients:
- 1/2 cup sea salt
- 1/2 cup olive oil
- 2 tablespoons honey
- 2 tablespoons cinnamon
- 2 tablespoons chili

- 2 tablespoons of the cumin
- 2 tablespoons fennel

Method:
- Mix sea salt and oil in a mixing bowl.

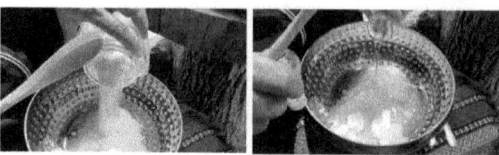

- Mix the herbal materials and grind well and then add to the mixture and put two spoons of honey in the mixture.

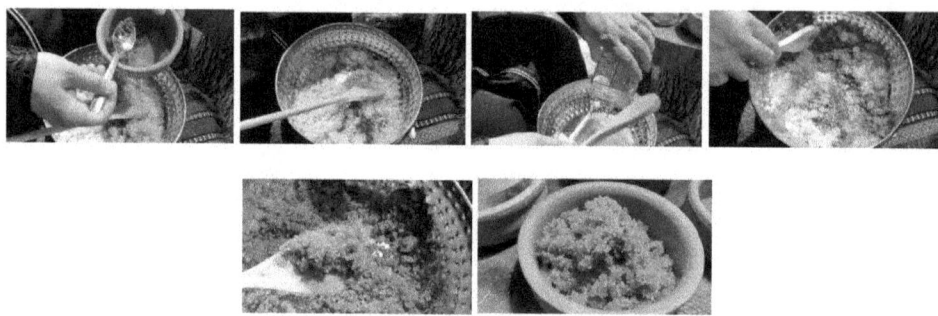

- Massage the painful area in circular motion with fingers.

Benefits:
- Relieves chronic pain
- Reduce Inflammation
- Activates blood circulation and nourishes the muscle
- Reduces skin infections.

Recipe 2
Peeled sugar with green tea

Ingredients:
- 2Bags of green tea
- 1 cup hot water
- 1 cup brown sugar
- 1/4 cup olive oil
- A teaspoon of Hyssopus, Ginseng, Chamomile, Clove, Rosemary.

Method:
- Add the tea bags and herbal ingredients to hot water.

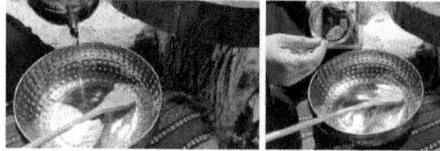

- Let the tea soak until cooled.
- Grind the cloves and mix it with the green tea. Mix well.

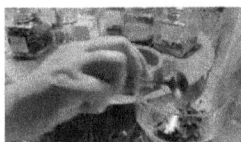 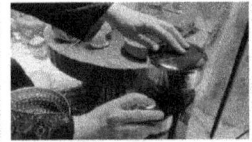 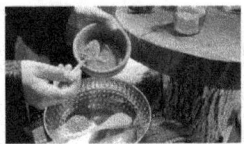 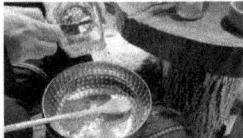

- Add the brown sugar with olive oil in a bowl.

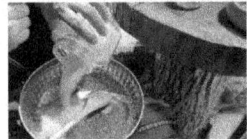 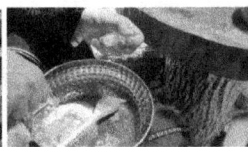 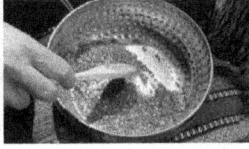 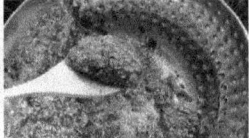

- Massage the mixture to the body with gentle circular movements.

Benefits:
- Relieves pain and stimulates nerves
- Reduce Inflammation
- Activates blood circulation and nourishes the muscle
- Reduces skin infections.

Recipe 3
Peeled sugar with honey
Honey repairs skin tissue and protects against UV rays, and also helps kill germs on the skin. Honey can be easily blended with granules and oil to make a beneficial peeler for the skin.

Ingredients:
- 1 cup brown sugar
- 1 cup olive oil
- A tablespoon honey
- 1/4 cup apple cider vinegar
- Sesame, mint, seed seeds, linden sunflower seed.

Method:
- Add brown sugar, oil, honey, and vinegar in the mixing bowl.

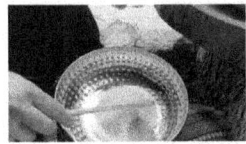 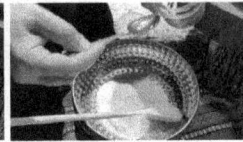 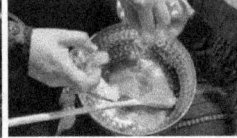 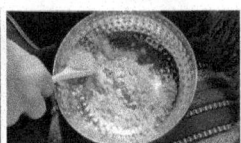

- Grind the herbal materials

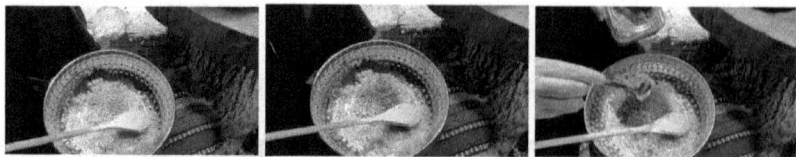

- Add to the oil mixture and mix well.

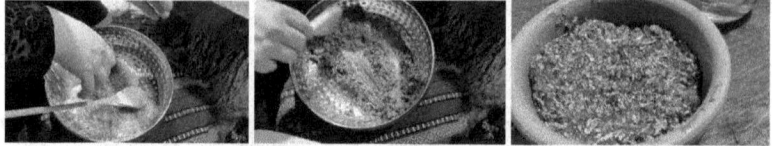

- Add more olive oil if the mixture is fragmented.
- Massage the mixture to the body with gentle circular movements

Recipes for chronic back pain
Recipe 1
Yogurt scrub: Yogurt scrub is suitable for dry skin, it contains ingredients that help clean the skin and get rid of dead cells, as it moisturizes the skin very well.

Ingredients:
- 1 tablespoon yogurt.
- A quarter cup of olive oil.
- A tablespoon of honey.
- ½ cup of salt or sugar
- Teaspoon of: Chamomile, basil, cinnamon, moringa and thyme

Method:
- Mix all the ingredients together until a rough paste is formed.

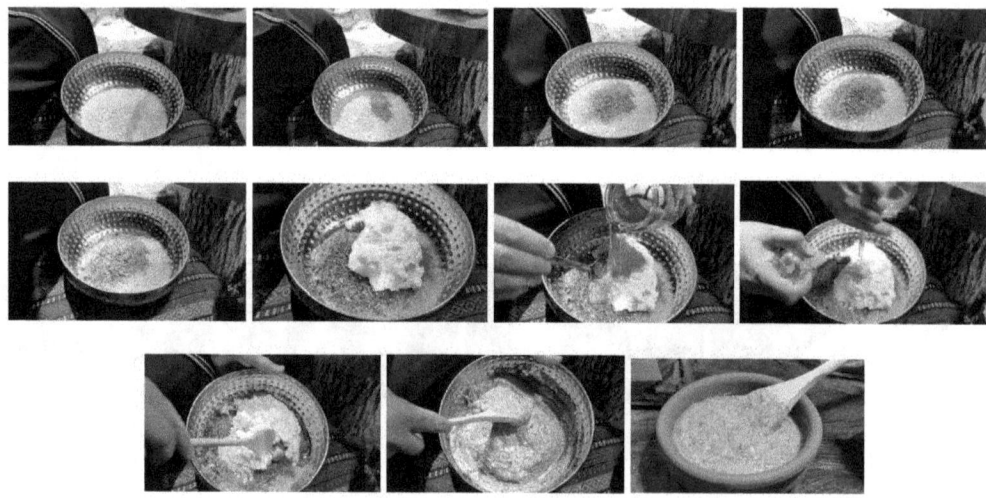

- Clean your skin, then apply the sugar mixture to it. Massage the place for 5-10 minutes.
- Then wash your body using a moisturizing peeler with warm water.

Benefits:
- Relieves pain and stimulates nerves
- Activates blood circulation and nourishes the muscle
- Reduces skin infections.

Recipe 2
Turmeric scrub: Turmeric is one of the most important elements used in natural cosmetics in India, it has antiseptic and antibacterial properties, and this keeps your skin young and can be prepared

Ingredients:
- 1 cup of salt
- 2 spoons honey.
- 2 teaspoons turmeric powder.
- 1/2 cup olive oil
- A teaspoon of the following ingredients: Fennel powder, coriander powder, black mustard powder, and cumin powder.

Method:
- Mix all the ingredients together until a rough paste is formed.

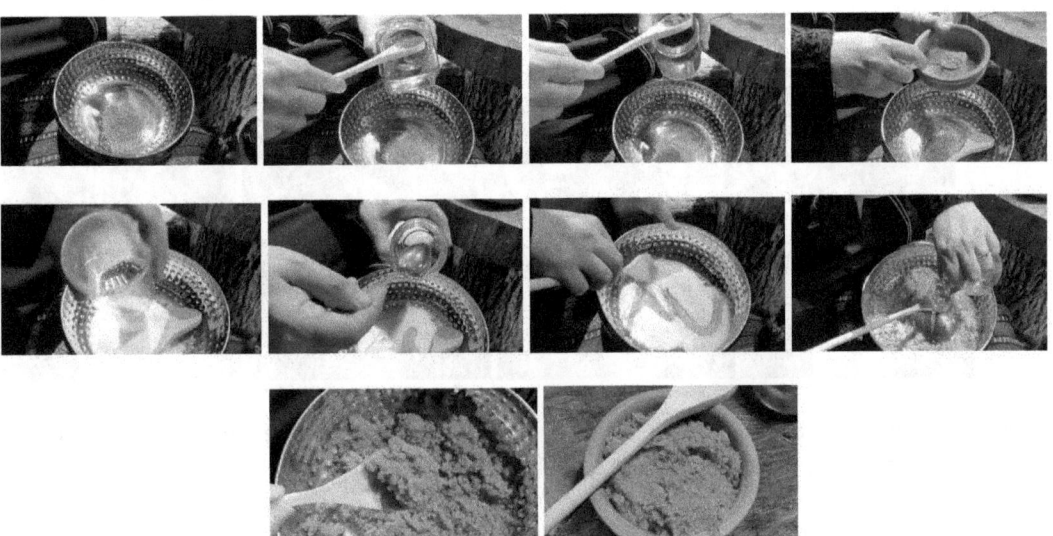

- Clean your skin, then apply the scrub mixture to it. Massage the place with your fingers with circular movement on the skin for 5-10 minutes.
- Wash your body using a moisturizing peeler with warm water.

Benefits:
- Relieves pain and stimulates nerves
- Activates blood circulation and nourishes the muscle
- Reduces skin infections and nerve infections

Recipe 3
Lemon sugar: Lemon contains large amounts of vitamin C, which is a nutrient for the skin, has a peeling effect, makes the skin soft, fresh, and can be prepared

Ingredients:

- Half a cup of sugar.
- A tablespoon of honey.
- Half a cup of lemon juice.
- Teaspoon of: Basil, Mint, camphor, chia seeds and fenugreek.

Method:
- Put the juice in a bowl and then add salt and honey then add ground herbs.

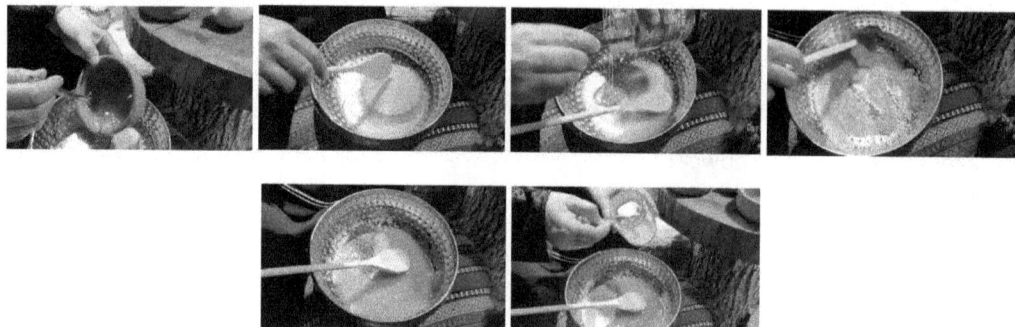

- Grind all the ingredients and mix all the rest of the ingredients together until a rough paste is formed and stir well.

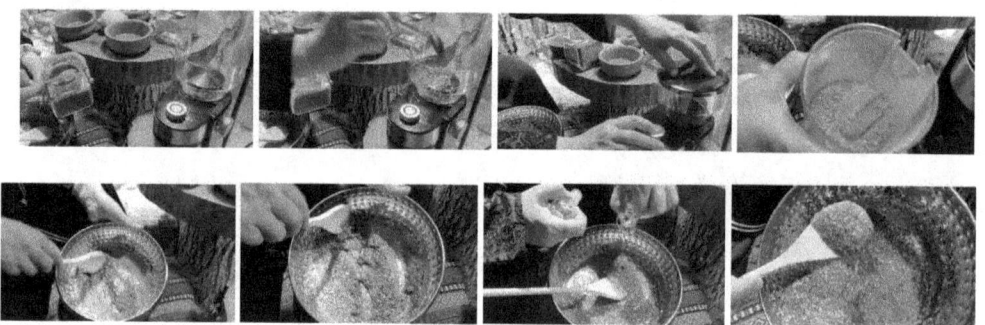

- Massage the place with your fingers with circular movement on the skin for 5-10 minutes.
- Wash your body using a moisturizing peeler with warm water.

Benefits:
- Relieves pain and stimulates nerves
- Activates blood circulation and nourishes the muscle
- Reduces skin infections and nerve infections

Recipe 4
Coffee scrub: Coffee is still a common ingredient in many of the body peelers you make at home.

Ingredients:
- 1/4 cup ground coffee
- 1 cup hot water
- ¼ cup of olive oil
- 1 tablespoon of lavender oil.
- 1 teaspoon of the following ingredients: Thyme, sage, dandelion, aloe-vera gel.

Method:
- Make a paste of aloe vera.

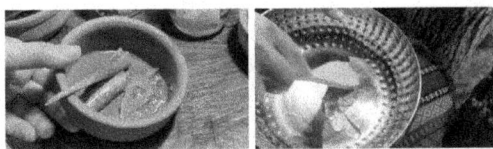

- Add ground coffee and hot water to the mixing bowl. Mix the coffee mixture with the aloe vera paste.

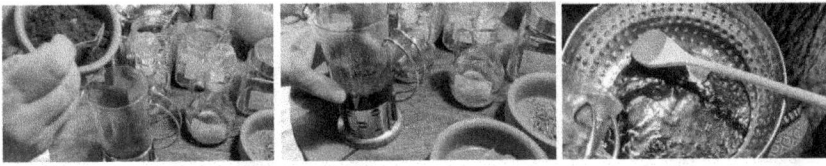

- Mix all the other ingredients with the coffee mixture together with a spoon until a rough paste is formed and stir well.

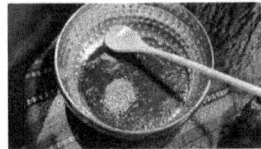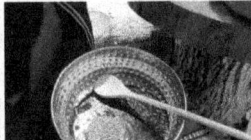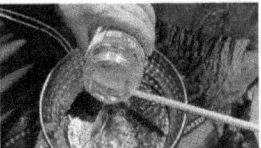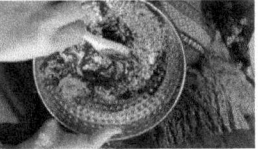

- Add olive oil at the last and mix well.

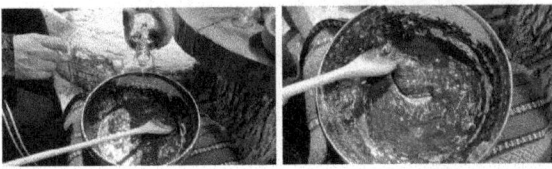

- Massage the place with your fingers with circular movement on the skin for 5-10 minutes.
- Wash your body using a moisturizing peeler with warm water.

Benefits:
- Relieves pain and stimulates nerves
- Activates blood circulation and nourishes the muscle
- Reduces skin infections and nerve infections

Recipe 5
Brown sugar Peeler
Brown Sugar is an available, inexpensive ingredient that peels off your skin greatly, and is gentler on the skin than sea salt or Epsom salt. This makes it an ideal ingredient for peeling sensitive skin. Brown sugar granules may make your skin a little sticky, so make sure to rinse them thoroughly after peeling.

Ingredients:
- 1 cup brown sugar or 2 tablespoons honey
- 1 cup oil of your choice such as coconut, jojoba, olive or almond oil.

- 3 tablespoons salt available preferably Himalayan
- 1 teaspoon of the following ingredients: Basil Thyme, Turmeric, fenugreek, and black seed.

Method:
- To make the peeled mix, add brown sugar and oil in the mixing bowl.

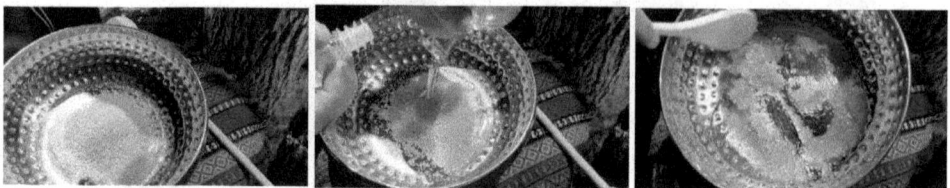

- Mix well and grind all dry ingredients into a powder form and put it over the previous mixture.

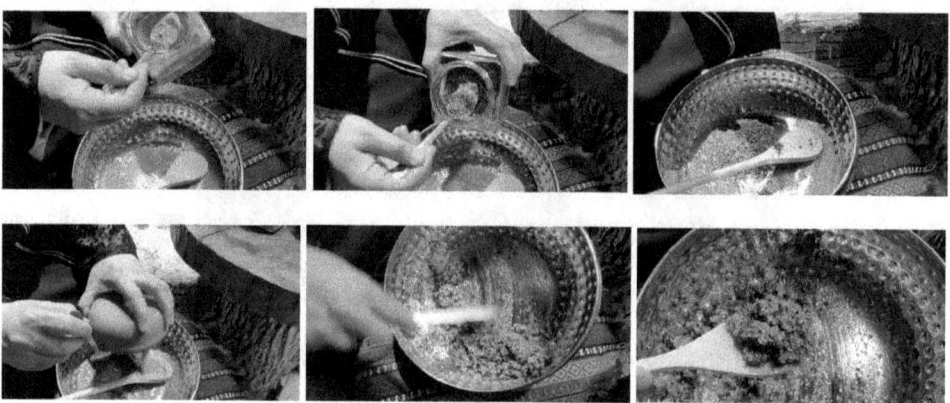

- Start the process of massage, add a drop or two of your favorite essential oil.

Benefits:
- Relieves pain and stimulates nerves
- Activates blood circulation and nourishes the muscle
- Reduces skin infections and nerve infections

How to do body scrub:

- When you are exfoliating, it's important to be gentle on your skin. You can make small, circular motions using your finger to apply a scrub or use your exfoliating tool of choice.
- If you use a brush, make short, light strokes. You can also use a thick cloth or a loofah. Avoid exfoliating if your skin has cuts, open wounds, or is sunburned.
- Always remember to clean the skin with lukewarm water or a wet towel and then apply the scrub mixture to the area.
- Massage your skin using your fingers with circular movements for 5-10 minutes.
- Wash your body and apply a moisturizing lotion afterwards.

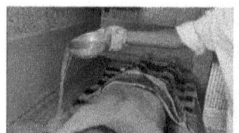 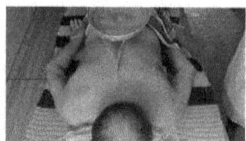 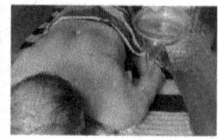 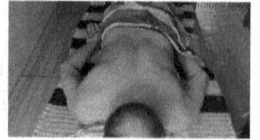

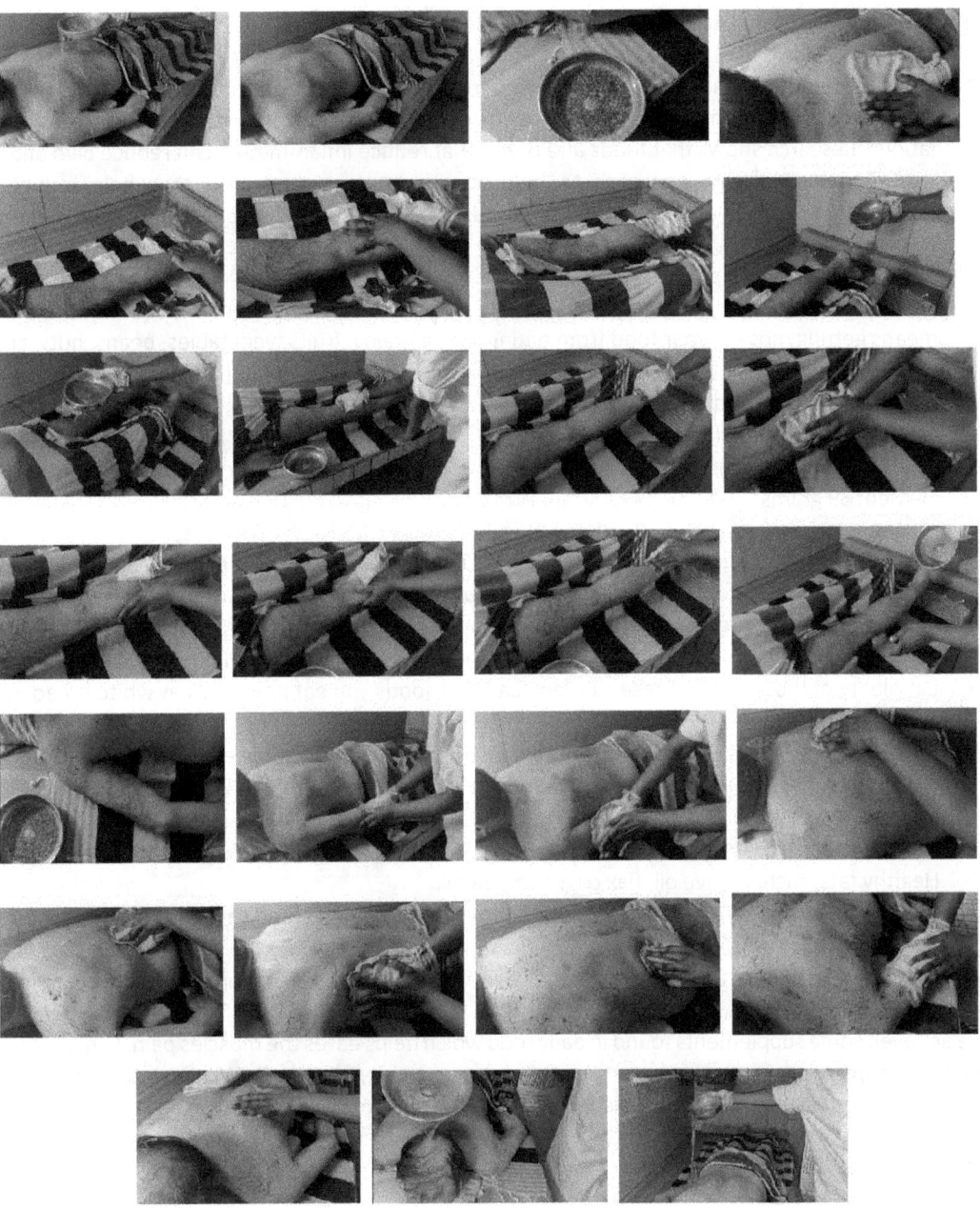

Benefits:
- Relieves pain and stimulates nerves
- Reduce Inflammation
- Activates blood circulation and nourishes the muscle
- Reduces skin infections.
- Nourishes and softens the skin.

CHAPTER 16: NUTRITIONAL FACTS AND BENEFITS OF BALANCE DIET TO REDUCE PAIN

It's been said that you are what you eat, and that's true when it comes to chronic pain. "A lot of pain is the result of inflammation, and the evidence is quite strong that your diet can contribute to increased systemic inflammation, "Research shows that foods and drinks that reduce inflammation can reduce pain and improve your mood. The best dietary approach to help your immune system, and thus help reduce chronic inflammation, is to cut out the bad inflammatory foods and adopt more of the good anti-inflammatory kinds.

Simple tips to lessen your pain,
- The best diet to lower inflammation and pain is based on healthy foods that come from plants. This means getting most of your food from eating whole grains, fruits, vegetables, beans, nuts, and seeds.
- Avoid foods that make your blood sugar go up quickly after a meal, including white bread, refined (processed) grains and other processed foods and sugary foods. If your blood sugar does this often, it creates inflammation in your body.
- Limit the amount of added sugar in your food each day. Daily limits for adults are:
  » Men: 39 grams
  » Women: 25 grams –

The limits don't mean you have to eat that much added sugar. You can eat less! But try to stick to that amount or less each day. You will need to read labels to check for how much sugar is in a serving of food. Most added sugar is already in the food, even foods you would not expect to have sugar. You might also need to measure the food to learn how many servings you have.
- Eat plenty of these foods. These can replace other foods you eat now, such as white bread, red meat, and packaged snacks.
- Fruits and vegetables - Most Americans eat just 1 fruit and 1 vegetable each day. Often, that vegetable is French fries—high in calories, salt, and fat and low in nutrition. Doctors and nutrition experts recommend eating 5 to 7 servings of fruits and vegetables every day.
- Herbs and spices—Use these to replace some of the salt you cook with.
- Healthy fats, such as olive oil, flax oil, or canola oil.
- Foods made from soy, such as tofu, roasted soy nuts, edamame, and soy milk, unless your doctor tells you to avoid soy.
- Fish—Two or 3 times a week. Look at the chart in this guide to learn more about the best types of fish.

There are even some supplements found in daily food which helps eases the muscles pain. It includes avocado-soybean oil, capsaicin, curcuma, ginger, melatonin, glucosamine, vitamin D. Will have brought to you some amazing recipes of soups and salads which you can include in your daily diet.

Recipes for salads
Recipe 1: Red beans Salad

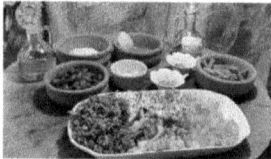

Ingredients - ¼ cup boiled red kidney beans, drained, ¼ 1 cup boiled and drained pinto beans, ½ cup chopped red onion, ½ cup chopped red pepper, ½ cup chopped yellow pepper, ½ cup chopped cucumber, ½ cup chopped parsley

For the dressing - ¼ cup olive oil, ¼ cup vinegar, 2 tablespoons lemon juice, 1 clove of minced garlic, 2 teaspoons ground cumin, 1 teaspoon ground coriander, ½ 1 teaspoon black pepper, ½ 1 teaspoon chili (optional), ¾ 1 teaspoon salt

Method - In a bowl, mix all the vegetables. Then, put all the ingredients for dressing gradually. Stir the salad and mix it well. Top it with fresh parsley and serve it directly. It can be used as a side dish with soup or main course.

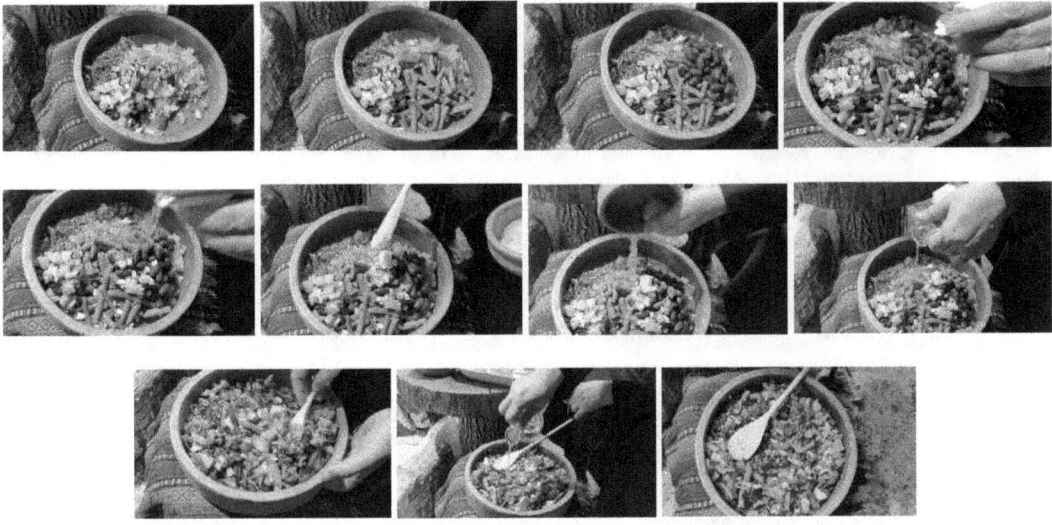

Recipe 2: Tuna Salad

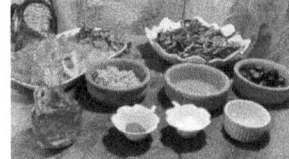

Ingredients - 1 cup chopped arugula, 2 cups of chopped salmon or tuna, 1 cup chopped tomatoes, ½ cup of colored capsicum, ¼ cup of black olives, 2 tablespoons of chopped parsley, ½ cup of chopped red cabbage

For dressing - 1 tablespoon olive oil, 1 clove of minced garlic, 2 teaspoons lemon juice, Pinch of chili, Pinch of salt.

Method - In a bowl, mix all the vegetables. Then, put all the ingredients for dressing gradually. Stir the salad and mix it well. Top it with fresh parsley and serve it directly. It can be used as a side dish with soup or main course.

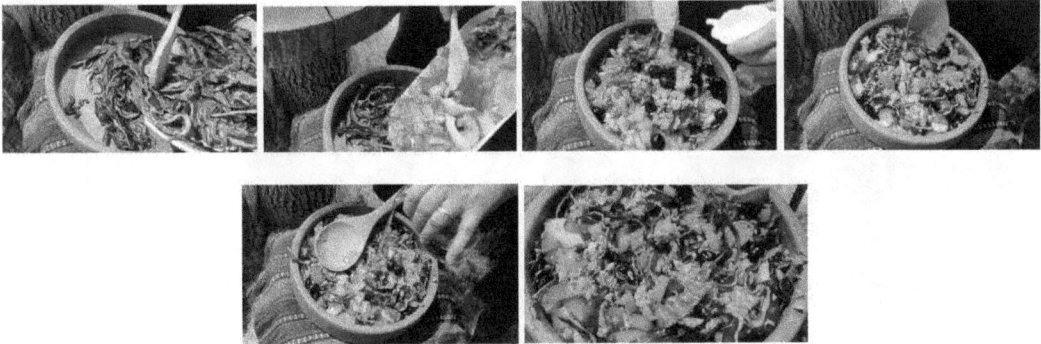

Recipe 3: Potato and herbs salad

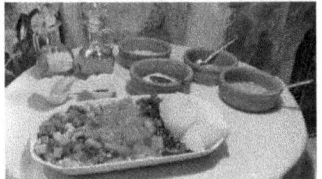

Ingredients - 3 medium potatoes boiled and diced, ½ cup chopped green onions, 2 tablespoons of chopped parsley, 2 tablespoons mayonnaise, a tablespoon of tahini, ¾ 1 teaspoon salt, and ½ 1 teaspoon black pepper

Method - Cover the potatoes with water in a deep bowl, add a tablespoon of salt, and boil them until a little tender. Peel the potatoes and cut them into medium cubes, then add half of the seasoning mixture. Add parsley and onions to the remaining seasoning, add to potatoes, squeeze a lemon, and then serve.

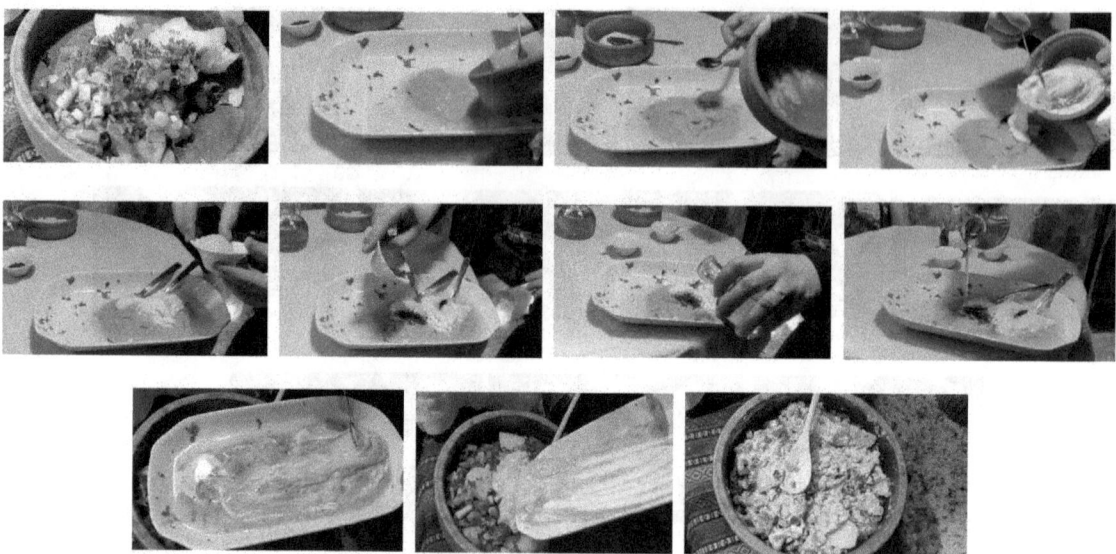

Recipe 4: Wheat and greens salad

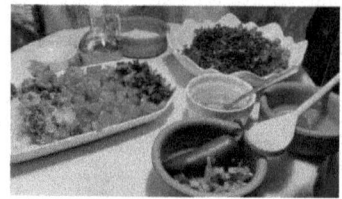

Ingredients : 2 cups of finely chopped parsley, 1 onion, finely chopped, 2 tablespoons of groats of wheat soaked in water, ¼ cup of pure olive oil, ½ cup of finely chopped tomatoes, 2 tablespoon of squeezed lemon, ¼ cup of finely chopped hot pepper - to taste, ½ cup of washed lettuce or any green leaves of your choice.

Method:
Put the soaked wheat, tomatoes, onions, mint, parsley and hot pepper and green leaves in a bowl and mix. Add lemon, salt, olive oil and mix until combined. Pour the salad into a large serving dish and serve fresh.

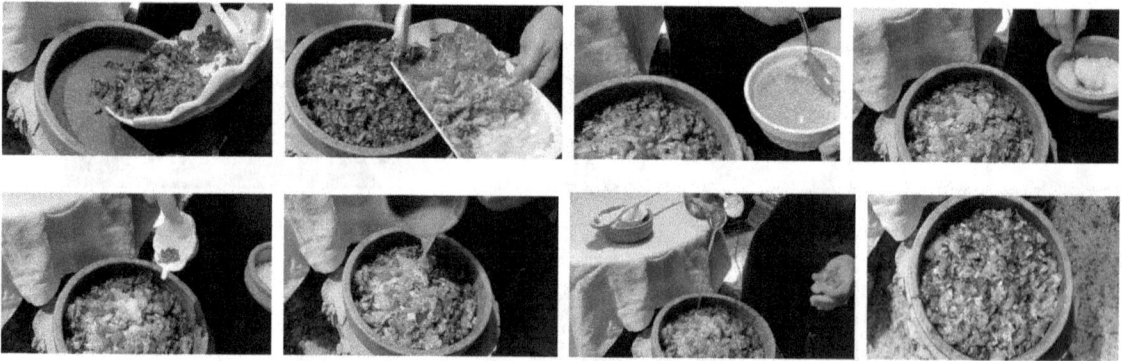

Recipe 5: Green Greek salad

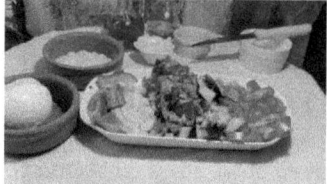

Ingredients – 2 cups of medium chopped tomatoes, 2 cups of chopped cucumbers, 1 cup medium chopped lettuce, 1 cup chopped onion, ½ cup chopped white cheese, 1 cup chopped sweet green pepper, few slices of black olives, ½ cup of lemon juice, pinch of salt, 1 tablespoon of vinegar, 2 tablespoons of olive oil, 1 tablespoon of thyme.

Method - Put all the ingredients together, and stir them except for the white cheese, onions, and black olives. Add salt, olive oil, thyme, vinegar, and lemon juice and mix well. Top the salad with cheese, onions and black olives while serving. It can be used as a side dish or main course.

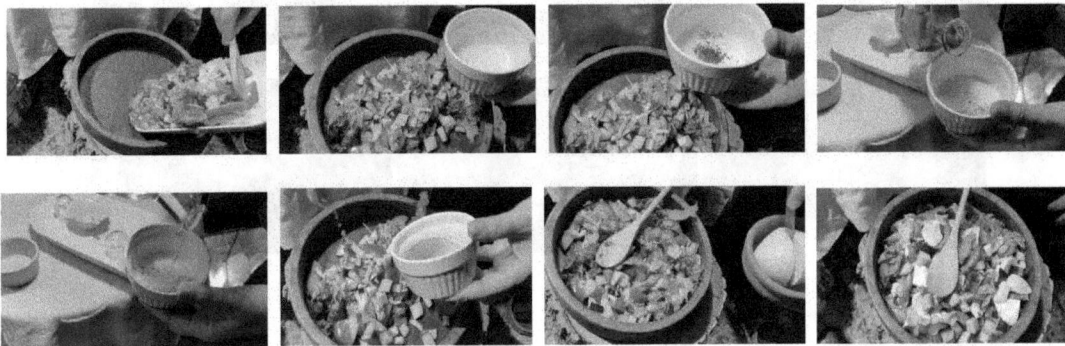

Recipe 6: Fruit bowl Salad

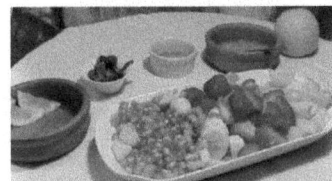

Ingredients - ¼ cup of chopped kiwi, ¼ cup of chopped strawberries, ¼ cup of chopped pineapple, ¼ cup of chopped bananas, ¼ cup of pomegranate, 1 teaspoon of finely chopped ginger, 1 teaspoon of honey, ¼ cup of orange juice, ¼ cup of lemon juice and ¼ cup chopped mint.

Method – Put the fruits in a bowl. Add honey, ginger, lemon juice, orange juice and mix well. Top it with freshly chopped mint and serve.

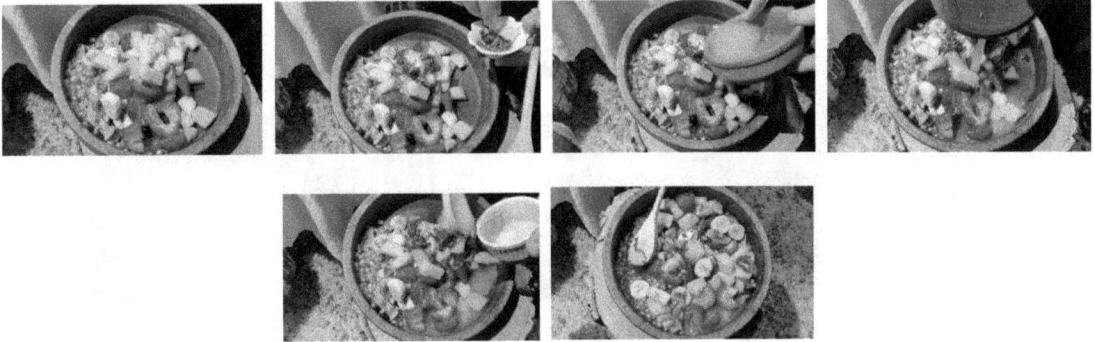

Recipes for juices
Recipe 1 – Green Juice

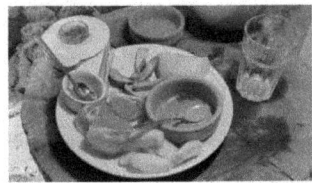

Ingredients - 1 orange, 2 cups of pineapple, a cup of chopped avocado, 2 sticks of celery, 2 pears, lemon juice, a piece of ginger, 2 spoons of turmeric, a little black pepper, half a spoon of honey

Method – take all the ingredients and blend it in a blender. Don't use the juicer machine as we want to keep the pulp for good results. Pour in a glass and consume fresh.

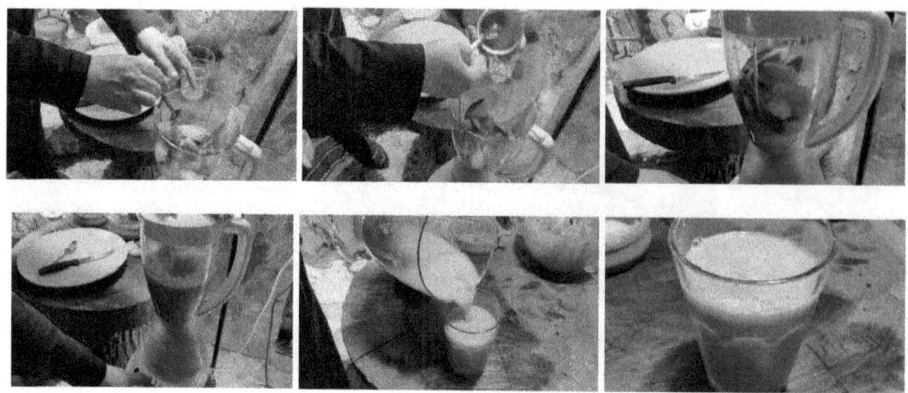

Recipe 2 – Hot Juice

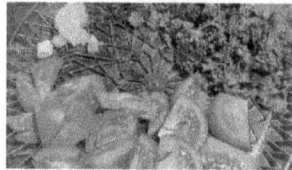

Ingredients – 5 medium chopped tomatoes, half a lemon, a bunch of parsley mixed with dill, a slice of garlic, and a glass of water (can be replaced with tomato juice)

Method – take all the ingredients and blend it in a blender. Don't use the juicer machine as we want to keep the pulp for good results. Pour in a glass and consume fresh.

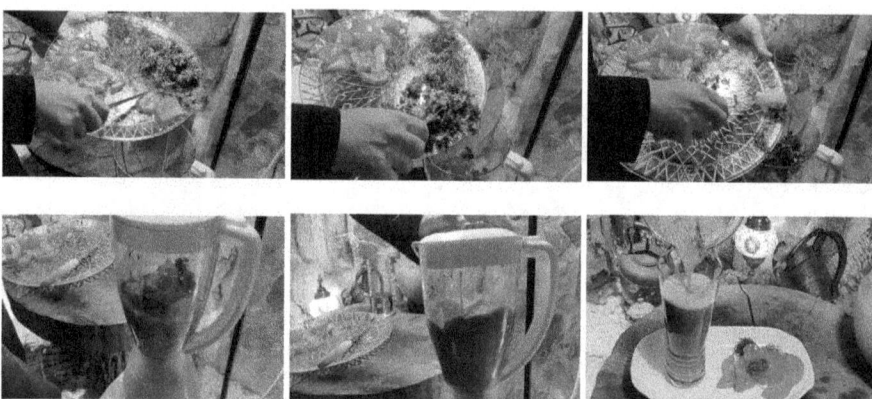

Benefits of this drink:
- Relieves pain, swelling and edema
- Reduces arthritis
- Reduces osteoporosis
- stimulates the nerves
- Stimulates blood circulation because it contains a large amount of vitamin C.

Recipe 3: Vitamin C juice

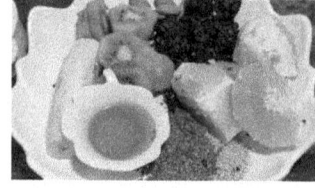

Ingredients: Half a banana, 1 orange, 2 pieces of kiwi, 2 teaspoons of flaxseed, 2 teaspoons of sesame, ¼ cup of pomegranate, 2 pieces of walnuts and almonds, 2 spoons of honey

Method:
Mix all together and bled it in a mixture. Drink it in the morning.

Benefits of this drink:
- It is a stimulant for the blood circulation.
- Stimulates the nerves.
- Reduces joint and respiratory infections.
- Lessens the pain.

Recipe 4: Pumpkin juice

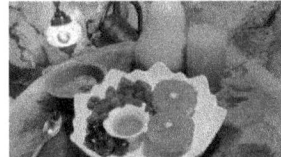

Ingredients - 1 cup of boiled red pumpkin, 1 cup of grapefruit, Quarter cup of lemon, ½ cup of cranberry, ¼ cup of cherries, ¼ teaspoon of turmeric, ½ teaspoon of flaxseed, ½ teaspoon of nigella, a teaspoon of cinnamon, 3 tablespoons of honey

Method: All materials are added to the mixer and drink two cups daily.

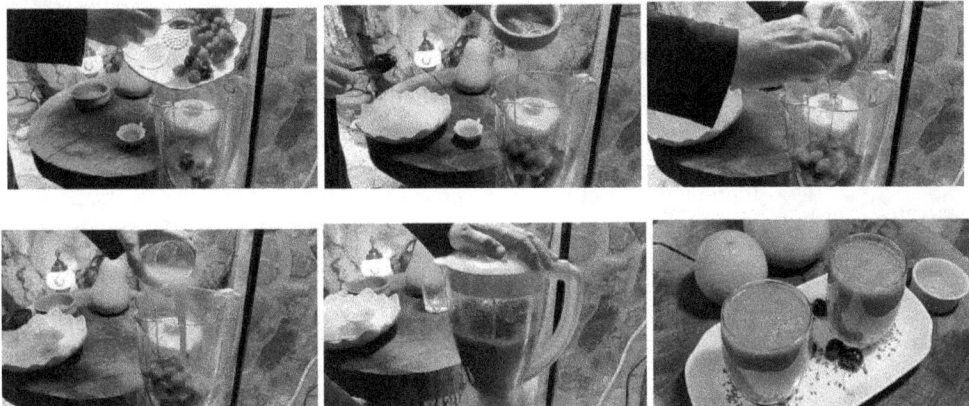

Benefits of this drink
- Activates blood circulation
- It stimulates the nerves
- Strengthens bones and relieves pain
- It is a rich source of many vitamins, such as folic acid, vitamin B3, and vitamin B, which are important for the functioning of various vital processes in the body, and the work of enzymes.
- Maintains the integrity and functions of nerves, in addition to contain important minerals, such as: potassium, calcium, copper, magnesium, and phosphorous.

Recipe 5: Milk cocktail with chia and flax seed

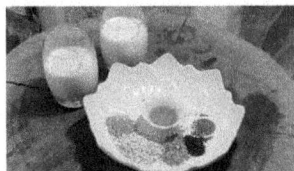

Ingredients: Two cups of milk, 1 teaspoon of chia seed, 1 teaspoon of nigella, a teaspoon of flaxseed, a teaspoon of honey
1 teaspoon of turmeric, a teaspoon of honey, 2 tablespoons of oats

Method: Mix everything in a blender and drink daily.

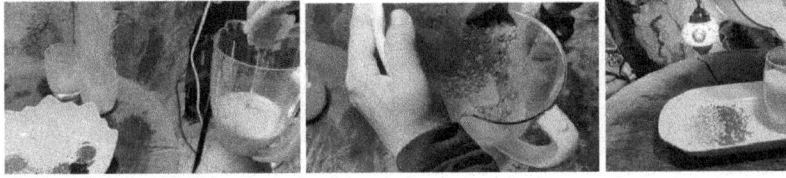

Benefits of drinking this mixture:
- Helps relieve pain

- Repairs bones
- Relieves osteoporosis and pain
- Relaxes muscles
- Reduces inflammation
- Stimulates blood circulation.

Recipes for soup
Recipe 1 – Bone broth soup

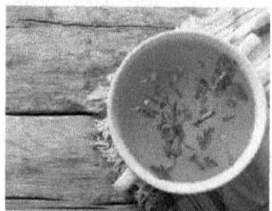

Ingredients – 1 liter water, Bones of meat, fish, or poultry, preferably meat, 1 teaspoon of vinegar, Pinch of salt and pepper

Method - Boil the ingredients in a suitable size pot over medium heat for 4 to 6 minutes, stir occasionally. After the water boils, reduce the flame and add Onions, Celery, Carrots, Parsley, Thyme and Garlic to add some flavours. Now cook with covered lid for 10 to 24 minutes. After that, turn off the flame and let it cool down. Once cooled, filter the broth with a cheesecloth or strainer. Add salt and pepper according to your taste.

Recipe 2: Mushroom soup

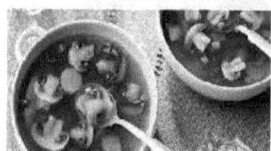

Ingredients – 1 cup of sliced potatoes, 1 cup of chopped carrots, 1 cup of chopped onions, 2 cups of chopped brown or white mushrooms, 3 tablespoons of olive oil, ¼ cup chopped parsley, 1 teaspoon of shredded ginger, 1 teaspoon of salt and pepper, 1 cup chopped pot

Method - Sautee onions and carrot with butter in a suitable size pot over medium heat for 4 to 6 minutes, then add mushrooms to it and sauté it for another 5mins. Now add salt and pepper to it. Add 3 cups of lukewarm water or you can use vegetable broth instead and bring it to boil. Add the shredded ginger, parsley and serve.

Recipe 3: Meat curry

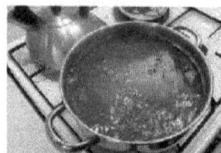

Ingredients – 2 medium sized onions finely chopped, 2 kg of yogurt, 1 kg of lamb meat, 3 leaves of laurel, 1 teaspoon of ginger chopped finely, ½ cup of carrot chopped, 1 cinnamon sick, 6 grains of cardamom, 4 teaspoons of starch dissolved in ½ cup of water and Salt to taste.

Method - Put the meat in a liter of water pot and boil. Put another pot with 1 and ½ liter of water and bring it to boil. After 10 minutes, transfer the meat to the second pot with water and add carrots, ginger, cinnamon, cardamom, bay leaves and salt (as per your taste). Simmer the mixture until it boils and cook it on low flame for 90 minutes. Now the meat is tender. Take a pan add 2 cups of water, onions and boil it for 5 minutes. Drain it and set it aside. Take a bowl add yogurt, water, and whisk it well until it comes smooth. Put this mixture on a low flame and stir well. Add salt in batches at interval of every 3 minutes and stir well. Remove the pot from the heat and set aside. Put the boiled meat and onions in a saucepan at low flame, add the milk and stir the ingredients from time to time with a wooden spoon for five minutes. Pour the mixture into a plate and serve with rice.

Recipe 4: Wheat soup

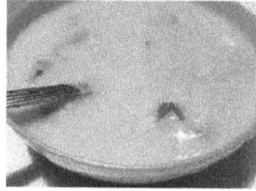

Ingredients - 2 tablespoons of olive oil, 1 medium chopped onion, 2 medium chopped sweet red pepper, 1 teaspoon of salt, 1 teaspoon of pepper, 3 cloves of crushed garlic, 1 teaspoon of dried and ground mint, ½ teaspoon smoked paprika, 1 tablespoon of tomato paste, 1 can of tomato pulp, 4 cups of chicken stock, 2 cups of water, ¾ cup of wheat and ½ cup of chopped fresh mint

Method – In a saucepan add oil, onions, red pepper, salt, and sauté over a medium heat for 6-8 minutes until the color changes to brown. After that add garlic, mint, smoked paprika and stir it until this mixture starts releasing oil. Add tomato paste and simmer for 1 minute. Put on the tomato pulp and cook for 10 minutes. After that add chicken stock, water, and wheat until it starts boiling. Cook until the wheat becomes soft. At last, add salt and pepper up to the taste and garnish with fresh mint.

Recipe 5: Lentil Soup

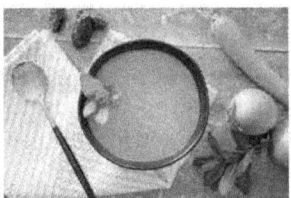

Ingredients – 1 and ½ cup of lentils, 4 cups vegetable broth, 2 tablespoons vegetable oil, 1 tablespoon butter grated onion, 1 chopped bell pepper, half a grated tomato, 2 cloves garlic minced, 1 celery stick, chopped, half a teaspoon of cumin, half a teaspoon of curry, half a teaspoon of turmeric, half a teaspoon of sweet pepper, Quarter of a teaspoon of ginger, salt and pepper as needed Toast with butter and herbs

Method - Heat a saucepan, add oil, butter, onions, leeks, celery and garlic and fry for 5 minutes. Add bell pepper, tomatoes and stir for 5 minutes more. Add the lentils, stirring constantly, then add the turmeric, curry, paprika, cumin, pepper, salt, and ginger, and stir well for two minutes. Add the broth, stir, and leave it on the fire until it boils. Cover the pot and leave for 35 minutes, until the lentils are well cooked. Blend the soup with a hand mixer until smooth. Return the soup to the pot and cook until boiled. Serve hot.

CHAPTER 17: CERVICOGENIC HEADACHE AND ITS MANAGEMENT

- Do you have a headache after a whiplash injury?
- Do you experience pain that seems to start in the neck and then spread to one side of your head or arm?
- Does moving your head seem to start your headache or exacerbate your pain when you have a headache?

If you answered yes to any of those questions, there's a high chance you have a type of headache known as a cervicogenic headache. There is unilateral pain, diffuse shoulder pain and arm pain also confirms the diagnosis. But Don't Worry! There are extremely effective interventions for you including cervicogenic headache stretching, exercises, massage techniques and herbal recipes! When you wake up and feel the pain with stiffness surrounding your neck then follow this 24-hour guide to help maintain your pain.

Step 1: Before starting activity, you can use the neck scrub to reduce the stress of on your neck and surrounding muscles, which will increase the blood circulation of that part and soothes your skin. It also helps in relieving tension. You can use recipe from chapter Scrubs and peeling recipes under the section for head and neck.

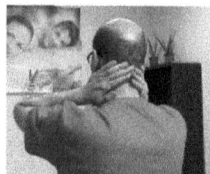 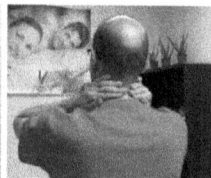 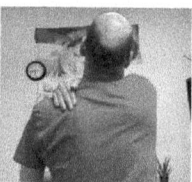 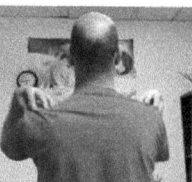

Step 2: After this, take a sip of hot herbal teas and caffeinated drinks. This will help reduce the effect of headache and make you able to carry out your routine activities as normal. Ginger tea can help with headaches. To drink ginger, add a half teaspoon of ground ginger to warm water or simply enjoy a cup of brewed ginger tea.

Step 3: After this, relax yourself in the way you are comfortable and then use the heat or cold compression to reduce the stiffness and pain of muscles. Selection of heat and cold therapy depends upon the onset of pain. For instance, if you are suffering from the pain from longer duration then you can use heat and if the pain is acute then you can use the cold.

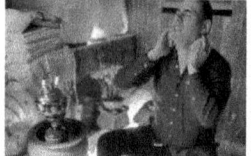 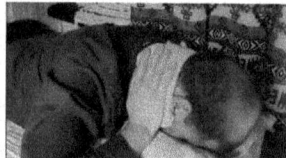

It can be applied directly to the neck and upper back area for 10-15 minutes. Repeat the application of heat or cold therapy 3-4 times a day. Details of application are described in the chapters for Heat and Cold therapy.

Step 4: Followed by heat and cold, start neck stretches and mobility exercises, which will help improve your range of motion of neck and will also make the neck muscles more flexible. Stiffness will be gradually released. Stretches which work best for cervicogenic headache are side stretch to your neck, posterior stretch to your neck, diagonal stretch. The procedure and other details have already been described in the chapter for stretching.

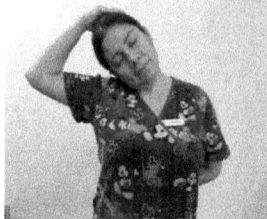 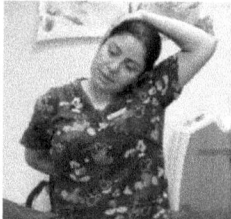 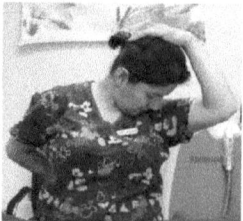 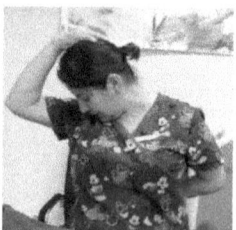

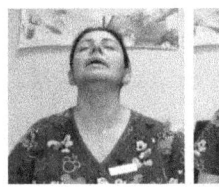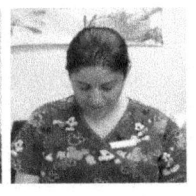

You must feel a slight pull on the tight muscle. It will pain initially, but don't panic. Gradually when the muscle loosens up it will feel better. When you do the movements make sure you don't pull your neck more as it can aggravate the symptom. Mobility exercises useful in this condition are neck movements. Please refer to chapter mobility exercise.

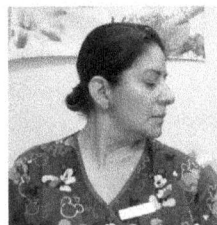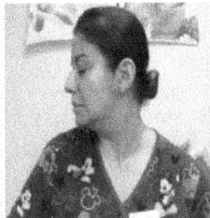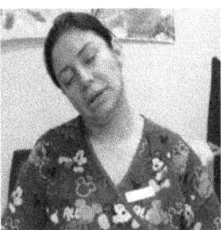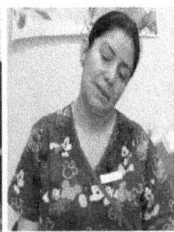

Step 5: Once you are relaxed, release your stiffness with massage. This works best with infused herbal oil recipes.

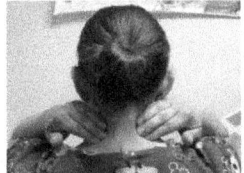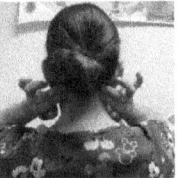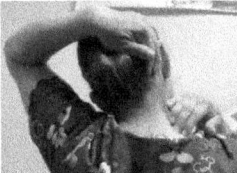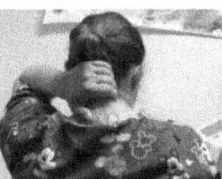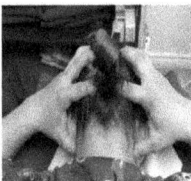

The recipe which works best for cervicogenic headache are given in chapter Herbs and herb infused oil under the section recipes for neck and upper back. Use different recipes each day so that you get more benefits.

Step 6: Once your symptoms are relieved to 50%, start with the strengthening exercises. As poor neck posture causes muscle weakness and leads to cervicogenic headache. Once you start with exercises you will feel discomfort in the muscles, but don't worry that is just because we are strengthening the weak muscles. Gradually this discomfort goes away. Exercises suitable for this condition are, isometric neck exercises, seated shoulder shrugs, backward shoulder shrugs, standing shoulder crunches.

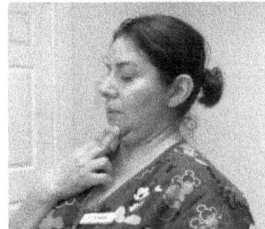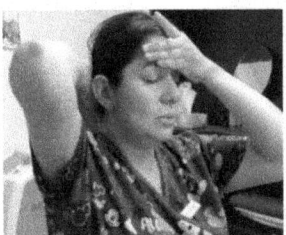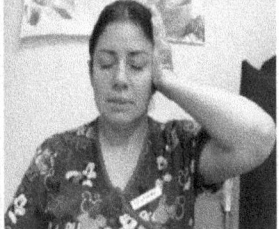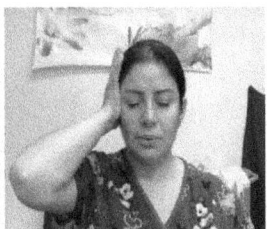

Step 7: Take a balanced diet which should include food rich in vitamins, omega 3, and magnesium in your diet. Green leafy vegetables like spinach, kale, swish charred, collard greens can be consumed. The recipes which is useful are described in chapter Nutritional facts and benefits of balanced diet. There are different sections including recipes for soups, salads and juices which you can include at least one in your daily diet.

Step 8: You can use homemade pastes on your neck to relieve the severe pain. These patches work on relieving stress and reduces the inflammation. The details and application are given in chapter Herbal poultices (paste) recipes under the section neck and shoulder pain.

Step 9: Use proper resting position and make sure your neck is in a relaxed position. These positions are used while resting or when you have applied the patches.

Step 10: Again, you can use the herbal teas to relieve your cervicogenic headache. The recipes are already described above in step 4.

Step 11: At the end of the day, indulge yourself in foot soak and body soak with herbs. This will relax your body senses and rejuvenate it. The recipes and application are already described in chapter Body and foot soak recipes for relaxation.

Step 12: "TAKEAWAY MESSAGE"

Cervicogenic headache are major due to poor posture alignment. Make sure you improve your posture while working. For details about posture correction refer to chapter Prophylactics.

If you are working on computers, make sure the screen is at eye level. Take break for neck movements and stretches after every 30 minutes.

CHAPTER 18: MIGRAINE HEADACHE AND ITS MANAGEMENT

- Has a headache limited your activities for a day or more in the last three months?
- Are you nauseated or sick to your stomach when you have a headache?
- Does light bother you when you have a headache?

If you answered yes to any of these questions, there's a high rate of having a specific type of headache known as a migraine headache. We will give you lifestyle modifications that promote overall good health can also reduce the frequency and severity of your migraines. Here is a 24-hour guide with a stepwise approach to manage your migraine headache

Step 1: At the first sign of a migraine, take a break and step away from whatever you're doing if possible. Turn off the lights. Migraines often increase sensitivity to light and sound. Relax in a dark, quiet room. Sleep if you can.

Step 2: Exfoliate your skin of neck with scrubs which will activate all the tissues and helps in relieving stress. You can use recipe from chapter Scrubs and peeling recipes under the section for head and neck.

Step 3: Relax yourself in a proper resting position and apply heat or cold compress to your head or neck. This will relax your muscles and the surrounding tension. Select the hot and cold temperature based on your triggering factor.

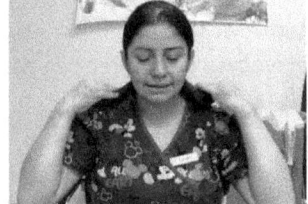

- Take a bowl filled with ice cubes and water. Soak a towel in it. Drain the extra water, roll it, and keep it on your shoulder and neck.
- If you are sensitive to cold, you can use Lukewarm water and repeat the same process.
- Also, keep the compress on your forehead with head rested.
- Put it in place until the temperature goes down and repeat it for 3 times.

Step 4: After this, take sip of hot herbal teas and caffeinated drinks. This will help reduce the effect of migraine and make you able to carry out your routine activities as normal. Ginger tea can help with headaches. To drink ginger, add a half teaspoon of ground ginger to warm water or simply enjoy a cup of brewed ginger tea. Here are the options for preparing ginger tea,

- Ginger tea bags: The simplest way to enjoy ginger tea. Choose a brand known for high-quality herbal teas and brew yourself a cup.
- Fresh ginger root tea: You simply boil peeled and sliced fresh ginger in water for about five minutes. Go a few extra minutes for more spice. Add honey or maple syrup to taste (optional).
- Black tea with ginger: Brew tea to your liking and add fresh ginger grated with a microplate.
- Iced ginger tea: Brew black or herbal tea and add sliced fresh ginger. Let cool and transfer to a glass pitcher for storage in the refrigerator.

Coffee and black tea can also be useful. These are brewed beverages which contain caffeine and constricts blood vessels.

Step 5: Next, use herb infused oil for massaging your pressure points which will relieve your headache. The recipe which works best for cervicogenic headache are given in chapter Herbs and herb infused oil under the section recipes for neck and upper back. You can choose any of those recipes depending on your triggering factor. Use this self-massage techniques to relieve your pressure points.

- Use your fingertips and massage with gentle pressure.
- Do not over press the points as this can trigger your headache.
- Circular motions can be done at each point for 30 seconds.

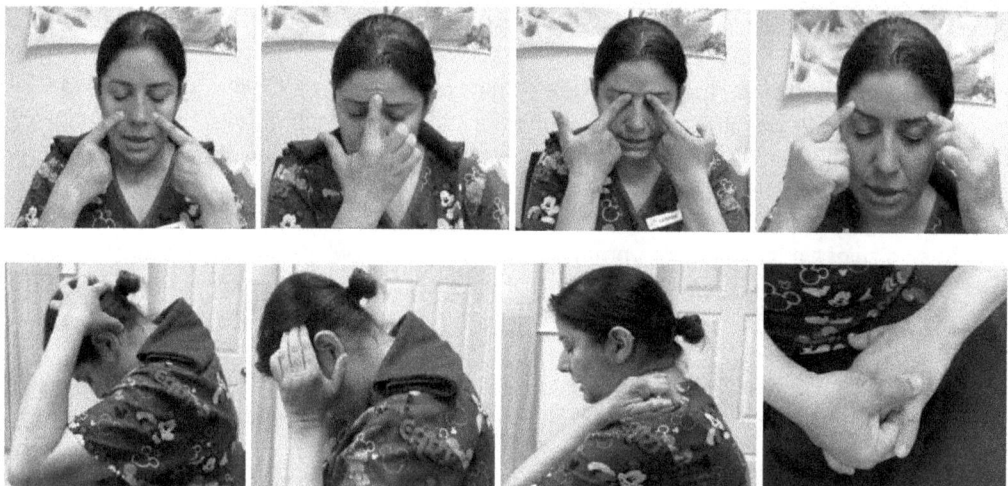

Step 6: If you feel your headache is reduced, continue your household chores as regular. Avoid going in areas where there is excessive wind, light, or typical smell. This can trigger your migraine again.

Step 7: At the end of the day, indulge yourself in foot soak with herbs. This will relax your body senses and rejuvenate it. The recipes and application are already described in chapter Body and foot soak recipes for relaxation.

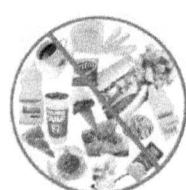

Step 8: Take a balanced diet which should include food rich in vitamins, omega 3, magnesium in your diet. Green leafy vegetables like spinach, kale, swish charred, collard greens can be consumed. The recipes which is useful are described in chapter Nutritional facts and benefits of balanced diet. Avoiding processed food is important for those with migraines. Processed foods have chemicals that are foreign to the human body (xenobiotics) and have negative effects on our physiology. These include food preservatives and food dyes.

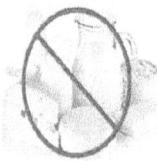

Many migraine sufferers do well when they avoid dairy products and grains, including gluten. Others with migraines are sensitive to corn and soy.

Step 9: Use proper sleeping positions which will relieve tension form your head and neck. For neck positioning, refer to chapter resting positions, Position 4.

CHAPTER 19: VERTIGO

Dizziness can be characterized as either vertigo with disequilibrium or light-headedness associated with feeling faint or the potential to lose consciousness or "pass out." It is a neck-related sensation in which a person feels like either they're spinning or the world around them is spinning.

Cervical vertigo is associated with dizziness from sudden neck movement, specifically from turning your head. Other symptoms of this condition include:
- headache
- nausea
- vomiting
- ear pain or ringing
- neck pain
- loss of balance while walking, sitting, or standing
- weakness
- problems concentrating

SELF TEST FOR BENIGN PEROXYSMAL POSITIONAL VERTIGO:
- Get in what we call the long sitting position with two or three pillows behind you. Turn your head 45 degrees to the right or left. It doesn't matter which way you do first.
- Quickly lower yourself down over those pillows. You're still turned to the right and your head is tipped over the pillows.
- Stay there for thirty seconds. If you're feeling dizzy during this time, or the room is actually spinning, then you may have benign paroxysmal positional vertigo (BPPV) in your posterior canal in your inner ear.
- After thirty seconds, wait about one minute, then test the other ear to make sure it's not in the other ear.
- Sit with your head turned 45 degrees to the left (or the opposite way you went last time). Go back quickly, and make sure your head is tipped over these pillows. Be sure to use enough pillows to make sure you're tipped back, it's very important.
- Stay there for thirty seconds and you're looking for the same thing, if you get dizzy in this position.
- After thirty seconds, you come up.

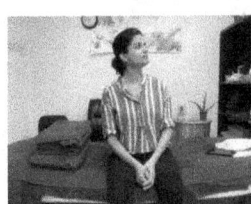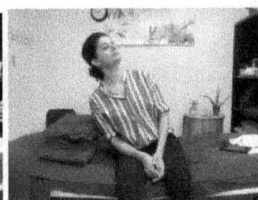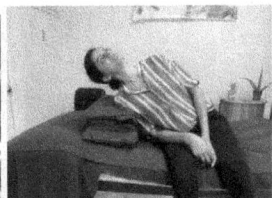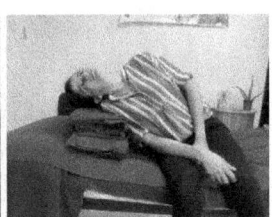

Usually, you'll be dizzy coming down in one position, but not the other position. Also, most people will get actual spinning of the room in this position. This will, in other words, reproduce your symptoms.

Step 1: At the first sign of your vertigo or dizziness, take a break and step away from whatever you're doing if possible. Relax yourself.

Step 2: Apply an ice pack to the upper part of the neck between the ears at the base of the skull. A soft ice pack is the best since it conforms to the contour of that area, but even a bag of frozen corn or peas wrapped in a towel will work. Do not to apply ice for longer than 20 minutes at a time. Applying ice to the upper neck between the ears helps to calm down the nervous system. It can be helpful to reduce both vertigo and nausea.

Step 3: Keep your head as still as possible. The vestibular system is stimulated by movement, so if the vestibular system is part of the problem causing vertigo symptoms, then reducing head movement will likely quiet that system down and reduce the discomfort. Also, you can keep your head upright, either sitting up or propped up on at least two pillows. The reason for this is because the most common inner ear cause of vertigo, or BPPV, is usually triggered by lying down or rolling in bed.

Step 4: Breathe through your nose into your belly. Mouth breathing into the upper chest can make vertigo symptoms feel worse and last longer, so belly breathing through the nose, deep into the belly, is ideal to reduce vertigo symptoms.

Step 5: After this when you feel better, take a sip of hot herbal teas or caffeinated drinks. This will help reduce the effect of dizziness and make you able to carry out your routine activities as normal. Ginger or peppermint tea can help with dizziness.

Step 6: To reduce the symptoms, stare at a vertical line when you are moving around. This gives you an external reference for "upright" and may help your brain re-orient itself but some people with acute inner ear infections may need to close their eyes to get relief.

Step 7: One of the most common ways to manage vertigo is a technique called the Epley maneuver. This involves a set of steps done before bed each night until the symptoms of vertigo resolve for at least 24 hours. If symptoms of vertigo occur from the left side and left ear, the Epley maneuver can be done by:

- sitting on the edge of a bed and turning the head 45 degrees to the left
- lying down quickly and facing head up on the bed at a 45-degree angle
- maintaining the position for 30 seconds
- turning the head halfway — 90 degrees — to the right without raising it for 30 seconds
- turning the head and entire body to the right side, looking downward for 30 seconds
- slowly sitting up but remaining sitting for at least a few minutes.
- If vertigo starts on the right side in the right ear, these directions should be done in reverse.

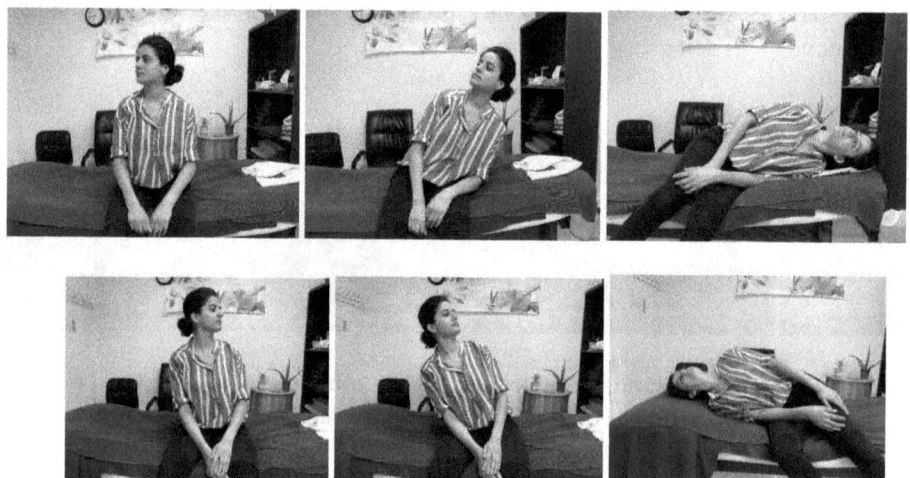

Step 8: Once you are relaxed, release your stiffness with massage. This works best with infused herbal oil recipes. The recipe which works best for neck stiffness are given in chapter Herbs and herb infused oil under the section recipes for neck and upper back.

Step 9: Take a balanced diet which should include food like almonds which are rich sources of vitamins A, B, and E. Eating a daily handful of almonds can help with vertigo symptoms. Apple cider vinegar and honey are believed to have curative properties to relieve blood flow to the brain. Two parts honey and one part apple cider vinegar can prevent and treat vertigo symptoms. Staying hydrated can help minimize dizziness and balance issues. The body needs 8 to 12 cups of liquid per day.

Step 10: You can use homemade pastes on your neck to relieve the severe stiffness. These patches work on relieving stress and reduces the inflammation. The details and application are given in chapter Herbal poultices (paste) recipes under the section neck and shoulder pain.

Step 11: Use proper resting position and make sure your neck is in a relaxed position. These positions are used while resting or when you have applied the patches.

Step 12: At the end of the day, indulge yourself in inhalation with essential oils. Essential oils are natural and affordable options for managing the symptoms of vertigo, including nausea, headaches, and dizziness. Some of the options available for managing vertigo include peppermint, ginger, lavender, and lemon essential oils. Essential oils are inhaled through an infuser or diluted in a carrier oil before being applied topically. This will relax your body senses and rejuvenate it.

CHAPTER 20: NECK TENDONITIS

Tendonitis, which is also commonly spelled tendinitis, is a type of inflammation that occurs within a tendon, especially when repetitive motion happens. Tendons connect the muscles to the bones. This is what allows the muscles to move the body. But if a tendon becomes inflamed, it can result in every little movement becoming painful.

- Do you feel pain in or around your neck?
- Does your pain radiate down to your shoulder blade which is making you difficult to move your neck?
- Do you have swelling around your neck area?

Here is a 24-hour guide to relieve neck tenonitis.

Step 1: Before starting activity, you can use the neck scrub to reduce the stress of on your neck and surrounding muscles, which will increase the blood circulation of that part and soothes your skin. It also helps in relieving tension. You can use recipe from chapter Scrubs and peeling recipes under the section for head and neck.

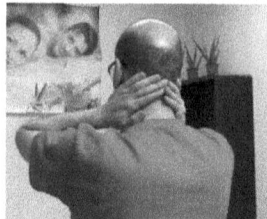 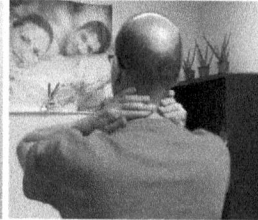 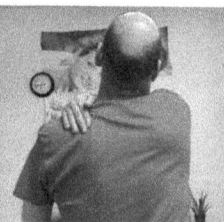 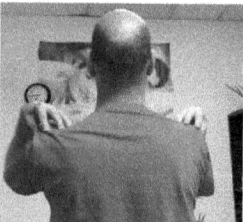

Step 2: After this, take a sip of hot herbal teas and caffeinated drinks. This will help reduce the effect of neck pain and make you able to carry out your routine activities as normal. Ginger tea can help with headaches. To drink ginger, add a half teaspoon of ground ginger to warm water or simply enjoy a cup of brewed ginger tea.

Step 3: After this, relax yourself in the way you are comfortable and then use the cold compression to reduce the stiffness and pain of muscles.

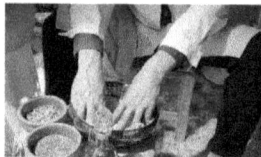 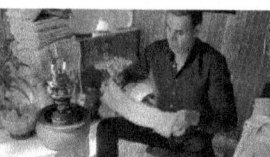 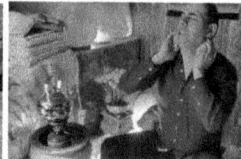 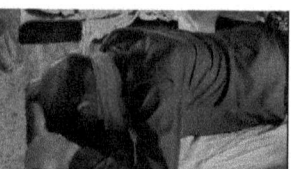

As this is an acute condition always choose cold compress. It can be applied directly to the neck and upper back area for 10-15 minutes. Repeat the application of cold therapy 3-4 times a day. Details of application are described in the chapters for Heat and Cold therapy.

Step 4: Followed by cold, start gentle neck stretches and mobility exercises, which will help improve your range of motion of neck and will also make the neck muscles more flexible. Stiffness will be gradually released. Stretches which work best for neck pain are side stretch to your neck, rotational stretch. The procedure and other details have already been described in the chapter for stretching.

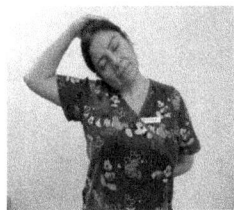 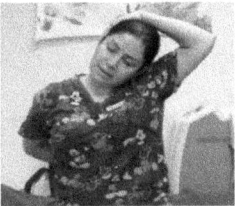 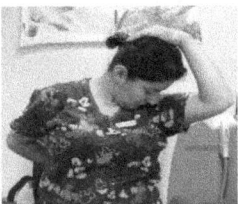 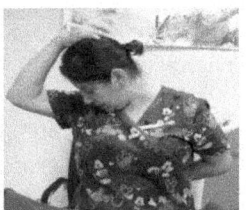

You must feel a slight pull on the tight muscle. It will pain initially, but don't panic. Gradually when the muscle loosens up it will feel better. When you do the movements make sure you don't pull your neck more as it can aggravate the symptom. If you have the pain radiating down to your arm or hands use the nerve stretches. If the pain is radiating down to your thumb, index and middle finger stretch median nerve.

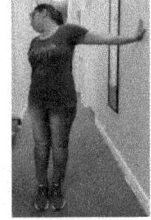

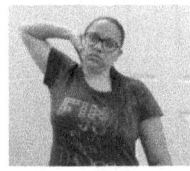 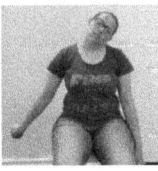

If the pain is radiating down to your pinky finger do the ulnar nerve stretch.

And if it is going on dorsal part of hand do the radial nerve stretch.

Mobility exercises useful in this condition are neck movements.

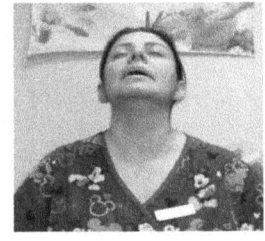 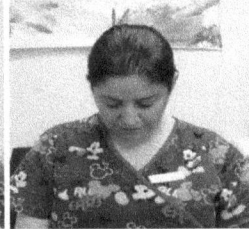 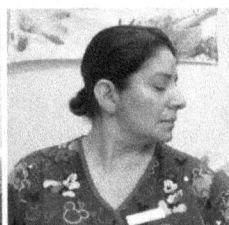 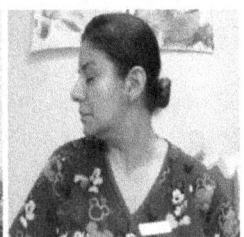

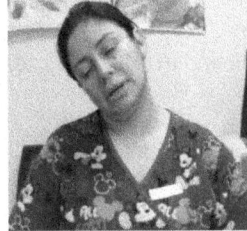 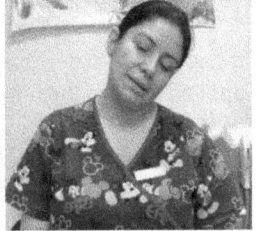

Step 5: Once you are relaxed, release your stiffness with massage. This works best with infused herbal oil recipes.

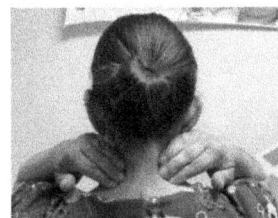 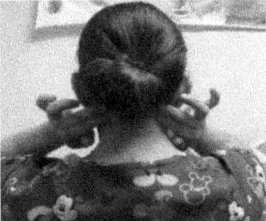 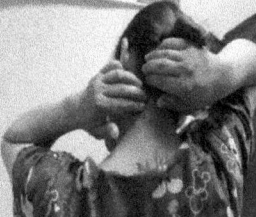 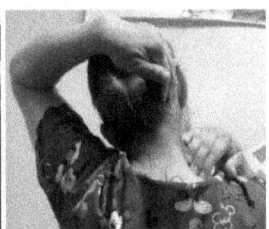

The recipe which works best for neck pain are given in chapter no Herbs and herb infused oil under the section recipes for neck and upper back. Use different recipes each day so that you get more benefits.

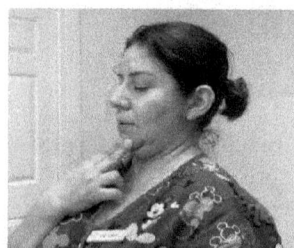

Step 6: Once your symptoms are relieved to 50%, start with the strengthening exercises. As poor neck posture causes muscle weakness and leads to cervicogenic headache. Once you start with exercises you will feel discomfort in the muscles, but don't worry that is just because we are strengthening the weak muscles. Gradually this discomfort goes away. Exercises suitable for this condition are, isometric neck exercises, seated shoulder shrugs, backward shoulder shrugs, standing shoulder crunches. For the exercises you need to refer chapter General Strengthening exercise.

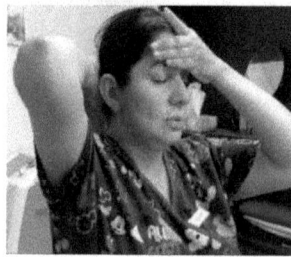 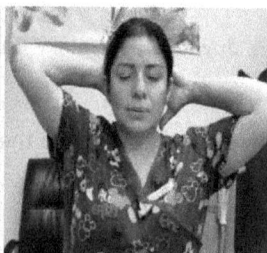 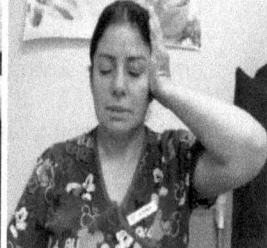 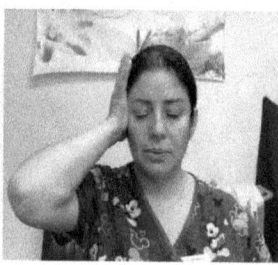

Step 7: Take a balanced diet which should include food rich in vitamins, omega 3, and magnesium in your diet. Green leafy vegetables like spinach, kale, swish charred, collard greens can be consumed. The recipes which is useful are described in chapter Nutritional facts and benefits of balanced diet. There are different sections including recipes for soups, salads, and juices which you can include at least one in your daily diet.

Step 8: You can use homemade pastes on your neck to relieve the severe pain. These patches work on relieving stress and reduces the inflammation. The details and application are given in chapter Herbal poultices (paste) recipes under the section neck and shoulder pain.

Step 9: Use proper resting position and make sure your neck is in a relaxed position. These positions are used while resting or when you have applied the patches.

Step 10: Again, you can use the herbal teas to relieve your cervicogenic headache. The recipes are already described above in step 4.

Step 11: At the end of the day, indulge yourself in foot soak and body soak with herbs. This will relax your body senses and rejuvenate it. The recipes and application are already described in chapter Body and foot soak recipes for relaxation.

CHAPTER 21: NECK PAIN ASSOSICATED WITH DISK HERNIATION

Disk herniation in neck is due to bulging of disc outside and compressing your nerve. It also narrows the spinal canal. Symptoms usually over a long period of time.

- Does your pain in neck radiates to the shoulder, arm or the hand and fingers?
- Is your neck pain, in the back and on the sides of the neck?
- Do you have spasm in your neck muscles?

If you answered yes to any of these questions, there's a high rate you are having a disk herniation. If you feel pain which increases when bending or turning your neck confirms the diagnosis that you have cervical disk herniation.

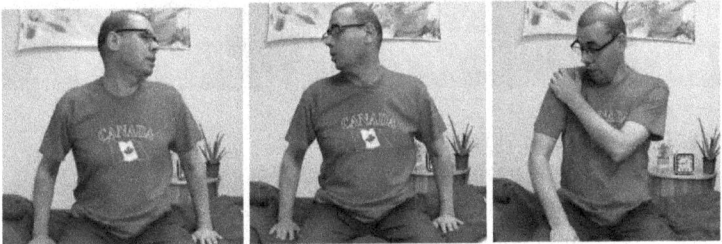

We will show you the exercises to follow, the positions while doing activity, resting positions, herbal recipe tips and nutritional tips. The purpose here is to align your bones and disc which is pressing your nerves.

Here is 7-day protocol to follow which will help reduce your symptoms.

Day 1:

- Starts with waking up in the morning and moving out of the bed in correct position. Make sure you turn to your side and push your body up with head straight. After getting up cover your neck with a warm scarf before you start any activity.

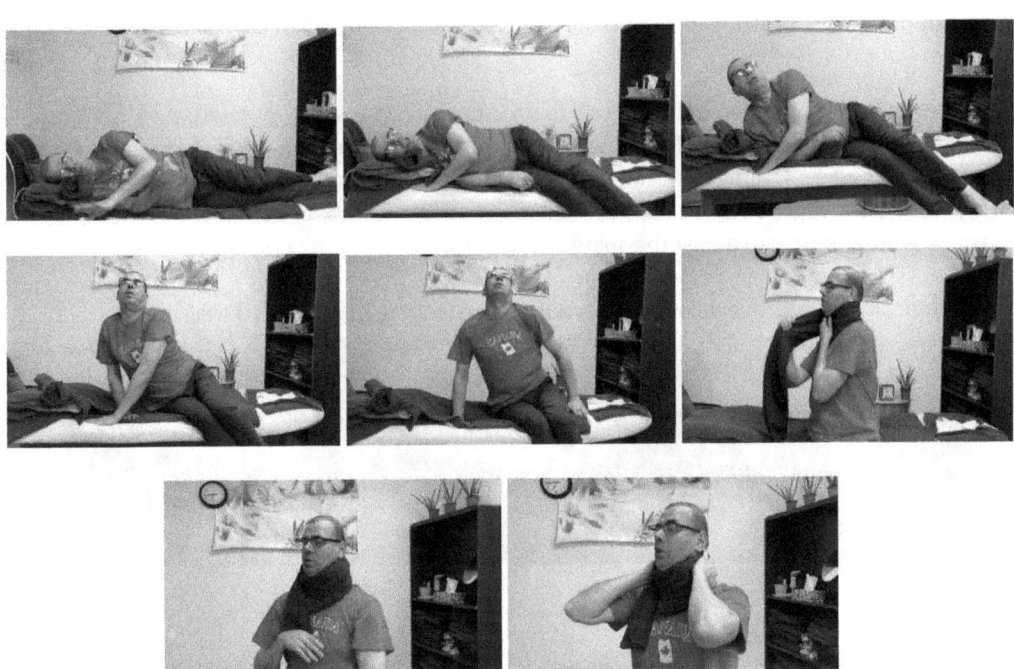

- After that, go to the washroom and do scrubbing to your neck and shoulder. This will help in relieving pain and stiffness which is more intense in the morning. Neck scrub which works best is recipe 1 which contain sea salt, Epsom or normal salt, olive oil, lemon, turmeric, mint, green tea, honey and dill. Recipe 2 which contains chamomile, star-anise, salt, caraway, sage, vinegar and honey. The 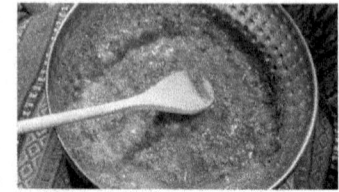 details of recipe preparation and application are already described in the chapter for body scrub. It relaxes the muscle. Wash the scrub with warm shower followed by a cold shower for 2 minutes.

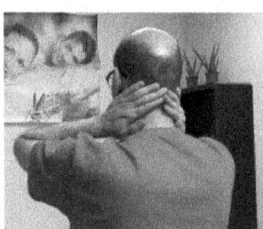 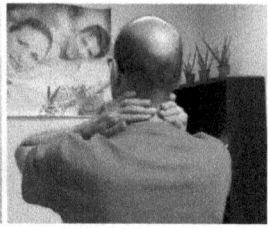 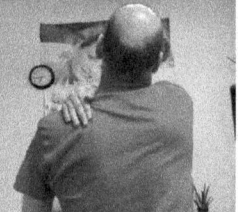 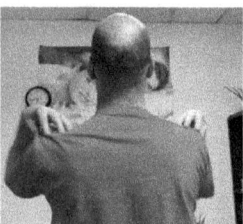

- Once you are done with scrubbing, put the scarf again around your neck and take hot beverages as normal. Take herbal ashwagandha or barley tea. Also, add the special juices to your drink. Try recipe 1 (Green Juice). The details of recipe preparation and application are already described in the chapter for nutritional facts

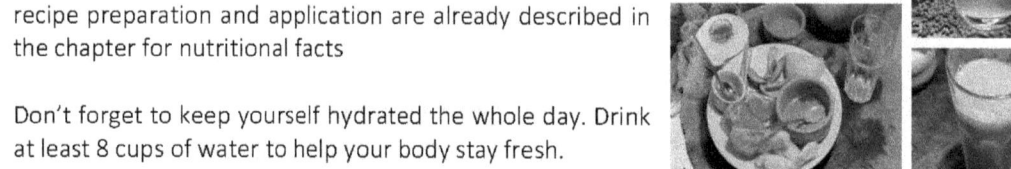

- Don't forget to keep yourself hydrated the whole day. Drink at least 8 cups of water to help your body stay fresh.

- You can continue with your breakfast after beverages. Sit with back supported in erect position. Make sure you don't bend your neck. Add a healthy salad and soup to your meal. The recipe 1 (Red beans) for salad and recipe 1 (Bone broth) for soup will work best.

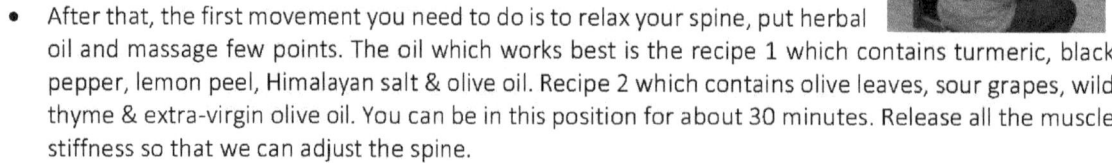

- After that, the first movement you need to do is to relax your spine, put herbal oil and massage few points. The oil which works best is the recipe 1 which contains turmeric, black pepper, lemon peel, Himalayan salt & olive oil. Recipe 2 which contains olive leaves, sour grapes, wild thyme & extra-virgin olive oil. You can be in this position for about 30 minutes. Release all the muscle stiffness so that we can adjust the spine.

Position: Lie down with a pillow under your tummy and head relaxed to the side.

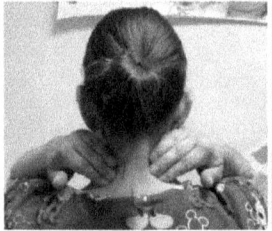 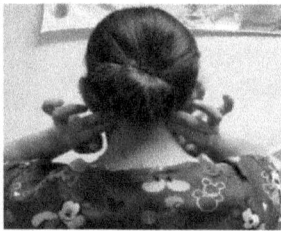 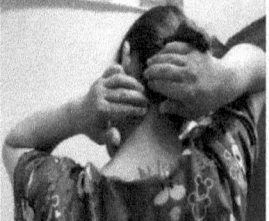 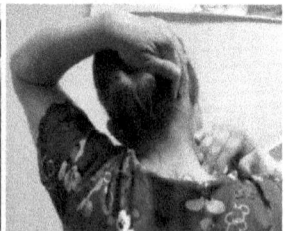

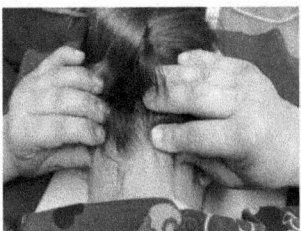
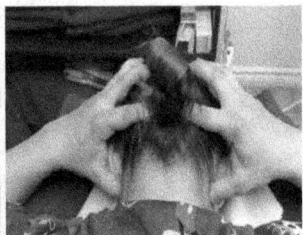

- After massage, you will feel more relaxed. Start with day-1 exercise protocol. To do the exercise, you need to lie down on your back with knees bent. Put a towel roll and place it under your neck to support your spine. Extend your neck back slowly, hold and relax.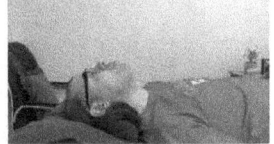

- Also, you can put your hands on the jaw which will help you to push upwards. This movement helps to put disc down in its position and reduce pain.

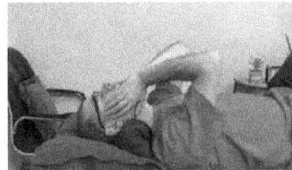
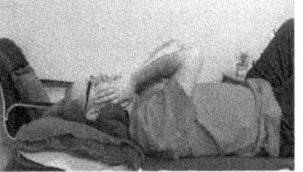

- You need to feel pain coming up from your hands to you shoulder or your neck then – this is a **sign of IMPROVEMENT**. If you feel your pain is going down than the compression is increasing with increase disc bulging. Stop the movement.

- Repeat the exercise for 10 times. Take a break and again repeat it for every 15 minutes. Don't take any pain killer while doing these exercises. If taken you will not feel the difference in pain.

- Once you feel less pain keep doing the movement for 10-15 minutes, every hour. If you feel pressure or tension in your neck – that's NORMAL.

- Also, to relieve stiffness use hot or cold compress while doing this movement. Use only ice if you feel there is swelling, redness or severity in your symptoms. Ice can be used for 15-20 minutes every hour. But if your symptoms are manageable with no swelling or redness always use the heat.

- After certain repetitions, you will feel the pain going in intensity and coming up from hands to neck – **"GOOD SYMPTOMS"**.

- Use herbal paste. The best herbal paste for this condition is Recipe 1 which contains figs, milk, oats, and turmeric. The detail for this recipe is already described in chapter 9 (Herbal paste and poultices) under the heading pastes for neck and shoulders.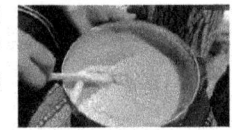

- If this movements are helpful, continue every hour for 2-3 times. Also, if you are doing any activity this movements can be done in sitting with a scarf wrap around your neck. Progress it slowly, stop if you feel more pain.

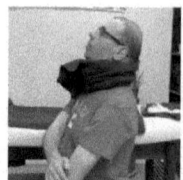 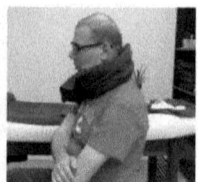

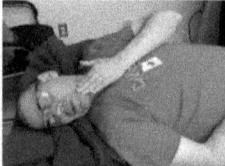 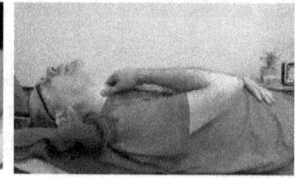

- If you feel the pain is going down progress the exercise by adding rotation to the movement. Lie down on your back with a towel placed under your head. Rotate your head to one side, hold and relax. If you feel the pain is getting better repeat it with head extension for 10 times every hour.

- Pain is not going down in this position than rotate the head to the other side, hold and relax. Repeat the movement for 10 times for every hour. The pain will subside gradually.

- Once you find the movement which relieves the pain, stick to that, and repeat it regularly.

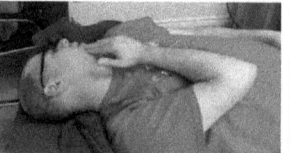 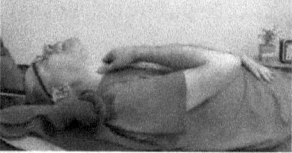

- In the evening to relax yourself do the foot soaking method. This helps relieve tension. Use recipe 1. The details and procedure are explained in chapter earlier

- Use inhalation method for relaxation. This will help relieving the stress and help in pain relief. Followed by inhalation do the gargling. Use Inhalation recipe 1 which contains vinegar, rosemary, thyme and also gargling recipe 1 which contains salt, chamomile and honey. Details are already described in chapter.

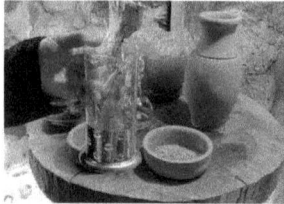 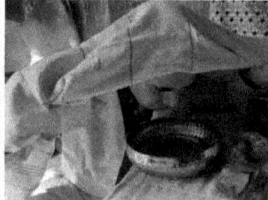 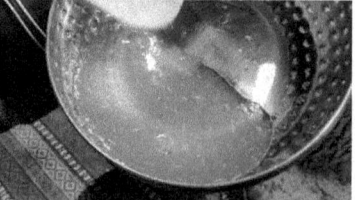

- Also do the body soaking for relaxation. Use recipe 1 for body soak. The recipe and procedure are already described in chapter earlier. The ideal position to soak your body is lying down on your tummy. Try doing some back extensions while body soak. This will give best results. Make sure you support your head with a scarf while doing the body soak.

- Before going to bed, apply herbal oil and leave it overnight. Cover the body area with thin linen this will help absorption of oil better.

Day 2:

- Next day you may feel more discomfort and muscle pain. Don't worry continue with the same sequence as above. The recipes for scrubs, juices, salads, soups, herbal oils, herbal pastes, foot soaks, body soaks, inhalation and gargling will be different for each day.

- Here are the recipes for day 2: Scrubs – use recipe 3 which contains sugar, honey, salt, oats, lemon , olive oil, cress seeds, sesame, flax seeds, sage and mint. Recipe 4 which contains olive oil, mint, sugar, green tea, turmeric, salt. Followed by scrub do the hot shower and end with cold shower for 2 minutes.
    - Juices/Tea – Drink chamomile and cinnamon tea. Use recipe 2 (Hot Juice). Details are given in chapter earlier.
    - Salads and soups – Use recipe 2 (Tuna salad) and (mushroom soup). Details are given in chapter earlier.
    - Herbal oils – Use recipe 3 which contains hot pepper, green tea, sesame, salt & extra virgin oil and recipe 4 which contains turmeric, sage, cinnamon & olive oil.
    - Herbal paste – Use recipe 2 which contains banana, avocado, cinnamon, and yogurt. Details are given in chapter under the heading neck and shoulder.
    - Foot soak – Recipe 2. Details are given in chapter earlier
    - Body soak – Recipe 2. Details are given in chapter earlier.
    - Inhalation and gargling – Recipe 2 for inhalation which contains lavender, chamomile, lemon oil and recipe 2 for gargling which contains mint, green tea, sage and salt.

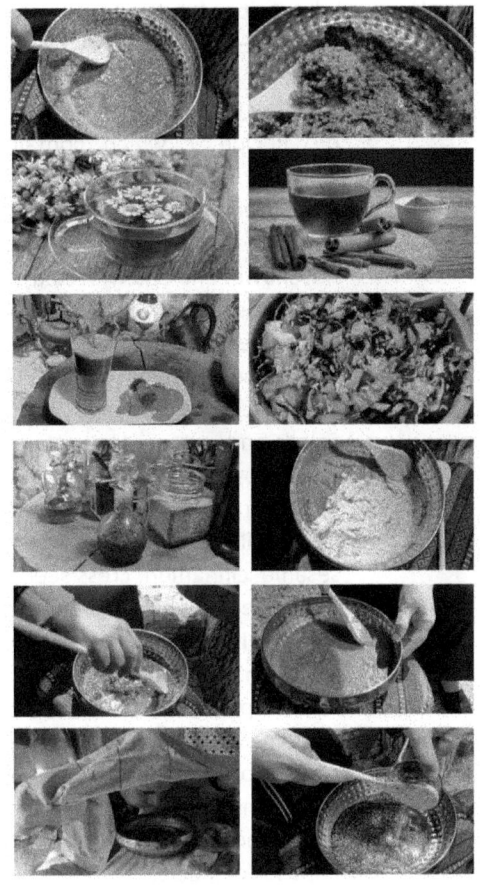

- Continue with the same sequence after getting up in the morning for above mentioned recipes. But on day 2 if you feel there is less pain, we will progress the exercise pattern.

- Lie down on your back. Put one hand on chin and another hand on forehead. Push your chin down. Hold the position for 5 seconds and relax. You will feel stretch pain at neck but if you feel pain going down to hands – STOP the movement.

- Also do the same movement in sitting. Place the hand on chin and straighten your neck up. The best way to do this exercise is sitting in front of mirror. Continue the movements if the symptoms are reduced. Repeat the movement for 10 times.

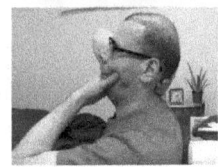

Day 3:
- You will feel improvement in your symptoms. There might be no pain or less pain radiating to your arms, or the pain will be only present on your neck. The recipes for scrubs, juices, salads, soups, herbal oils, herbal pastes, foot soaks, body soaks, inhalation and gargling will be different for each day.

- Here are the recipes for day 3:
    - Scrubs – Recipe 5 which contains oatmeal, brown sugar, honey, thyme, lavender, glow powder, ginger, and olive oil. Recipe 1 which contains which contains salt, olive oil, lemon, turmeric, mint, green tea, honey and dill. (Brown sugar peeler). Followed by scrub do the hot shower and end with cold shower for 2 minutes.
    - Juices/Tea – Use cranberry or ginger tea. Use recipe 3 (Vitamin C Juice). Details are given in chapter earlier.
    - Salads and soups – Use recipe 3(potato and herbs salad) and (meat curry soup). Details are given in chapter earlier.
    - Herbal oils – Use recipe 5 which contains sesame, cinnamon, cress seeds, olive oil & recipe 6 which contains mustard, sesame, bay leaves and olive oil. Details are given in chapter earlier.
    - Herbal paste – Use recipe 3 which contains eggshells, lemon juice, cress seeds, honey, pepper & olive oil. Details are given in chapter under the heading pastes for neck and shoulder
    - Foot soak – Recipe 3
    - Body soak – Recipe 3.
    - Inhalation and gargling – Recipe 3 for inhalation which contains water, camphor. Recipe 3 for gargling which contains salt and water.

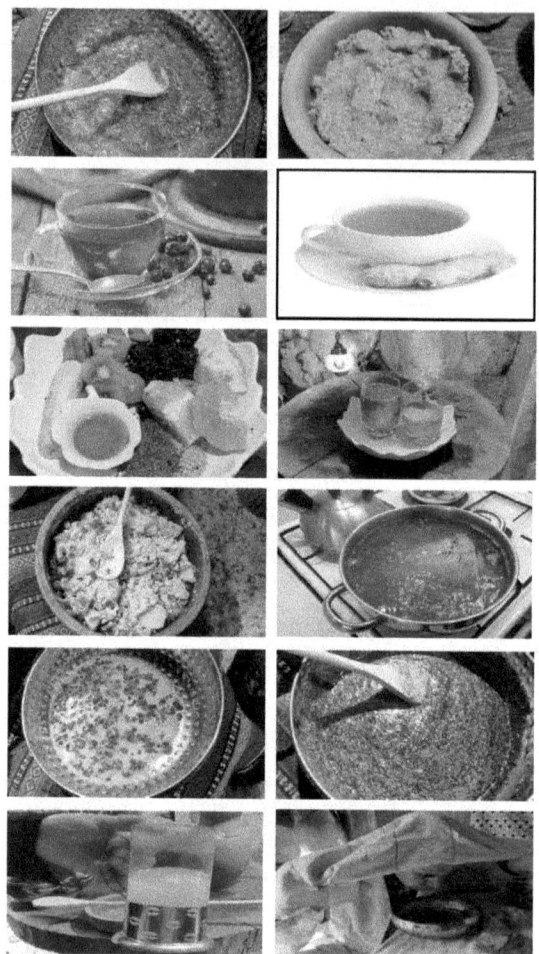

- Continue with the same sequence as of day-1 and day-2 after getting up in the morning for above mentioned recipes. But on day 3 there will be less pain, so you need to add more exercise.

- Lie down on your back and wrap a towel around your temporals with holding the edges of towel in your hand. Use assistance as you may feel dizzy or have headache. Move down slowly taking the head out of bed.

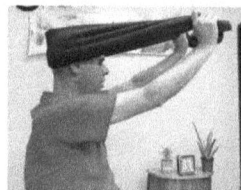 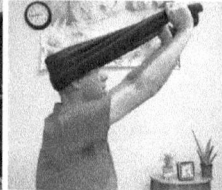 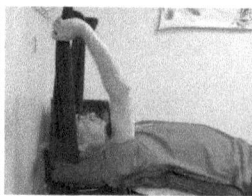 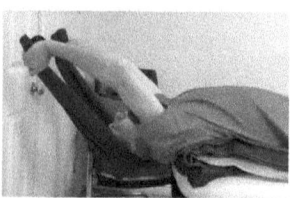

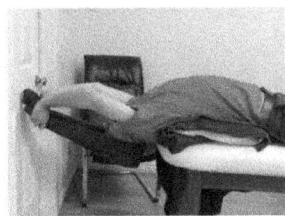

- Control the movements with towel. I you feel good continue further. If you feel dizzy, stop the movement, hold the position, and then go further. When you reach the end, range hold the position for 10 seconds. This will adjust your spine. The pain is reduced but we need more pressure to fix the herniation. Repeat the exercise for 10 times.

Day 4:

- You will feel improvement in your symptoms and comfortable in extending your neck in sitting we need to try retraction and extension. The recipes for scrubs, juices, salads, soups, herbal oils, herbal pastes, foot soaks, body soaks, inhalation and gargling will be different for each day.

- Here are the recipes for day 4:
    o Scrubs –Recipe 2 which contains chamomile, star anise, salt, caraway, sage, vinegar and honey. Recipe 3 which contains sugar, honey, salt, oats, lemon, olive oil, cress seeds, sesame, flax seeds, sage and mint. Followed by scrub do the hot shower and end with cold shower for 2 minutes
    o Juices/tea – Lemon or turmeric tea. Use recipe 4 (Pumpkin Juice). Details are given in chapter earlier.
    o Salads and soups – Use recipe 4 (Wheat and greens salad) and (wheat soup).
    o Herbal oils – Use recipe 7 which contains turmeric, chilli powder, chamomile, extra virgin olive oil and recipe 8 which contains mustard, black seeds, chia seeds & olive oil.
    o Herbal paste – Use recipe 1 which contains figs, milk, oats and turmeric.
    o Foot soak – Recipe 4.
    o Body soak – Recipe 4.
    o Inhalation and gargling – Recipe 4 for inhalation which contains orange peel, lemon peel and vinegar and recipe 1 for gargling which contains salt, chamomile and honey.

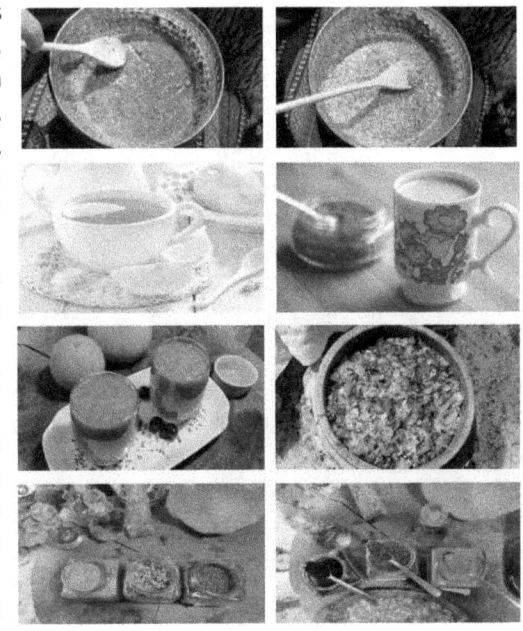

- Continue with the same sequence as of day-1 after getting up in the morning for above mentioned recipes. But on day 4 there will be less pain, so you need to change the exercise protocol.

- Sit with back erect. Place hand on your chin and push your head backwards. Maintain the position and extend your back until the end. Repeat it for 10 times.

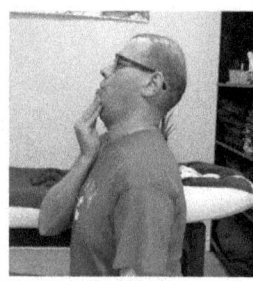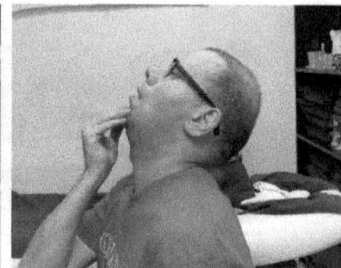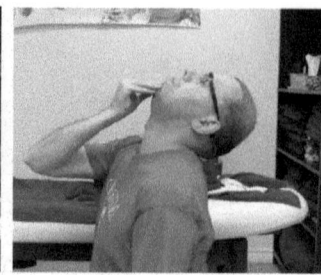

- Also, you can use both hands for supporting and pushing hand backwards. If this position worsens your symptoms – STOP, we don't want to aggravate the condition. But continue other exercises as before.

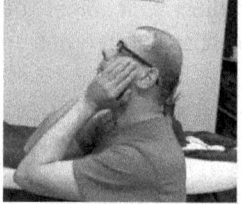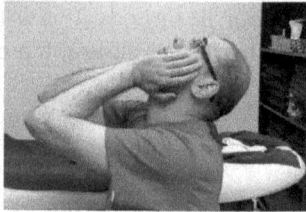

Day 5:

- You will feel improvement in your symptoms. The recipes for scrubs, juices, salads, soups, herbal oils, herbal pastes, foot soaks, body soaks, inhalation and gargling will be different for each day.

- Here are the recipes for day 5:
    - Scrubs – Recipe 4 which contains olive oil, mint, sugar, green tea, turmeric, salt. Recipe 5 which contains oatmeal, brown sugar, honey, thyme, lavender, glow powder, ginger and olive oil. Followed by scrub do the hot shower and end with cold shower for 2 minutes.
    - Juices/tea – Lemongrass or sage tea. Use recipe 5(Milk cocktail with chia seeds and flax seeds).
    - Salads and soups – Use recipe 5 (Greek green salad) and (lentil soup).
    - Herbal oils – Use recipe 9 which contains ground ginger, fenugreek, bay leaves, olive oil and recipe 10 which contains apple cider vinegar, salt, turmeric, garlic powder & olive oil.
    - Herbal paste – Use recipe 2 which contains banana, avocado, cinnamon and yogurt.
    - Foot soak – Recipe 1.
    - Body soak – Recipe 5.
    - Inhalation and gargling – Recipe 1 for inhalation which contains vinegar, rosemary, thyme and recipe 2 for gargling. Details are given in chapter

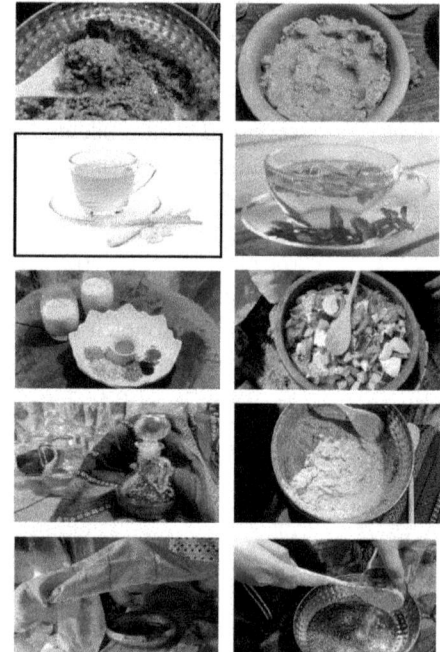

- Continue with the same sequence as of day-1 after getting up in the morning for above mentioned recipes. But on day 5 there will be less pain, so you need to change the exercise protocol.

- Repeat the exercise sequence from day 1 to 4. While doing this you need to only feel a stretch pain in back. There should be no radiating pain.

Day 6:
- You will feel improvement in your symptoms. The recipes for scrubs, juices, salads, soups, herbal oils, herbal pastes, foot soaks, body soaks, inhalation and gargling will be different for each day.

- Here are the recipes for day 6:
    - Scrubs – Recipe 1 which contains salt, olive oil, lemon, turmeric, mint, green tea, honey and dill. Recipe 2 which contains chamomile, star anice, salt, caraway, sage, vinegar and honey. Followed by scrub do the hot shower and end with cold shower for 2 minutes.
    - Juices/tea – Rosemarry or rooibos tea. Use recipe 1(Green Juice).
    - Salads and soups – Use recipe 6 for salad (Fruit bowl salad) and recipe 1 (bone broth) for soup.
    - Herbal oils – Use recipe 11 which contains wheat bran, cinnamon,wild thyme, laurel powder, olive oil and recipe 1 which contains turmeric, black pepper, lemon peel, Himalayan salt and olive oil.
    - Herbal paste – Use recipe 3 which contains egg shells, lemon juice, cress seeds, honey, pepper and olive oil.
    - Foot soak – Recipe 2.
    - Body soak – Recipe 1.
    - Inhalation and gargling – Recipe 2 for inhalation which contains lavender, chamomile, lemon oil and recipe 3 for gargling.

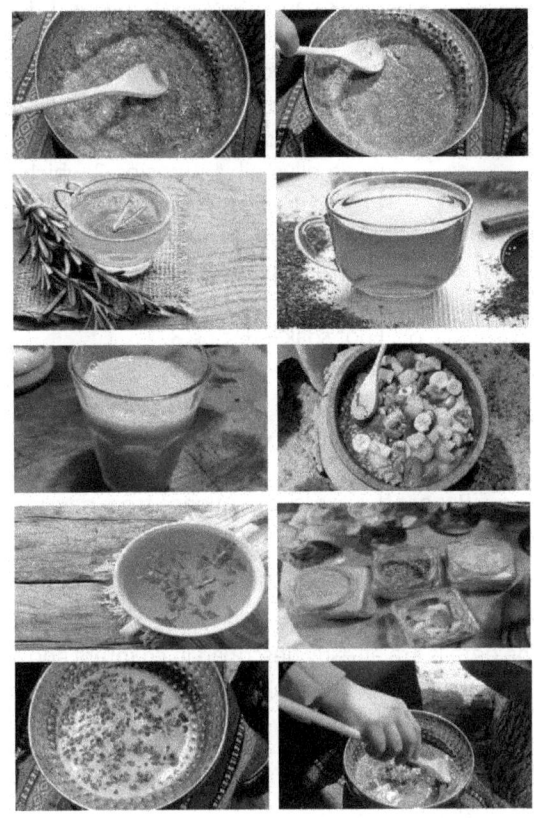

- Continue with the same sequence as of day-1 after getting up in the morning for above mentioned recipes. But on day 6 there will be a sequence of exercise you will need to follow.

- Repeat the exercise sequence from day 1 to 4. While doing this you need to only feel a stretch pain in back. There should be no radiating pain.

- Repeat the sequence throughout the day.

Day 7:
- At this day you will feel 80-90% of relief in your symptoms.

- Here are the recipes for day 6:
    - Scrubs – Use recipe 3 which contains sugar, honey, salt, oats, lemon, olive oil, cress seeds, sesame, flax seeds, sage and mint. Recipe 4 which contains olive oil, mint,

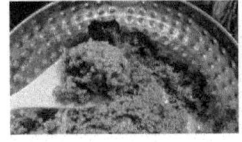 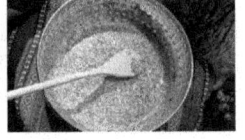

sugar, green tea, turmeric, salt. Chapter 12. Followed by scrub do the hot shower and end with cold shower for 2 minutes.
- o Juices/tea – peppermint or olive leaves tea. Use recipe 2 (Hot Juice).
- o Salads and soups – Use recipe 1 (Red beans salad) for salad and recipe 2 (mushroom soup) for soup.
- o Herbal oils – Use recipe 2 which contains olive leaves, sour grapes, wild thyme, extra-virgin olive oil and recipe 3 which contains hot pepper, green tea, sesame seeds, salt and extra virgin olive oil.
- o Herbal paste – Use recipe 1 which contains figs, milk, oats and turmeric.
- o Foot soak – Recipe 3.
- o Body soak – Recipe 2.
- o Inhalation and gargling – Recipe 3 for inhalation which contains water, camphor and recipe 1 for gargling.

- Repeat the exercise sequence from day 1 to 4. While doing this you need to only feel a stretch pain in back. There should be no radiating pain.

After this 7-day protocol there will be relieve in your symptoms.

If the pain is manageable after 7 days start with the stretching and strengthening techniques for neck pain. The details are already described in chapters above. After 2 weeks start with intense strengthening exercises like scapular strengthening, shoulder strengthening also. All the exercises are described in chapter before.

If the pain persists or there is no improvement after 7 days, consult your doctor as you may have any another underlying condition.

CHAPTER 22: NECK PAIN ASSOCIATED WITH CERVICAL SPINAL STENOSIS

Cervical spinal stenosis is the narrowing of the spinal canal in the neck. Symptoms usually cause over a long period of time.

- Do you feel pain in your neck or surrounding structures?
- Does your pain radiate to your arms or hands with "pins and needles" kind of sensation on both upper limb or one any one side?
- Do you feel weakness in your shoulder or hands on both sides or on one side?

If you answered yes to these questions, there's a high rate that your spinal canal is getting narrow. If you are feeling the symptoms on both hands then there is a chance that you are having central stenosis and it is only limited to one side of hand then it is a lateral stenosis. It can be because of many reasons like herniated disc, posture, injury, or tumor. The purpose here is to align your bones and disc which is pressing your spinal cord.

When you wake up and feel the pain with stiffness surrounding your neck or "pins and needle sensation" through your arm then follow this 24-hour guide to help maintain your pain.

Step 1: Before starting activity, you can use the neck scrub to reduce the stress of on your neck and surrounding muscles, which will increase the blood circulation of that part and soothes your skin. It also helps in relieving tension. You can use recipe from chapter Scrubs and peeling recipes under the section for head and neck.

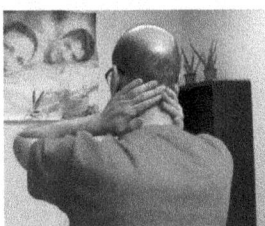 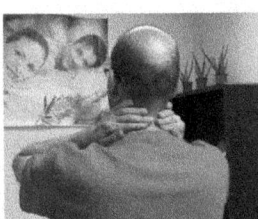 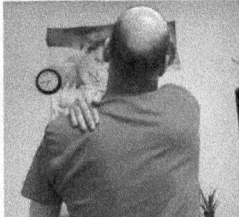 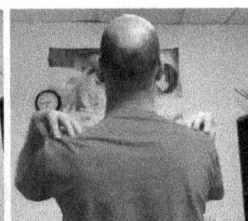

Step 2: After this, take a sip of hot herbal teas and caffeinated drinks. This will help reduce the effect of neck pain and make you able to carry out your routine activities as normal.

Step 3: After this, relax yourself in the way you are comfortable and then use the heat or contrast compress with heat-cold compression to reduce the stiffness and pain of muscles. It can be applied directly to the neck and upper back area for 10-15 minutes. Repeat the application of heat or contrast therapy 3-4 times a day. Details of application are described in the chapters for Heat and Cold therapy.

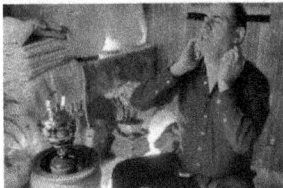 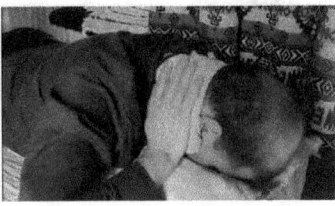

Step 4: Followed by heat once the area is relaxed, start gentle neck stretches and mobility exercises, which will help improve your range of motion of neck and will also make the neck muscles more flexible. Stiffness will be gradually released.

Stretches which work best for neck pain are side stretch to your neck, posterior stretch to your neck, diagonal stretch. The procedure and other details have already been described in the chapter for stretching.

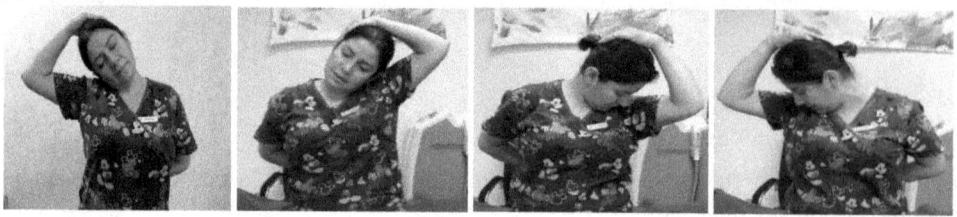

You must feel a slight pull on the tight muscle. It will pain initially, but don't panic. When you do the movements make sure you don't pull your neck more as it can aggravate the symptom.

Mobility exercises useful in this condition are neck movements.

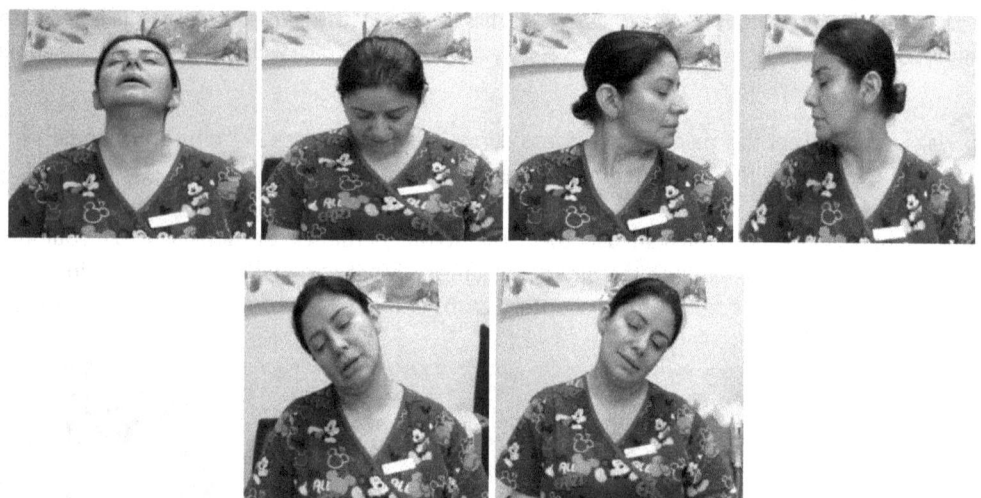

Step 5: Once you are relaxed, release your stiffness with massage. This works best with infused herbal oil recipes.

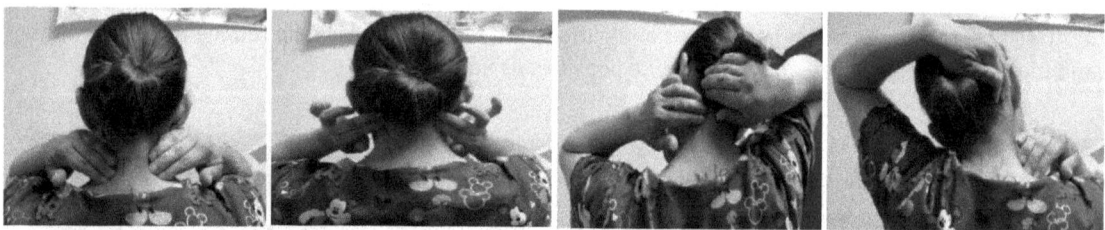

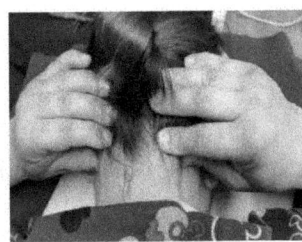
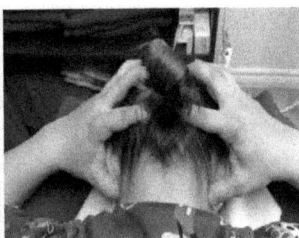

The recipe which works best for neck pain are given in chapter Herbs and herb infused oil under the section recipes for neck and upper back. Use different recipes each day so that you get more benefits.

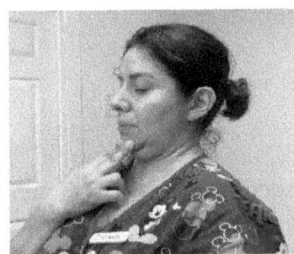

Step 6: Once your symptoms are relieved to 50%, start with the strengthening exercises. As poor neck posture causes muscle weakness and leads to cervicogenic headache. Once you start with exercises you will feel discomfort in the muscles, but don't worry that is just because we are strengthening the weak muscles. Gradually this discomfort goes away. Exercises suitable for this condition are, isometric neck exercises, seated shoulder shrugs, backward shoulder shrugs, standing shoulder crunches. For the exercises you need to refer chapter General Strengthening exercise.

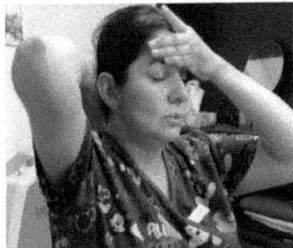
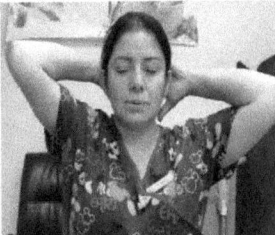
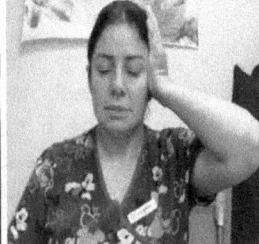
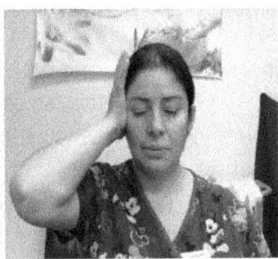

Step 7: Take a balanced diet which should include food rich in vitamins, omega 3, and magnesium in your diet. Green leafy vegetables like spinach, kale, swish charred, collard greens can be consumed. The recipes which is useful are described in chapter Nutritional facts and benefits of balanced diet. There are different sections including recipes for soups, salads and juices which you can include at least one in your daily diet.

Step 8: You can use homemade pastes on your neck to relieve the severe pain. These patches work on relieving stress and reduces the inflammation. The details and application are given in chapter Herbal poultices (paste) recipes under the section neck and shoulder pain.

Step 9: Use proper resting position and make sure your neck is in a relaxed position. These positions are used while resting or when you have applied the patches.

Step 10: Again, you can use the herbal teas to relieve your cervicogenic headache. The recipes are already described above in step 4.

Step 11: At the end of the day, indulge yourself in foot soak and body soak with herbs. This will relax your body senses and rejuvenate it. The recipes and application are already described in chapter Body and foot soak recipes for relaxation.

Step 12: Use can also do the inhalation therapy with herbal recipes which will help reduce the stress. Before sleeping apply herbal oil to your neck and wrap it with a linen cloth. This helps in pain relief.

CHAPTER 23: CERVICAL SPONDYLOSIS – DEGENERATION OF BONES

Cervical spondylosis is the natural wearing down of cartilage, disks, ligaments, and bones in your neck.

You may have cervical spondylosis and not even know it. It's common to have no symptoms related to this condition.

If you experience symptoms which typically include:

- Neck pain or stiffness. This may be the main symptom. Pain may get worse when you move your neck.
- A nagging soreness in the neck.
- Muscle spasms.
- A clicking, popping, or grinding sound when you move your neck.
- Dizziness.
- Headaches.

Then, there are high chances of spinal degeneration which is leading to cervical spondylosis. The treatment strategy for cervical spondylosis depends on the severity of a patient's signs and symptoms. The goals of treatment are to relieve pain, improve functional ability in day-to-day activities, and prevent permanent injury to neural structures. Symptomatic cervical spondylosis is approached in a stepwise fashion which include,

Step 1: Before starting activity, you can use the neck scrub to reduce the stress of on your neck and surrounding muscles, which will increase the blood circulation of that part and soothes your skin. It also helps in relieving tension. You can use recipe from chapter Scrubs and peeling recipes under the section for head and neck.

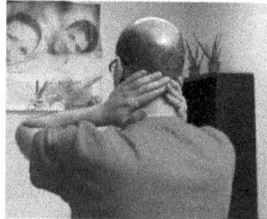 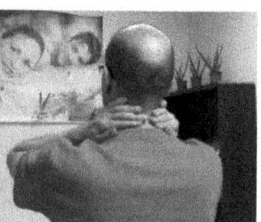

Step 2: After this, take a sip of hot herbal teas and caffeinated drinks. This will help reduce the effect of neck pain and make you able to carry out your routine activities as normal.

Step 3: After this, relax yourself in the way you are comfortable and then use the heat or cold compression to reduce the stiffness and pain of muscles. Selection of heat and cold therapy depends upon the onset of pain. For instance, if you are suffering from the pain from longer duration then

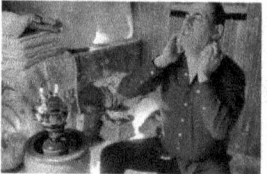 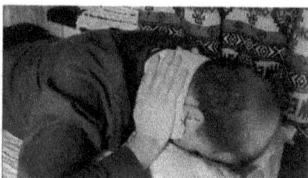

you can use heat and if the pain is acute then you can use the cold. It can be applied directly to the neck and upper back area for 10-15 minutes. Repeat the application of heat or cold therapy 3-4 times a day. Details of application are described in the chapters for Heat and Cold therapy.

Step 4: Followed by heat or cold, start gentle neck stretches and mobility exercises, which will help improve your range of motion of neck and will also make the neck muscles more flexible. Stiffness will be gradually released.

Stretches which work best for cervicogenic headache are side stretch to your neck, posterior stretch to your neck, diagonal stretch. The procedure and other details have already been described in the chapter for stretching.

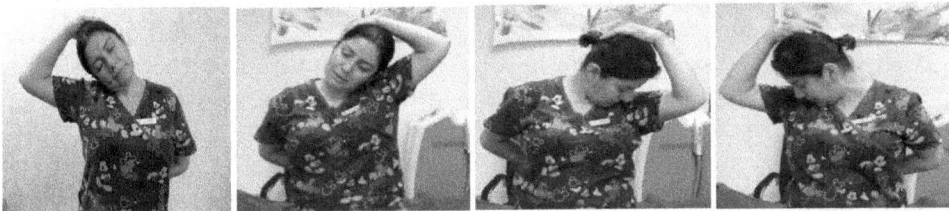

You must feel a slight pull on the tight muscle. It will pain initially, but don't panic. Gradually when the muscle loosens up it will feel better. When you do the movements make sure you don't pull your neck more as it can aggravate the symptom.

Mobility exercises useful in this condition are neck movements.

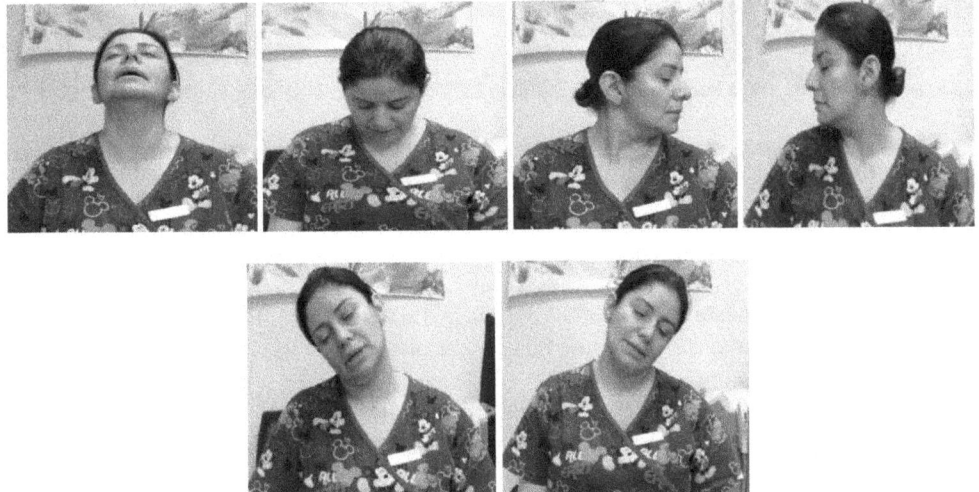

Step 5: Once you are relaxed, release your stiffness with massage. This works best with infused herbal oil recipes.

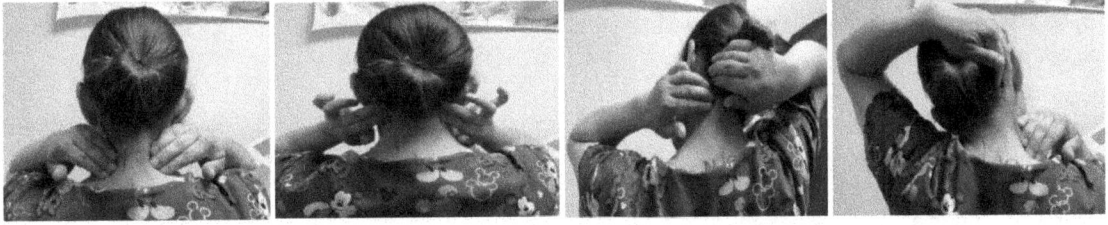

The recipe which works best for neck pain are given in chapter Herbs and herb infused oil under the section recipes for neck and upper back. Use different recipes each day so that you get more benefits.

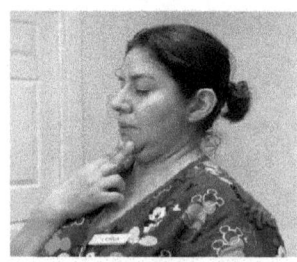

Step 6: Once your symptoms are relieved to 50%, start with the strengthening exercises. As poor neck posture causes muscle weakness and leads to cervicogenic headache. Once you start with exercises you will feel discomfort in the muscles, but don't worry that is just because we are strengthening the weak muscles. Gradually this discomfort goes away. Exercises suitable for this condition are, isometric neck exercises, seated shoulder shrugs, backward shoulder shrugs, standing shoulder crunches. For the exercises you need to refer chapter General Strengthening exercise.

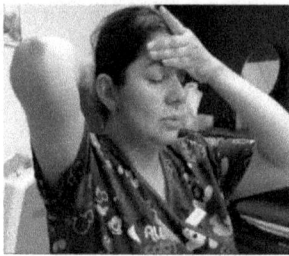
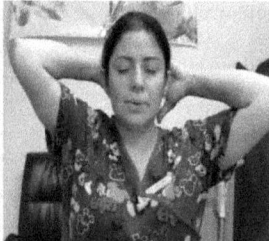
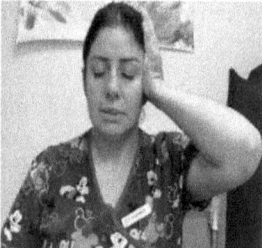
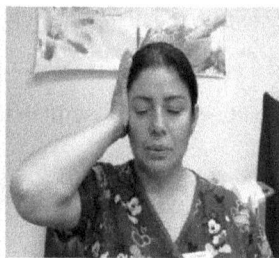

Step 7: Take a balanced diet which should include food rich in vitamins, omega 3, and magnesium in your diet. Green leafy vegetables like spinach, kale, swish charred, collard greens can be consumed. The recipes which is useful are described in chapter Nutritional facts and benefits of balanced diet. There are different sections including recipes for soups, salads and juices which you can include at least one in your daily diet.

Step 8: You can use homemade pastes on your neck to relieve the severe pain. These patches work on relieving stress and reduces the inflammation. The details and application are given in chapter Herbal poultices (paste) recipes under the section neck and shoulder pain.

Step 9: Use proper resting position and make sure your neck is in a relaxed position. These positions are used while resting or when you have applied the patches.

Step 10: Again, you can use the herbal teas to relieve your cervicogenic headache. The recipes are already described above in step 4.

Step 11: At the end of the day, indulge yourself in foot soak and body soak with herbs. This will relax your body senses and rejuvenate it. The recipes and application are already described in chapter Body and foot soak recipes for relaxation.

Step 12: Use can also do the inhalation therapy with herbal recipes which will help reduce the stress. Before sleeping apply herbal oil to your neck and wrap it with a linen cloth. This helps in pain relief.

Always remember as there is degeneration process, we cannot reverse the condition but prevent it from further progressing.

CHAPTER 24: MIDDLE BACK (THORACIC) PAIN DUE TO DISK HERNIATION

Thoracic spinal stenosis occurs when the spine at the middle of the back has become narrowed. It's a degenerative spinal condition that affects any of the 12 thoracic vertebrae (T1 – T12).

Symptoms of thoracic spinal stenosis:

Individuals experience different symptoms, and some people may not have any symptoms. The most common symptoms of spinal stenosis include:

- Intermittent pain
- Pain around the spine area or radiating pain to chest
- Numbness and tingling
- Breathing difficulties

To confirm the diagnosis, cross your hands over the shoulder and extend your back. If the pain goes down in intensity, then it confirms the diagnosis for thoracic disk herniation. We need to do exercise to put the disk bulge inside again. This will reduce the symptoms and help you relieve pain.

Treatment protocol for 7 days:

Here is 7-day protocol to follow which will help reduce your symptoms.

Day 1:

- Starts with waking up in the morning and moving out of the bed in correct position. Make sure you turn to your side and push your body up with head straight.

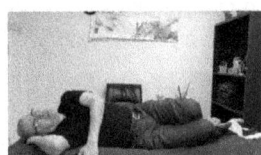 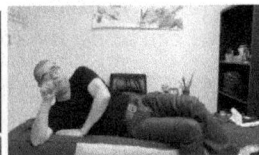 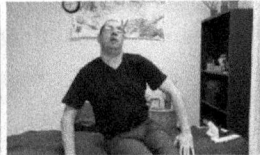 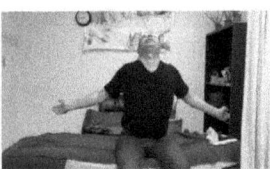

- After that, go to the washroom and do scrubbing to your middle back. This will help in relieving pain and stiffness which is more intense in the morning. Body scrub which works best is recipe 1 (yogurt scrub) and recipe 2 (Turmeric scrub). The details of recipe preparation and application are already described in the chapter for body scrub.

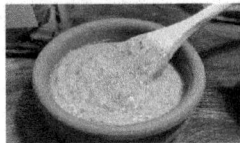 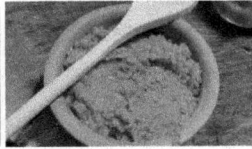 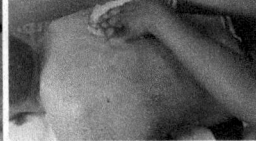 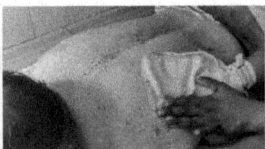

- Once you are done with scrubbing, Take herbal ashwagandha and barley tea. Also, add the special juices to your drink. Try recipe 1 (Green Juice). The details of recipe preparation and application are already described in the chapter for nutritional facts.

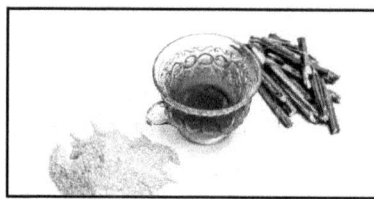 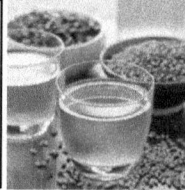 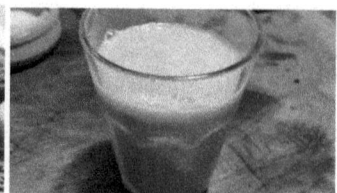

- Don't forget to keep yourself hydrated the whole day. Drink at least 8 cups of water to help your body stay fresh.

- You can continue with your breakfast after beverages. Add a healthy salad and soup to your meal. The recipe 1 (Red beans) for salad and recipe 1 (Bone broth) for soup will work best. While eating if you are in sitting position make sure you are supported or seated upright.

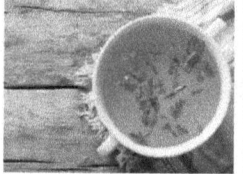 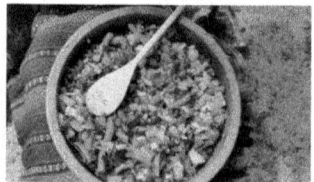

- After that, the first movement you need to do is to relax your spine. Lie down with a pillow under your chest and head relaxed. Gently breathe in and out in this position. You can be in this position for about 30 minutes.

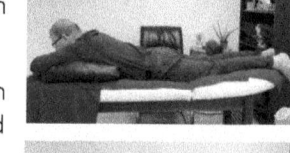

- If you feel pain is not going down or getting worse in this position, you can take the pillow out and rest your head on your hands. Gently breathe in and out in this position. This will give a traction feeling to the spine.

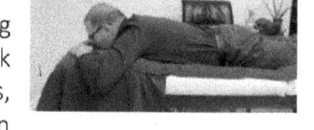

- Once you feel relaxed, you need to massage your mid back in resting position described above. Use recipe 1 which contains turmeric, black pepper, lemon peel, salt, olive oil and recipe 2 which contains olive leaves, dried sour grape leaves, wild thyme, olive oil from chronic upper back pain section. The details for recipes and application are already described in chapter 8 (herbs and herbs infused oils). This will help remove the stiffness so we can adjust the spine in a proper way.

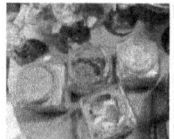 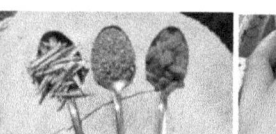 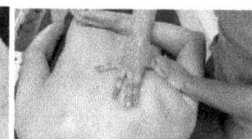 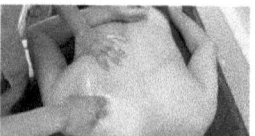

- After massage, you will feel more relaxed. Start with day-1 exercise protocol. To do the exercise, you need to lie down on your tummy with elbows bend and hands rested properly. Push up your body in this position slowly, hold and relax.

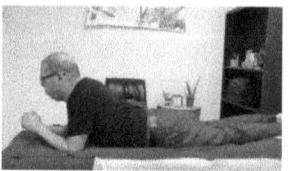 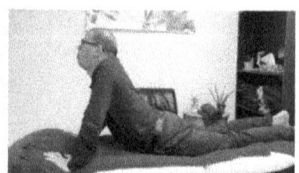

- Halfway if you feel pain in your back, stop at that position and hold for few seconds. Breath in and breathe out in this position and progress it forward.

- Make sure you only do up to your available range. Of course, you will not achieve the full range right away. You need to feel pain coming up from your legs to the back – this is a sign of IMPROVEMENT.

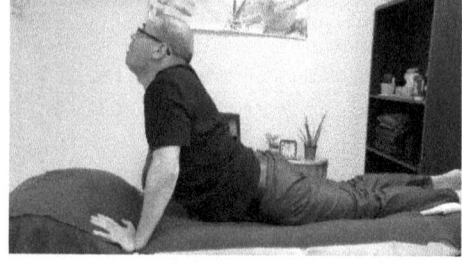

- Repeat the exercise for 5 times. Take a break and again repeat it for 5 times. Make sure you do it in a correct manner. Do this movement throughout the day. If you feel pressure or tension in your middle back – that's **NORMAL**.

- Also, to relieve stiffness use hot or cold compress while doing this movement. Use only ice if you feel there is swelling, redness or severity in your symptoms. Ice can be used for 15-20 minutes every hour. But if your symptoms are manageable with no swelling or redness always use the heat.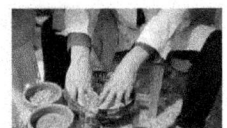

- Use herbal paste recipe 1 which contains ginger, cloves, cinnamon and vinegar on your lower back. Keep the paste on your back for about 15-20 minutes. This will help reduce the stiffness. The detail for recipe is already described in chapter (Herbal paste and poultices).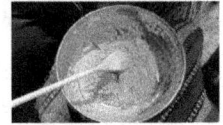

- Continue this exercise protocol even though you feel pain or discomfort. You may feel more stiffness or muscle pain the next day but that is okay!

- While working you can put a pillow under your chest and keep your spine in extended position. This will help relieve pressure on your back.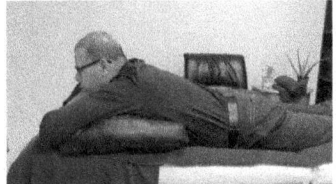

- In the evening if you feel pain in your legs do the foot soaking method. This helps relieve tension. Use recipe 1

- Use inhalation method for relaxation. This will help relieving the stress and help in pain relief. Followed by inhalation do the gargling. Use Inhalation recipe 1 which contains vinegar, rosemary, thyme and gargling also recipe 1 which contains salt, chamomile and honey. Details are already described in chapter.

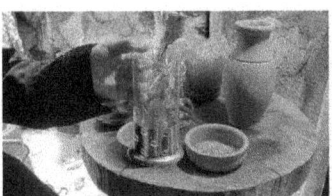 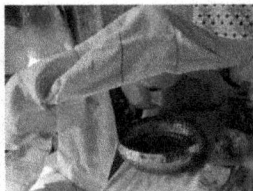 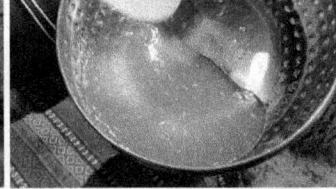

- Also do the body soaking for relaxation. Use recipe 1 for body soak. The recipe and procedure are already described in chapter earlier. The ideal position to soak your body is lying down on your tummy. Try doing some back extensions while body soak. This will give best results. If you are not comfortable lying on your tummy, lie flat on your back. **Don't do body soaking in sitting – "not recommended".**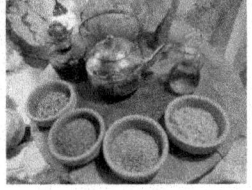

- Before going to bed, apply herbal oil and leave it overnight. Cover the body area with thin linen this will help absorption of oil better.

Day 2:

- Next day you may feel more discomfort and muscle pain. Don't worry continue with the same sequence as above. The recipes for scrubs, juices, salads, soups, herbal oils, herbal pastes, foot soaks, body soaks, inhalation and gargling will be different for each day.

- Here are the recipes for day 2:
    - Scrubs – use recipe 3 (Lemon sugar) and recipe 4(Coffee scrub). Followed by scrub do the hot shower and end with cold shower for 2 minutes.
    - Juices – Chamomile or cinnamon tea. Use recipe 2 (Hot Juice).
    - Salads and soups – Use recipe 2 (Tuna salad) and (mushroom soup).
    - Herbal oils – Use recipe 3 which contains hot pepper, green tea, sesame seeds, salt, olive oil and recipe 4 which contains turmeric, sage, cinnamon, olive oil.
    - Herbal paste – Use recipe 2 which contains camphor, black seed, thyme, lavender, mint, basil, honey and oatmeal.
    - Foot soak – Recipe 2.
    - Body soak – Recipe 2.
    - Inhalation and gargling – Recipe 2 for inhalation which contains lavender, chamomile, lemon oil and recipe 2 for gargling which contains mint, green tea, sage and salt.
- Continue with the same sequence after getting up in the morning for above mentioned recipes. But on day 2 if you feel there is no improvement in symptoms you need to change the exercise pattern.
- Lie down on your tummy. Put a pillow under your mid back. Take a towel and wrap it around your neck and hold straight with your hands. Put your head up and go down slowly. Breath in and breath out. If you feel pain at any range while going down hold at that position and continue forward. If this helps, continue with same movement for 10 times.

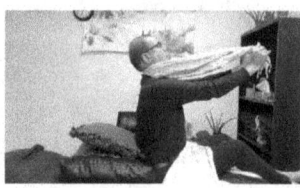 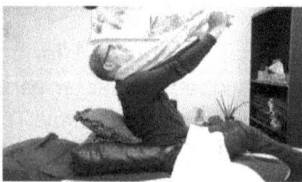 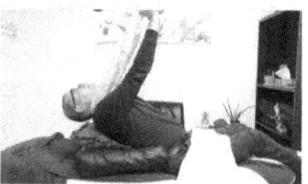

- To come up again hold on the towel and support your hand. Slowly come up without bending your neck. Repeat the whole process for 8-10 times.

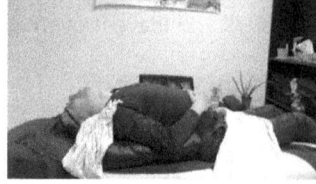 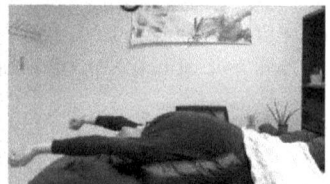

- If the above position is not comfortable stretch your arms out and above. Hold the position with gently breath in and breathe out.

Day 3:

- You will feel improvement in your symptoms. There might be no pain or less pain radiating to your legs, or the pain will be only present on your back. The recipes for scrubs, juices, salads, soups, herbal oils, herbal pastes, foot soaks, body soaks, inhalation and gargling will be different for each day.

- Here are the recipes for day 3:

    - Scrubs – Recipe 1 (yogurt scrub) and recipe 5 (Brown sugar peeler). Followed by scrub do the hot shower and end with cold shower for 2 minutes.

    - Juices – Cranberry or ginger tea. Use recipe 3 (Vitamin C Juice).

    - Salads and soups – Use recipe 3 (potato and herbs salad) and (meat curry soup).

    - Herbal oils – Use recipe 5 which contains sesame, cinnamon, cress seeds, olive oil and recipe 6 which contains mustard, sesame, bay leaves and olive oil.

    - Herbal paste – Use recipe 3 which contains wheat flour, ginger, fenugreek and chia seeds.

    - Foot soak – Recipe 3.

    - Body soak – Recipe 3

    - Inhalation and gargling – Recipe 3 for inhalation which contains water, camphor. Recipe 3 for gargling which contains salt and water.

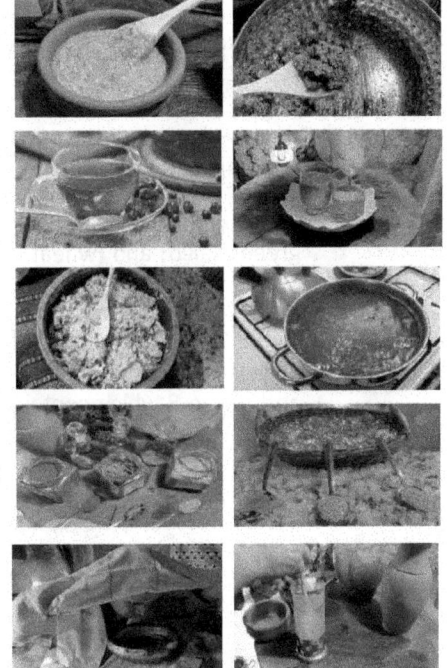

- Continue with the same sequence as of day-1 after getting up in the morning for above mentioned recipes. But on day 3 there will be less pain, so you need to change the exercise protocol.

- We will do some exercise in sitting. Sit with putting hands on your lap and extend your back. Repeat this for 5-10 times. You will feel pain going down in intensity. But you will still feel pain at mid back.

- For that, lie down on your tummy and wrap a towel around your lower back with holding the edges of towel in your hand. Extend your back while keep holding the towel. This will adjust your spine. The pain is reduced but we need more pressure to fix the herniation. Repeat the exercise for 10 times.

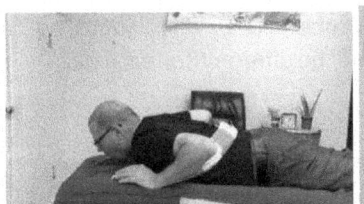 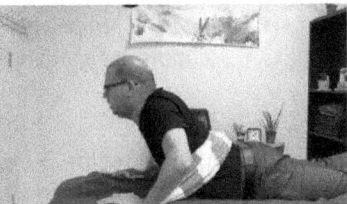 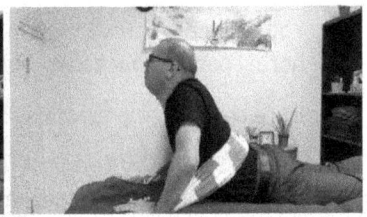

Day 4:
- You will feel improvement in your symptoms and comfortable in extending your back in standing we need to try shifting hips and side bending. The recipes for scrubs, juices, salads, soups, herbal oils, herbal pastes, foot soaks, body soaks, inhalation and gargling will be different for each day.
- Here are the recipes for day 4:
    - Scrubs – Recipe 2 (Turmeric scrub) and recipe 3 (Lemon sugar). Followed by scrub do the hot shower and end with cold shower for 2 minutes.
    - Juices – Lemon or turmeric tea. Use recipe 4 (Pumpkin Juice).
    - Salads and soups – Use recipe 4 (Wheat and greens salad) and (wheat soup). Details are given in chapter 13.
    - Herbal oils – Use recipe 7 which contains chilli powder, chamomile, turmeric, olive oil and recipe 8 which contains mustard, black seeds, chia seeds and olive oil.
    - Herbal paste – Use recipe 4 which contains garlic, aloe vera, cloves and honey. Details are given in chapter 9.

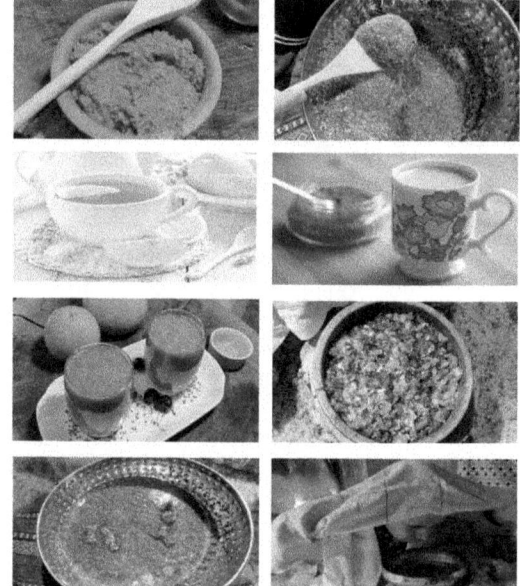

    - Foot soak – Recipe 4.
    - Body soak – Recipe 4.
    - Inhalation and gargling – Recipe 4 for inhalation which contains orange peel, lemon peel and vinegar and recipe 1 for gargling which contains salt, chamomile and honey.
- Continue with the same sequence as of day-1 after getting up in the morning for above mentioned recipes. But on day 4 there will be less pain, so you need to change the exercise protocol.

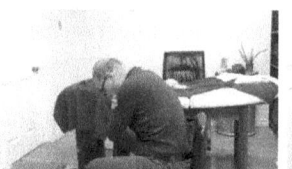 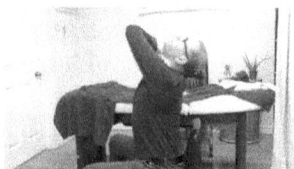

- Sit with your hands cross on shoulder. Maintain the position and extend your back. Repeat it for 5 times.
- If this position worsens your symptoms – STOP, we don't want to aggravate the condition. But continue other exercises as before.

Day 5:
- You will feel improvement in your symptoms. The recipes for scrubs, juices, salads, soups, herbal oils, herbal pastes, foot soaks, body soaks, inhalation and gargling will be different for each day.
- Here are the recipes for day 5:
    - Scrubs – Recipe 4 (coffee scrub) and recipe 5 (Brown sugar peeler). Chapter 12. Followed by scrub do the hot shower and end with cold shower for 2 minutes.

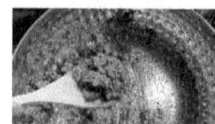 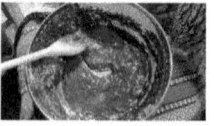

A 24-HOUR HOME REMEDY GUIDE TO YOUR BACK PAIN

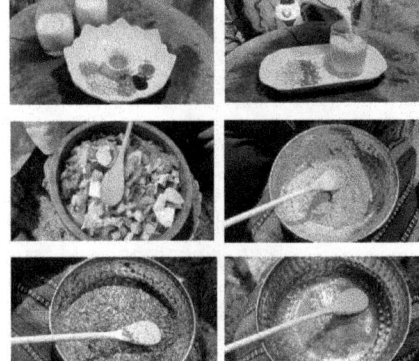

- Juices – Lemon grass or sage tea. Use recipe 5(Milk cocktail with chia seeds and flax seeds).
- Salads and soups – Use recipe 5 (Greek green salad) and (lentil soup).
- Herbal oils – Use recipe 9 which contains ground ginger, fenugreek, bay leaf, wild thyme, olive oil and recipe 10 which contains apple cider vinegar, salt, turmeric, garlic powder and olive oil.
- Herbal paste – Use recipe 1.
- Foot soak – Recipe 1.
- Body soak – Recipe 5.
- Inhalation and gargling – Recipe 1 for inhalation which contains vinegar, rosemary, thyme, and recipe 2 for gargling.

- Continue with the same sequence as of day-1 after getting up in the morning for above mentioned recipes. But on day 5 there will be less pain, so you need to change the exercise protocol.

- Sit erect with your hands crossed on shoulder. Rotate your body to one side and repeat it for 5-10 times. If you are comfortable with one side, you can repeat the same exercise on the other side. Make sure you breath in and breathe out. Repeat for 10 times. While doing this you need to only feel a stretch pain in back. There should be no radiating pain.

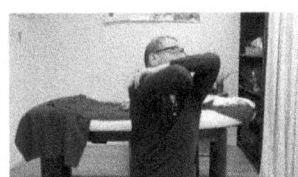 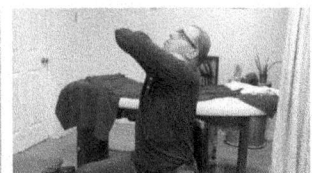

- Repeat the movement on each side with back extension for 10 times.

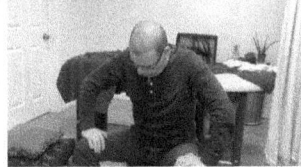 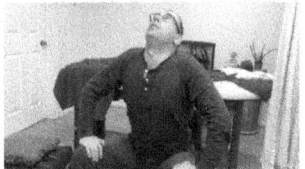

Day 6:

- You will feel improvement in your symptoms. The recipes for scrubs, juices, salads, soups, herbal oils, herbal pastes, foot soaks, body soaks, inhalation and gargling will be different for each day.

- Here are the recipes for day 6:
    - Scrubs – Recipe 1 (Yogurt scrub) and recipe 2 (Turmeric scrub). Followed by scrub do the hot shower and end with cold shower for 2 minutes.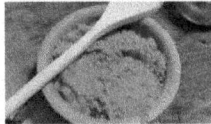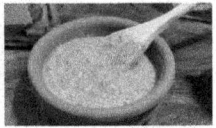

- Juices – Rose Mary and rooibos tea. Use recipe 1(Green Juice).
- Salads and soups – Use recipe 6 for salad (Fruit bowl salad) and recipe 1 (bone broth) for soup.
- Herbal oils – Use recipe 11 which contains wheat bran, cinnamon, wild thyme, olive oil and recipe 1 which contains black pepper, turmeric, lemon peel, salt and olive oil.
- Herbal paste – Use recipe 2.
- Foot soak – Recipe 2.
- Body soak – Recipe 1.
- Inhalation and gargling – Recipe 2 for inhalation which contains lavender, chamomile, lemon oil and recipe 3 for gargling.

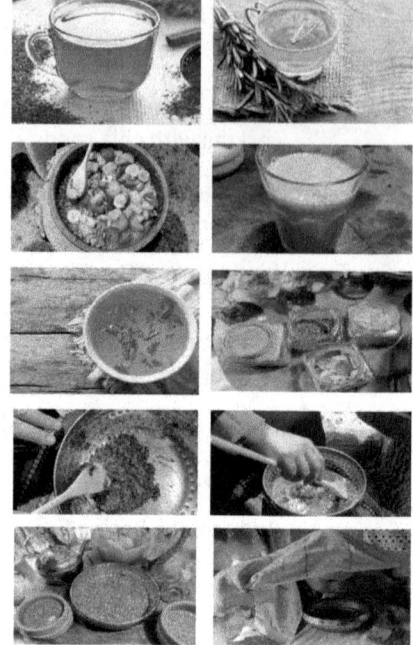

- Continue with the same sequence as of day-1 after getting up in the morning for above mentioned recipes. But on day 6 there will be a sequence of exercise you will need to follow.
- Start with back extensions (20 times), followed by supine back extension (10 times), sitting back extensions (10 times) and rotations (10 times) on each side.
- Repeat the sequence throughout the day.

Day 7:
- At this day you will feel 80-90% of relief in your symptoms.
- Here are the recipes for day 6:
    - Scrubs – Recipe 3 (Lemon sugar) and recipe 4 (coffee scrub). Followed by scrub do the hot shower and end with cold shower for 2 minutes.
    - Juices – Peppermint or olive leaves tea. Use recipe 2 (Hot Juice).
    - Salads and soups – Use recipe 1 (Red beans salad) for salad and recipe 2 (mushroom soup) for soup.
    - Herbal oils – Use recipe 2 which contains olive leaves, wild thyme, olive oil and recipe 3 which contains hot pepper, green tea, sesame seeds, salt and olive oil.

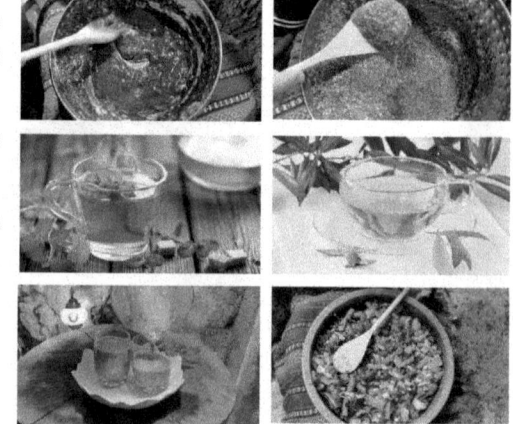

- Herbal paste – Use recipe 3.
- Foot soak – Recipe 3.
- Body soak – Recipe 2.
- Inhalation and gargling – Recipe 3 for inhalation which contains water, camphor and recipe 1 for gargling. Details are given in chapter

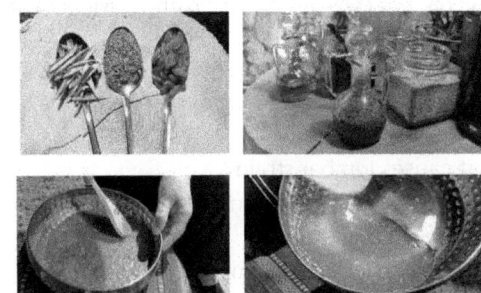

- For exercise, repeat the same sequence of exercise as of day 6. Increase the repetitions for each exercise. The disc goes inside and decreases the compression.

After this 7-day protocol there will be relieve in your symptoms.

If the pain is manageable after 7 days start with the stretching and strengthening techniques for thoracic pain. The details are already described in chapters above.

If the pain persists, consult your doctor as you may have any another underlying condition.

CHAPTER 25: LOW BACK PAIN DUE TO MUSCLE STRAIN

A lumbar strain is an injury to the lower back. This results in damaged tendons and muscles that can go in spasm and feel sore. The lumbar vertebra makes up the section of the spine in your lower back.

What causes lumbar strain?
- Heavy lifting, twisting the spine, lifting from the ground, or an item overhead are common causes of low back strain
- Sudden impact from a car accident or a fall is another common contributor to back muscle strain
- Impact from jarring motions can place heavy, immediate stress on the low back muscles. For example, high-impact sports such as football and lacrosse place excessive pressure on joints and muscles.
- It may be due to deconditioned, stiff muscles
- Stressful, repeated motions can cause muscles to tighten or tear
- Sports such as rowing, golf, or baseball may cause chronic strain due to repeated, forceful motions
- Chronic strain may gradually become painful over time, or pain can suddenly worsen if a muscle is already sore and then put under intense stress.
- It may be due to low back and core abdominal muscles are weak, the lower back becomes more susceptible to injury.
- Symptoms
- pain in the lumbar muscles or nonspecific pain
- pain could be exacerbated during standing and twisting motions, with active contractions and passive stretching of the involved muscle increasing the pain
- point tenderness, muscle spasm, possible swelling in and around the involved musculature, a possible lateral deviation in the spine with severe spasm and a decreased range of motion

Step 1: Before starting activity, you can use the back scrub to reduce the stress of on your lower back and surrounding muscles, which will increase the blood circulation of that part and soothes your skin. It also helps in relieving tension. You can use recipe from chapter scrubs and peeling recipes under the section for lower back.

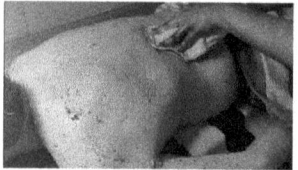 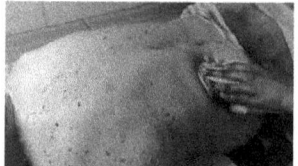

Step 2: After this, take a sip of hot herbal teas and caffeinated drinks. This will help reduce the effect of back pain. You can get the options for herbal teas in the chapter Herbal teas for relaxation. While doing your daily activities make sure you support your lower back with a brace or wrap a towel around it. This will limit the movements and promote healing of structures fast.

Step 3: After this, relax yourself in the way you are comfortable and then use the cold compression to reduce the stiffness and pain of muscles. As this is an acute condition always choose cold compress. It can be applied directly to the lower back area for 10-15 minutes. Repeat the application of cold therapy 3-4 times a day. Details of application are described in the chapters for Heat and Cold therapy.

Step 4: Once your pain is subsided, start gentle lower back stretches and mobility exercises, which will help improve your range of motion of back and will also make the back muscles more flexible. Stiffness will be gradually released. Stretches which work best for back pain are hamstring stretch, calf stretch, Figure of four stretch, side stretch in standing and sitting. The procedure and other details have already been described in the chapter for General stretching.

A 24-HOUR HOME REMEDY GUIDE TO YOUR BACK PAIN

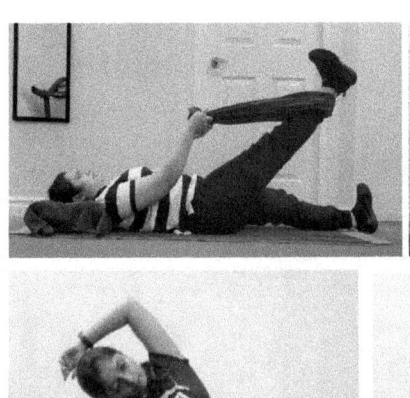
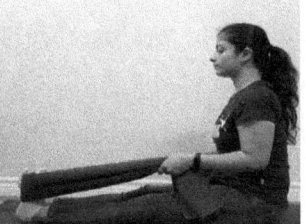

You must feel a slight pull on the tight muscle. It will pain initially, but don't panic. Gradually when the muscle loosens up it will feel better. When you do the movements make sure you don't pull your legs more as it can aggravate the symptom.

Mobility exercises useful in this condition are knee to chest, cat and camel pose, side-rotations in sitting, Lumbar rotation in lying and back extension on elbows.

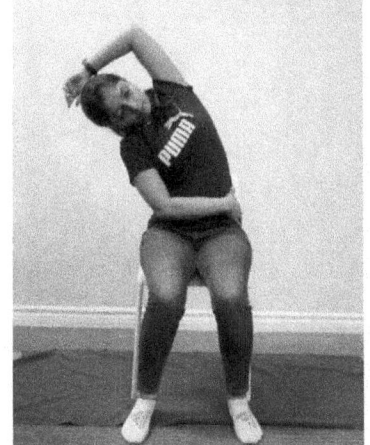
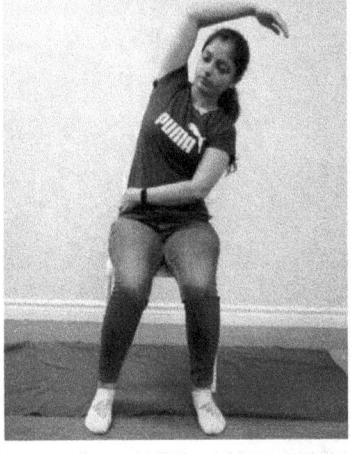
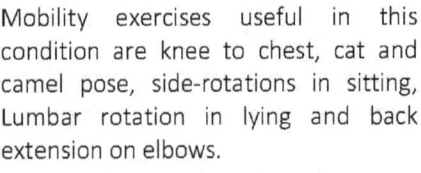
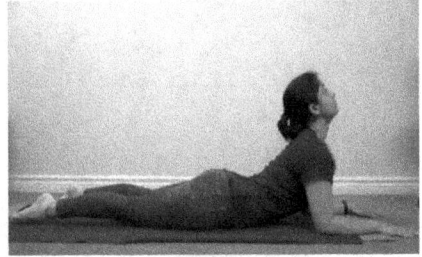
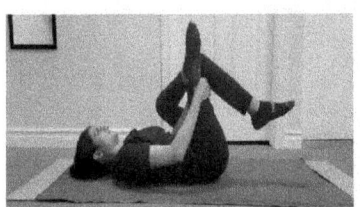
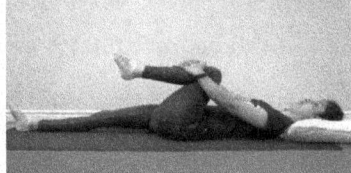
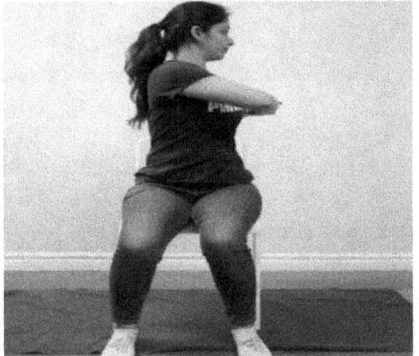
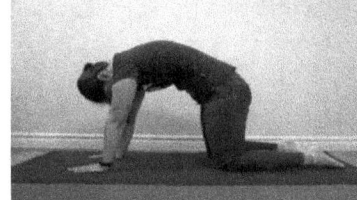
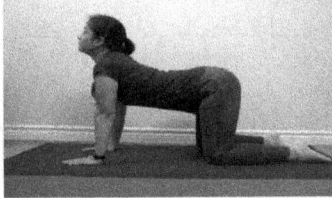
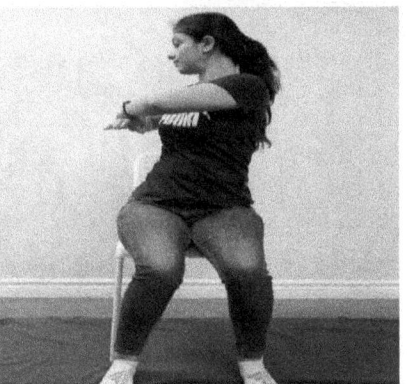
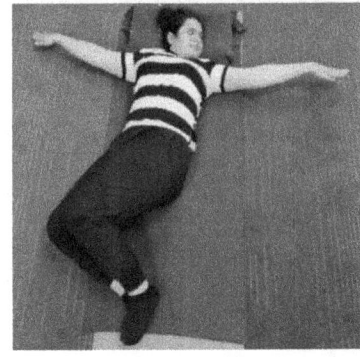
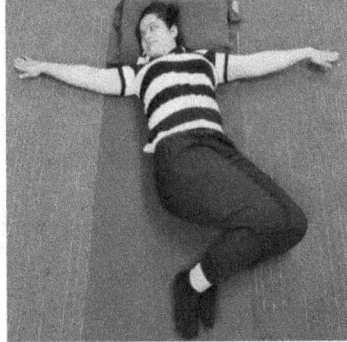

Step 5: Once you are relaxed, release your stiffness with massage. This works best with infused herbal oil recipes.

The recipe which works best for back pain are given in chapter Herbs and herb infused oil under the section recipes for acute lower back. Use different recipes each day so that you get more benefits.

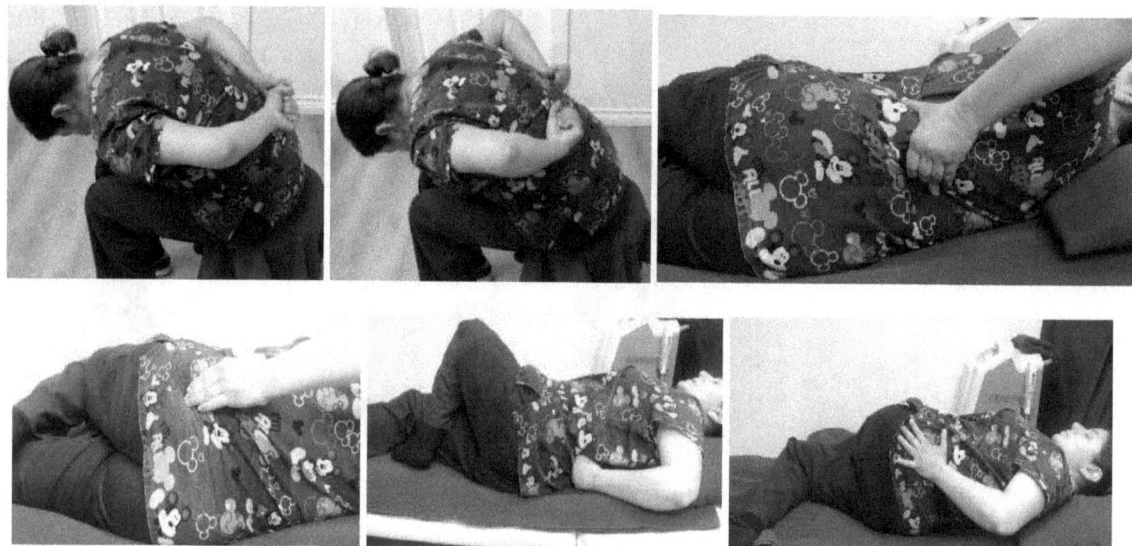

Step 6: Once your symptoms are relieved to 50%, start with the strengthening exercises. As poor back posture causes muscle weakness and leads to imbalance of muscles.

Once you start with exercises you will feel discomfort in the muscles, but don't worry that is just because we are strengthening the weak muscles. Gradually this discomfort goes away.

Exercises suitable for this condition are, Adductor squeeze, buttock squeeze, pelvic tilting, supine straight leg raise, side straight leg raise, modified plank. For the exercises you need to refer chapte General Strengthening exercise.

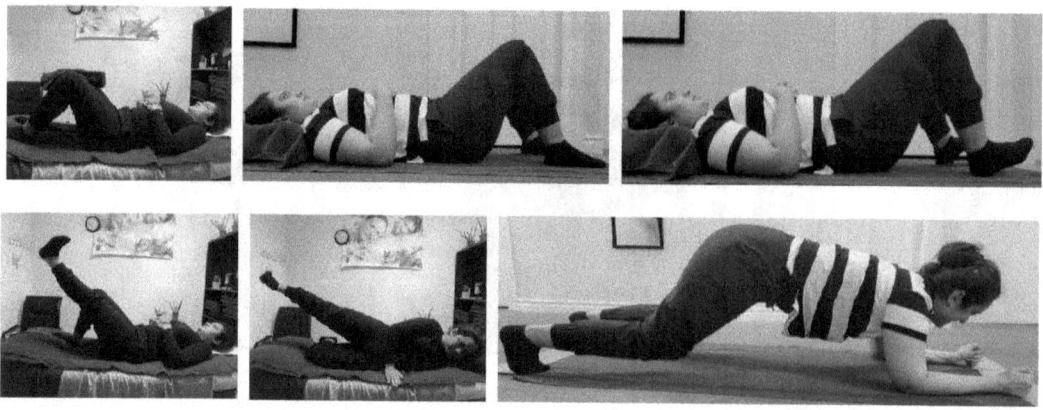

Step 7: Take a balanced diet which should include food rich in vitamins, omega 3, and magnesium in your diet. Green leafy vegetables like spinach, kale, swish charred, collard greens can be consumed. The recipes which is useful are described in chapter Nutritional facts and benefits of balanced diet. There are different sections including recipes for soups, salads, and juices which you can include at least one in your daily diet.

Step 8: You can use homemade pastes on your back to relieve the severe pain. These patches work on relieving stress and reduces the inflammation. The details and application are given in chapter Herbal poultices (paste) recipes under the section lower back.

Step 9: Use proper resting position and make sure your back is in a relaxed position. These positions are used while resting or when you have applied the patches or doing any activity.

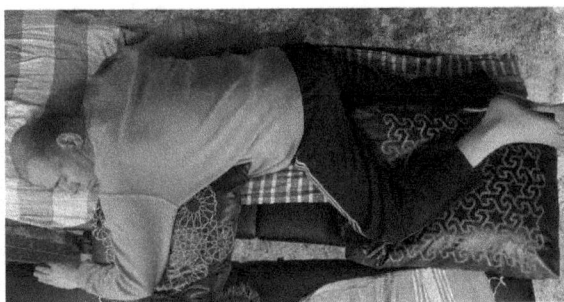 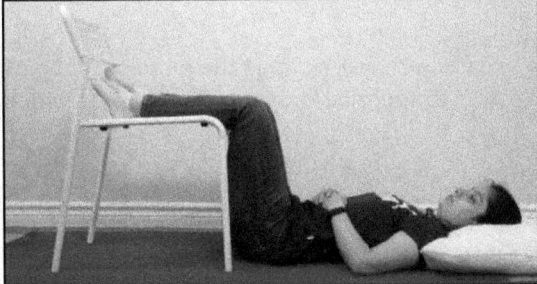

Step 10: At the end of the day, indulge yourself in foot soak and body soak with herbs. This will relax your body senses and rejuvenate it. The recipes and application are already described in chapter Body and foot soak recipes for relaxation.

Step 11: Also, do the inhalation therapy which will help reduce the stress induced by the pain. Before going to bed make sure you apply oil to your lower back and wrap it with a linen cloth. This fastens the process of tissue healing and pain relief.

CHAPTER 26: LOWER BACK PAIN BY DISK HERNIATION

Disk herniation in lower back is due to bulging of disc outside and compressing your nerve. It also narrows the spinal canal. Symptoms usually over a long period of time

- Do you feel stiffness, pain, numbness, or weakness in legs?
- Did you have trouble controlling yourself for urination or difficulty in your bowel control?

If you answered yes to any of these questions, there's a high rate you are having a disk herniation. If you feel pain sitting for prolong time or any bending activity, this confirms your diagnosis for disk herniation. We will show you the exercises to follow, the positions while doing activity, resting positions, herbal recipe tips and nutritional tips. The purpose here is to align your bones and disc which is pressing your nerves. Here is 7-day protocol to follow which will help reduce your symptoms.

Day 1:
- Starts with waking up in the morning and moving out of the bed in correct position. Make sure you turn to your side and push your body up with head straight.

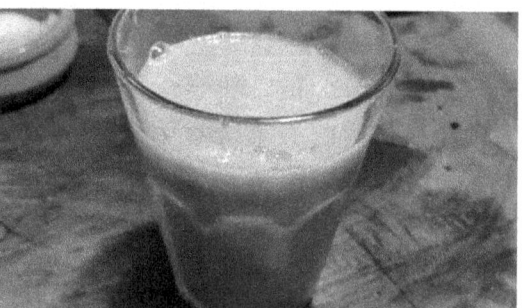
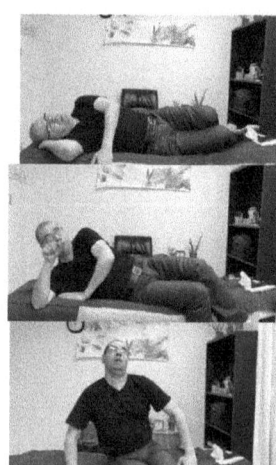
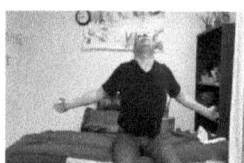

- After that, go to the washroom and do scrubbing to your lower back. This will help in relieving pain and stiffness which is more intense in the morning. Body scrub which works best is recipe 1 (yogurt scrub) and recipe 2 (Turmeric scrub). The details of recipe preparation and application are already described in the chapter 12 for body scrub.

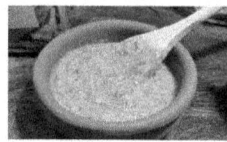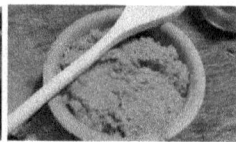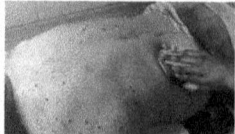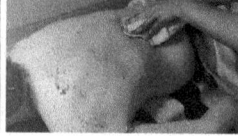

- Once you are done with scrubbing, take hot beverages as normal. Also, add the special juices to your drink. Try recipe 1 (Green Juice). The details of recipe preparation and application are already described in the chapter for nutritional facts.

- Don't forget to keep yourself hydrated the whole day. Drink at least 8 cups of water to help your body stay fresh.

- You can continue with your breakfast after beverages. Add a healthy salad and soup to your meal. The recipe 1 (Red beans) for salad and recipe 1 (Bone broth) for soup will work best. While eating if you are in sitting position make sure you are supported or seated upright.

- After that, the first movement you need to do is to relax your spine. There are 2 positions you can do which are mentioned below. You can be in this position for about 30 minutes.

    Position 1: Lie down with a pillow under your tummy and head relaxed to the side.

    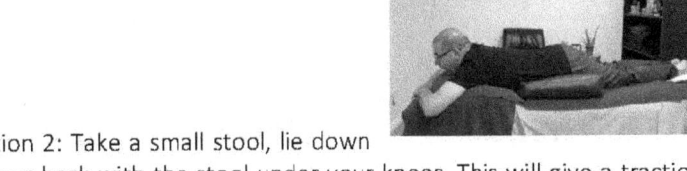

    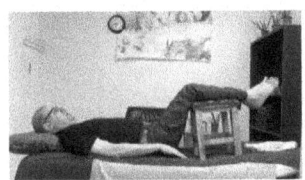 Position 2: Take a small stool, lie down on your back with the stool under your knees. This will give a traction feeling to the spine.

- Once you feel relaxed, you need to massage your lower back in resting position 1 described above. Use recipe 1 which contains sage, thyme, mint and chia seeds and recipe 2 which contains turmeric, basil, garden cress seeds and mint from chronic lower back pain section. The details for recipes and application are already described in chapter (herbs and herbs infused oils). This will help remove the stiffness so we can adjust the spine in a proper way.

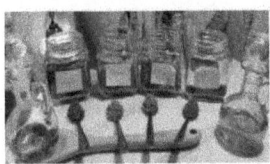 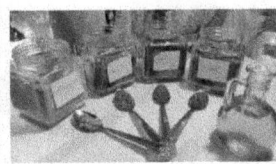 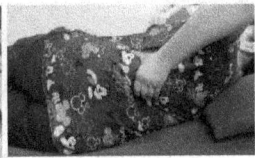 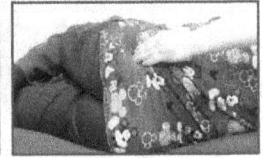

- After massage, you will feel more relaxed. Start with day-1 exercise protocol. To do the exercise, you need to lie down on your tummy with elbows bend and hands rested properly. Push up your body in this position slowly, hold and relax.

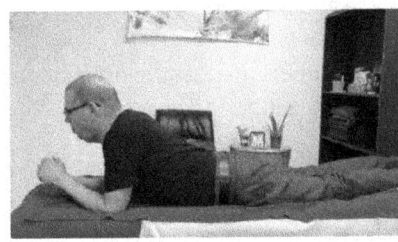 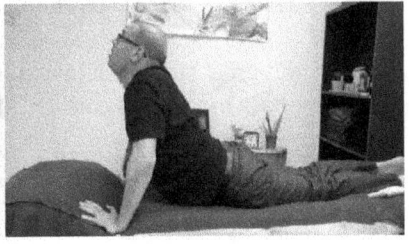

- Also, you can put your hands a bit forward which will help you to push upwards. This movement helps to put disc down in its position and reduce pain.

- Make sure you only do up to your available range. Of course, you will not achieve the full range right away. You need to feel pain coming up from your legs to the back – this is a sign of IMPROVEMENT.

- Repeat the exercise for 5 times. Take a break and again repeat it for 5 times. Make sure you do it in a correct manner. The hips must be in contact with the bed while you extend your back. Do this movement throughout the day. If you feel pressure or tension in your lower back – that's NORMAL.

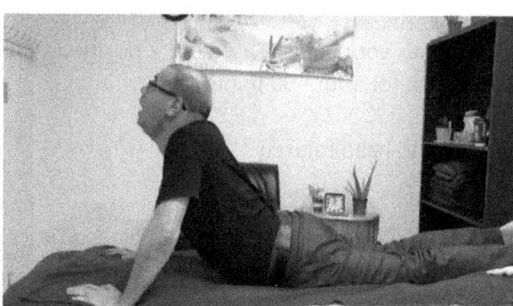 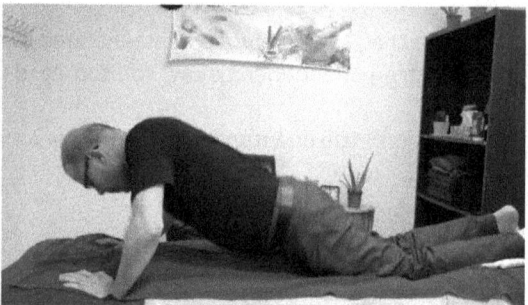

- Also, to relieve stiffness use hot or cold compress while doing this movement. Use only ice if you feel there is swelling, redness or severity in your symptoms. Ice can be used for 15-20 minutes every hour. But if your symptoms are manageable with no swelling or redness always use the heat.

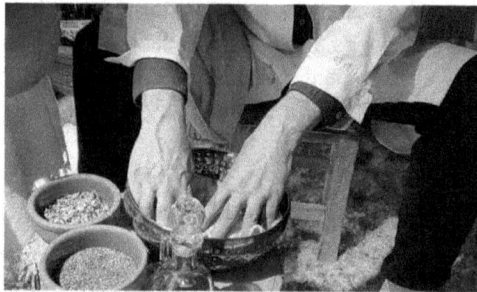 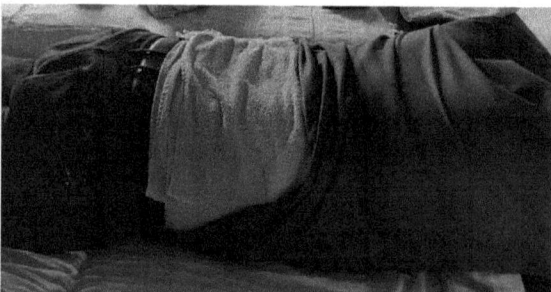

- After certain repetitions, you will feel the pain going in intensity and coming up from legs to back – **"GOOD SYMPTOMS"**.

- Use herbal paste recipe 1 which contains ginger, cloves, cinnamon, and vinegar on your lower back. Keep the paste on your back for about 15-20 minutes. This will help reduce the stiffness. The detail for recipe is already described in chapter (Herbal paste and poultices).

- While working always seat straight or take the back support. Repeat the exercises again. Once you are good extend your back in standing position. This position is good to align your spine.

- Continue this exercise protocol even though you feel pain or discomfort. You may feel more stiffness or muscle pain the next day but that is okay!

- In the evening if you feel pain in your legs do the foot soaking method. This helps relieve tension. Use recipe 1.

- Use inhalation method for relaxation. This will help relieving the stress and help in pain relief. Followed by inhalation do the gargling. Use Inhalation recipe 1 which contains vinegar, rosemary, thyme and gargling also recipe 1 which contains salt, chamomile and honey.

- Also do the body soaking for relaxation. Use recipe 1 for body soak. The ideal position to soak your body is lying down on your tummy. Try doing some back extensions while body soak. This will give best results. If you are not comfortable lying on your tummy, lie flat on your back. Don't do body soaking in sitting – "not recommended".

- Before going to bed, apply herbal oil and leave it overnight. Cover the body area with thin linen this will help absorption of oil better.

Day 2:

- Next day you may feel more discomfort and muscle pain. Don't worry continue with the same sequence as above. The recipes for scrubs, juices, salads, soups, herbal oils, herbal pastes, foot soaks, body soaks, inhalation and gargling will be different for each day.

- Here are the recipes for day 2:
    - Scrubs – use recipe 3 (Lemon sugar) and recipe 4 (Coffee scrub). Followed by scrub do the hot shower and end with cold shower for 2 minutes
    - Juices – Use recipe 2 (Hot Juice).
    - Salads and soups – Use recipe 2 (Tuna salad) and (mushroom soup).
    - Herbal oils – Use recipe 3 which contains lemon peel, chicory and fennel seeds and recipe 4 which contains honey, basil, turmeric, and white vinegar.
    - Herbal paste – Use recipe 2 which contains camphor, black seed, thyme, lavender, mint, basil, honey and oatmeal.
    - Foot soak – Recipe 2.
    - Body soak – Recipe 2.
    - Inhalation and gargling – Recipe 2 for inhalation which contains lavender, chamomile, lemon oil and recipe 2 for gargling which contains mint, green tea, sage and salt.

- Continue with the same sequence after getting up in the morning for above mentioned recipes. But on day 2 if you feel there is no improvement in symptoms you need to change the exercise pattern.

- Lie down on your tummy. You need to shift your hip to the opposite side of the pain and then extend your back. For e.g.: If you have pain down to left side, shift your hip to the right and extend your back. If this helps, continue with same movement for 10 times.

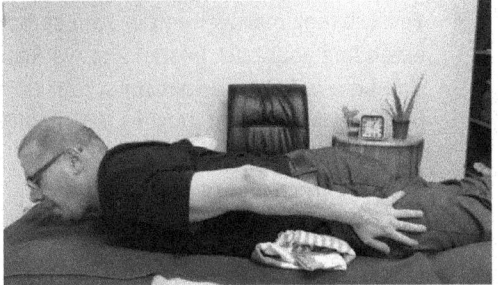

- Even if you don't feel any improvement with the above position put a towel roll under the hip on opposite side and do the back extensions. Continue the movements if the symptoms are reduced.

- But, if still the symptoms persist, put the towel roll on the other side and do back extensions. Repeat the movement for 10 times.

Day 3:

- You will feel improvement in your symptoms. There might be no pain or less pain radiating to your legs, or the pain will be only present on your back. The recipes for scrubs, juices, salads, soups, herbal oils, herbal pastes, foot soaks, body soaks, inhalation and gargling will be different for each day.

- Here are the recipes for day 3:
    - Scrubs – Recipe 1 (yogurt scrub) and recipe 5 (Brown sugar peeler). Followed by scrub do the hot shower and end with cold shower for 2 minutes.
    - Juices – Use recipe 3 (Vitamin C Juice).
    - Salads and soups – Use recipe 3(potato and herbs salad) and (meat curry soup).
    - Herbal oils – Use recipe 5 which contains violet, juniper, linden and oats and recipe 6 which contains milk powder, fenugreek, thyme, marjoram.
    - Herbal paste – Use recipe 3 which contains wheat flour, ginger, fenugreek and chia seeds.
    - Foot soak – Recipe 3.
    - Body soak – Recipe 3.
    - Inhalation and gargling – Recipe 3 for inhalation which contains water, camphor. Recipe 3 for gargling which contains salt and water.

- Continue with the same sequence as of day-1 after getting up in the morning for above mentioned recipes. But on day 3 there will be less pain, so you need to change the exercise protocol.

- Lie down on your tummy and wrap a towel around your lower back with holding the edges of towel in your hand. Extend your back while keep holding the towel. This will adjust your spine. The pain is reduced but we need more pressure to fix the herniation. Repeat the exercise for 10 times.

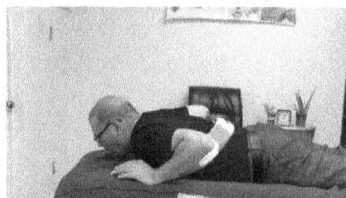 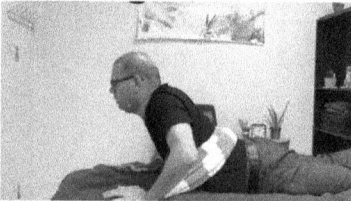 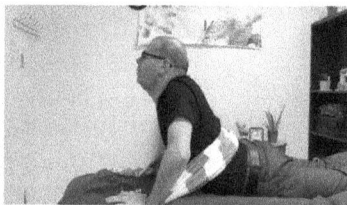

- Also, exercise in standing with same. A back support brace is recommended while you do any vigorous activities. If you don't have any wrap a towel around your lower back.

Day 4:

- You will feel improvement in your symptoms and comfortable in extending your back in standing we need to try shifting hips and side bending. The recipes for scrubs, juices, salads, soups, herbal oils, herbal pastes, foot soaks, body soaks, inhalation and gargling will be different for each day.

- Here are the recipes for day 4:
    - Scrubs – Recipe 2 (Turmeric scrub) and recipe 3 (Lemon sugar). Followed by scrub do the hot shower and end with cold shower for 2 minutes.
    - Juices – Use recipe 4 (Pumpkin Juice).
    - Salads and soups – Use recipe 4 (Wheat and greens salad) and (wheat soup).
    - Herbal oils – Use recipe 7 which contains turmeric, thyme and cumin and recipe 8 which contains cress seeds, turmeric, sesame and pepper cone.

    - Herbal paste – Use recipe 4 which contains garlic, aloe vera, cloves and honey.

-
    - Foot soak – Recipe 4.
    - Body soak – Recipe 4.
    - Inhalation and gargling – Recipe 4 for inhalation which contains orange peel, lemon peel and vinegar and recipe 1 for gargling which contains salt, chamomile, and honey.

- Continue with the same sequence as of day-1 after getting up in the morning for above mentioned recipes. But on day 4 there will be less pain, so you need to change the exercise protocol.

- Stand with hands supported at lower back. Shift your hip to the painful side and bend. Repeat it for 5 times.

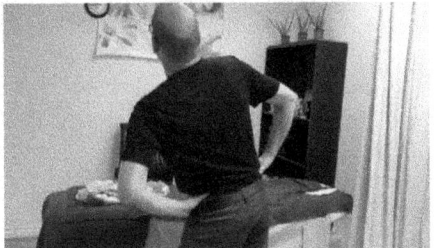

- Once you are comfortable with bending combine back extension with bending. If this position worsens your symptoms – STOP, we don't want to aggravate the condition. But continue other exercises as before.

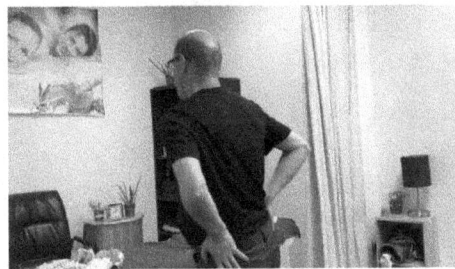 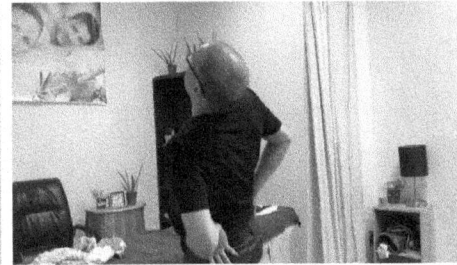

Day 5:
- You will feel improvement in your symptoms. The recipes for scrubs, juices, salads, soups, herbal oils, herbal pastes, foot soaks, body soaks, inhalation and gargling will be different for each day.

- Here are the recipes for day 5:
    - Scrubs – Recipe 4 (coffee scrub) and recipe 5 (Brown sugar peeler). Followed by scrub do the hot shower and end with cold shower for 2 minutes.
    - Juices – Use recipe 5 (Milk cocktail with chia seeds and flax seeds).
    - Salads and soups – Use recipe 5 (Greek green salad) and (lentil soup).
    - Herbal oils – Use recipe 9 which contains milk powder, camphor, wheat flour, cumin and mint and recipe 10 which contains cloves and olive oil.
    - Herbal paste – Use recipe 1.
    - Foot soak – Recipe 1.
    - Body soak – Recipe 5.
    - Inhalation and gargling – Recipe 1 for inhalation which contains vinegar, rosemary, thyme and recipe 2 for gargling.

- Continue with the same sequence as of day-1 after getting up in the morning for above mentioned recipes. But on day 5 there will be less pain, so you need to change the exercise protocol.

- Repeat back extension for 10 times. After that, lie on your back and slowly take your knees to the chest. While doing this you need to only feel a stretch pain in back. There should be no radiating pain.

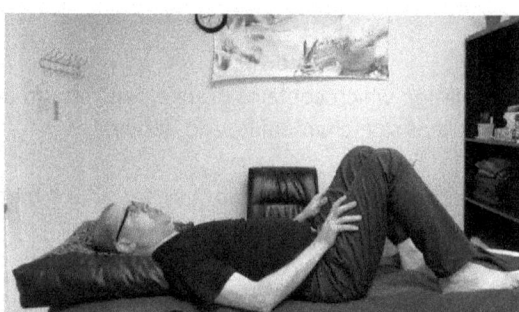 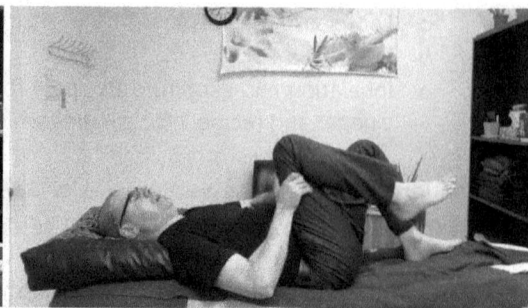

- Repeat the movement on each side for 10 times. Also, continue with the back extensions in standing. You can increase the intensity of exercise by pulling both knees to the chest.

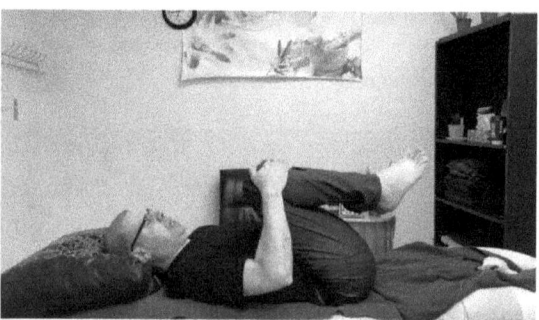

Day 6:

- You will feel improvement in your symptoms. The recipes for scrubs, juices, salads, soups, herbal oils, herbal pastes, foot soaks, body soaks, inhalation and gargling will be different for each day.

- Here are the recipes for day 6:
    - Scrubs – Recipe 1 (Yogurt scrub) and recipe 2 (Turmeric scrub). Followed by scrub do the hot shower and end with cold shower for 2 minutes.
    - Juices – Use recipe 1(Green Juice).
    - Salads and soups – Use recipe 6 for salad (Fruit bowl salad) and recipe 1 (bone broth) for soup.
    - Herbal oils – Use recipe 11 which contains levandor, camphor, coconut, peppercone, mint and olive oil and recipe 12 which contains salt, peppercone, black seeds, sesame and thyme.
    - Herbal paste – Use recipe 2.
    - Foot soak – Recipe 2.
    - Body soak – Recipe 1.
    - Inhalation and gargling – Recipe 2 for inhalation which contains lavender, chamomile, lemon oil and recipe 3 for gargling.

- Continue with the same sequence as of day-1 after getting up in the morning for above mentioned recipes. But on day 6 there will be a sequence of exercise you will need to follow.

- Start with back extensions (20 times), followed by supine knee to chest (10 times) on both sides and at last leg rotations while lying on back (10 times) on each side.

- Repeat the sequence throughout the day.

Day 7:

- At this day you will feel 80-90% of relief in your symptoms.
- Here are the recipes for day 6:
    - Scrubs – Recipe 3 (Lemon sugar) and recipe 4 (coffee scrub). Followed by scrub do the hot shower and end with cold shower for 2 minutes.
    - Juices – Use recipe 2 (Hot Juice).
    - Salads and soups – Use recipe 1 (Red beans salad) for salad and recipe 2 (mushroom soup) for soup.
    - Herbal oils – Use recipe 1 which contains sage, thyme, mint and chia seeds and recipe 2 which contains turmeric, basil, garden cress seeds.
    - Herbal paste – Use recipe 3.
    - Foot soak – Recipe 3.
    - Body soak – Recipe 2.
    - Inhalation and gargling – Recipe 3 for inhalation which contains water, camphor and recipe 1 for gargling.

- For exercise, repeat the same sequence of exercise as of day 6. Increase the repetitions for each exercise. The disc goes inside and decreases the compression.

After this 7-day protocol there will be relieve in your symptoms.

If the pain is manageable after 7 days start with the stretching and strengthening techniques for lower back pain. The details are already described in chapters above.

If the pain persists, consult your doctor as you may have any another underlying condition.

CHAPTER 27: LOW BACK PAIN DUE TO LUMBAR STENOSIS

Spinal stenosis is the narrowing of the spinal canal in the neck. Symptoms usually cause over a long period of time.
- Is there any aching pain in legs while you walk?
- Do you have stiff back which gradually getting worse as the day passes?
- Do you feel weakness in your back or legs?

If you answered yes to these questions, there's a high rate that your spinal canal is getting narrow and is compressing your spinal cord. This condition is known as Lumbar Stenosis. It can be because of many reasons like herniated disc, posture, injury, or tumor. The purpose here is to align your bones and disc which is pressing your spinal cord. Here is a 24-hour guide to your pain which will open up the spinal canal and ease the symptoms of stenosis.

Step 1: Starts with waking up in the morning and scrubbing your stiff back. This will help in relieving pain and stiffness and prevent your back from getting more worse throughout the day. Body scrub which works best is recipe 1 (yogurt scrub) and recipe 2 (Turmeric scrub). The details of recipe preparation and application are already described in the for body scrub.

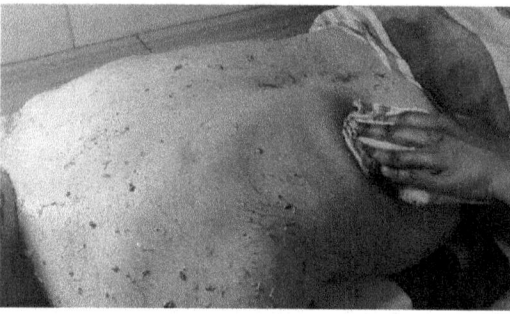
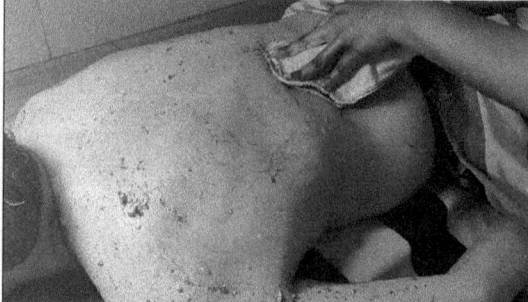

Step 2: Once you are done with scrubbing, take hot beverages as normal. You can take the herbal teas which have tremendous benefit in healing tissues. Also, add the special juices to your drink. Try recipe 1 (Green Juice). The details of recipe preparation and application are already described in nutritional facts.

Step 3: You can continue with your breakfast after beverages. Add a healthy salad and soup to your meal. The recipe 1 (Red beans) for salad and recipe 1 (Bone broth) for soup will work best. While eating make sure you support your lower back with a brace or wrap a towel around it so that it is supported.

Step 4: After about an hour of your breakfast, the first movement you need to do is to relax your spine lying down in a comfortable position and release stiffness in back muscles with gentle massage. Always do your massage with herb-infused oils. It will give you best results.

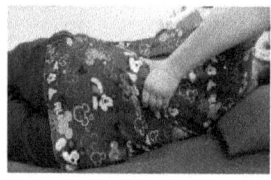
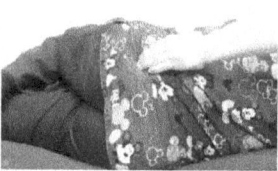
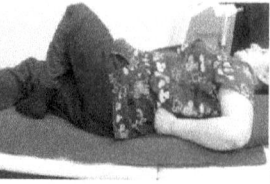
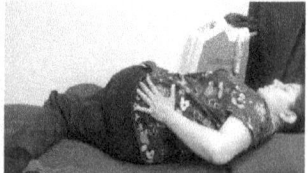

Also, you will feel pain in your lower legs and thigh. Release your stiffness in your legs also with gentle massage.

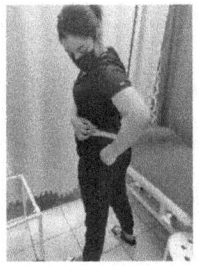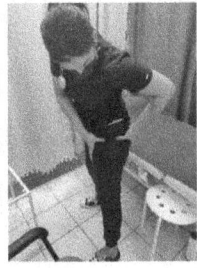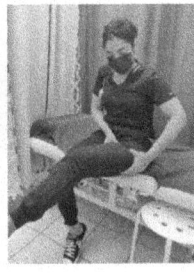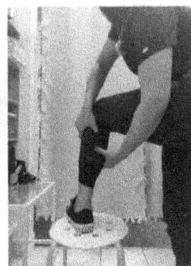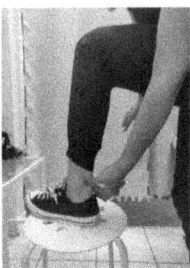

Use recipe 1 which contains sage, thyme, mint and chia seeds and recipe 2 which contains turmeric, basil, garden cress seeds and mint from chronic lower back pain section. The details for recipes and application are already described in (herbs and herbs infused oils).

Step 5: After massage, you will feel more relaxed. Start with gentle stretches in your lower back and leg muscles which will make the back muscles more flexible. Stiffness will be gradually released. Stretches which work best for this condition are hamstring stretch, calf stretch, Figure of four stretch, Child pose, forwards bending in standing, side stretch in standing and sitting.

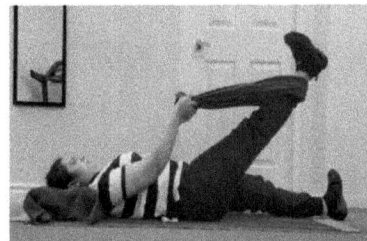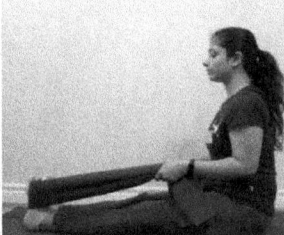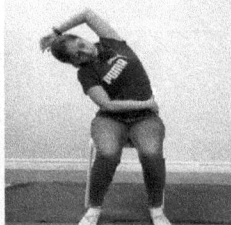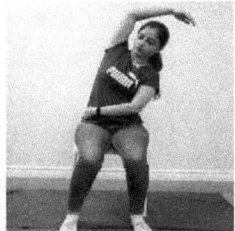

You must feel a slight pull on the tight muscle. Gradually when the muscle loosens up it will feel better. Hold each stretch for 30 seconds and repeat it for 3 times. For stretching of the legs, repeat it on both the sides. The procedure and other details have already been described in the chapter for General stretching.

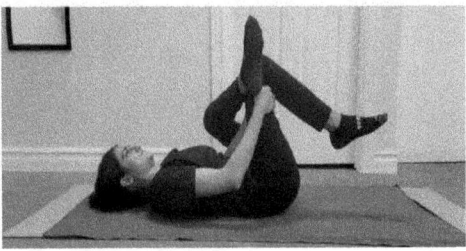

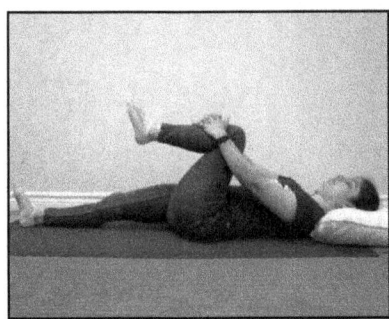

Step 6: After stretching you will feel relief in your symptoms to 50%. Start with mobility exercise to your spine and legs. This will help in alignment as well as improve the range of motion. Exercises which will be helpful in this condition are knee to chest, cat and cow, lumbar rotations in sitting as well as lying down. Initially when you start there will restrict range of motion and attempting these exercise will cause a discomfort.

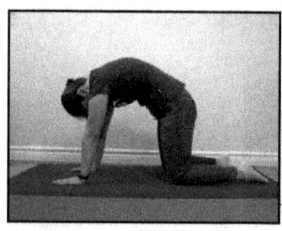 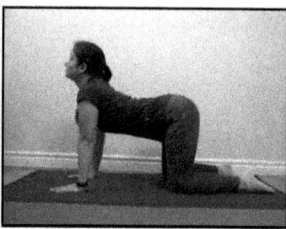 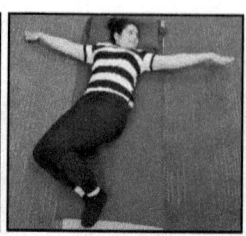 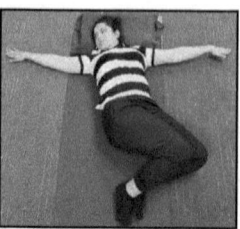

Don't stop the exercises and continue until you reach the full range. Repeat each movement for 10 times. The detail about the exercises is already described in chapter General mobility exercises.

Step 7: After this, relax yourself and use the heat or contrast compress with heat-cold compression to reduce the stiffness and pain of muscles. It can be applied directly to the lower back area for 10-15 minutes. Repeat the application of heat or contrast therapy 3-4 times a day. Details of application are described in the chapters for Heat and Cold therapy.

Step 8: Repeat only stretches and mobility exercises in initial days. Once the pain and symptoms ae subsided or manageable start with strengthening exercises As narrowing of the canal is due to weak spinal stability which resulted as a cause of weak core muscles. Exercises suitable for this condition are, Buttock squeeze, adductor squeeze, heel squeeze, Abdominal crunches, modified plank, straight leg raise, side leg raise, clam shells. For the exercises you need to refer chapter General Strengthening exercise.

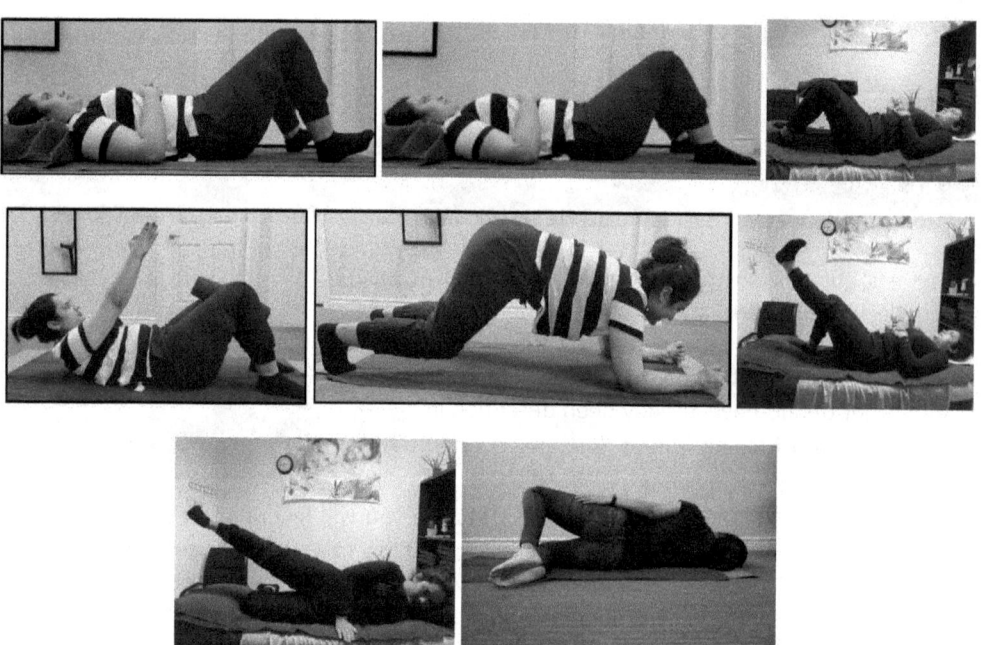

Once you start with exercises you will feel discomfort in the muscles, but don't worry that is just because we are strengthening the weak muscles. Gradually this discomfort goes away. Make sure you hold each exercise for 10 seconds and repeat it for 5-6 times initially.

Step 9: Many a time people are only prescribed with flexion-based exercises and asked to avoid extension exercises. Why? Because this position causes an increase in your spinal canal diameter, and this is thought to take pressure off spinal nerves. In addition to flexion exercises, however, people with lumbar spinal stenosis may also benefit from bending backward with an exercise called sustained standing lumbar extension. This exercise can gently press against your spinal discs, moving them away from your spinal canal and nerves to give them more room. Exercises are prone extension on elbows, standing extension and bridging.

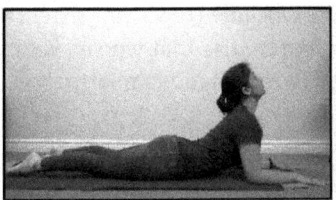 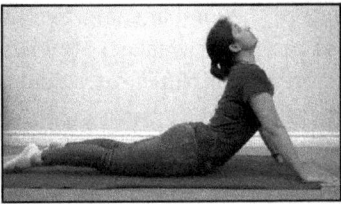 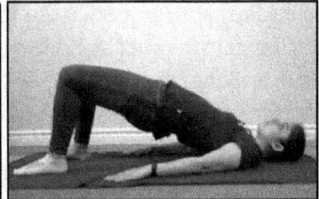

Step 10: Take a balanced diet which should include food rich in vitamins, omega 3, and magnesium in your diet. Green leafy vegetables like spinach, kale, swish charred, collard greens can be consumed. The recipes which is useful are described in chapter Nutritional facts and benefits of balanced diet. There are different sections including recipes for soups, salads and juices which you can include at least one in your daily diet.

Step 11: You can use homemade pastes on your back to relieve the severe pain. These patches work on relieving stress and reduces the inflammation. The details and application are given in chapter Herbal poultices (paste) recipes under the section lower back pain.

Step 12: Use proper resting position and make sure your back is in a relaxed position. These positions are used while resting or when you have applied the patches.

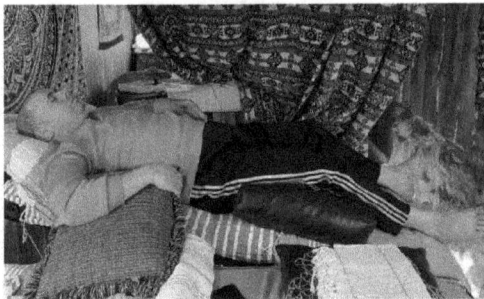 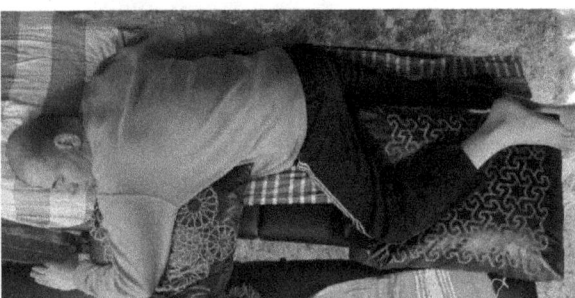

Step 13: At the end of the day, indulge yourself in foot soak and body soak with herbs. This will relax your body senses and rejuvenate it. The recipes and application are already described in chapter Body and foot soak recipes for relaxation.

Step 14: Use can also do the inhalation therapy with herbal recipes which will help reduce the stress. Before sleeping apply herbal oil to your lower back and wrap it with a linen cloth. This helps in pain relief.

TAKE AWAY MESSAGE: "If you are living with lumbar spinal stenosis, stop hoping it will just go away. Spinal stenosis is a progressive condition, but symptoms can be improved with the right exercises. It's important to do these exercises and not just use anti-inflammatory medications alone. "

CHAPTER 28: LOWER BACK PAIN BY DEGENERATIVE CHANGES

Spondylosis may be applied non-specifically to all degenerative conditions affecting the disks, vertebral bodies, and/or associated joints of the lumbar spine. Symptoms include (to varying extents) lower back pain, leg pain, as well as numbness and motor weakness to lower extremities that worsen with upright stance and walking and improve with sitting and supine positioning. Symptomatic lumbar spondylosis is approached in a stepwise fashion which include,

Here is a 24-hour guide to your pain which will reduce the stress on spine and improve muscle strength.

Step 1: Starts with waking up in the morning and scrubbing your stiff back. This will help in relieving pain and stiffness and prevent your back from getting more worse throughout the day. Body scrub which works best is recipe 1 (yogurt scrub) and recipe 2 (Turmeric scrub). The details of recipe preparation and application are already described in the chapter for body scrub.

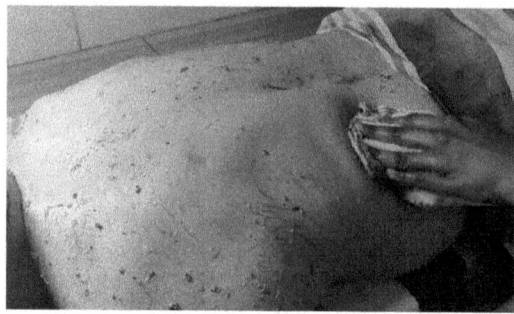
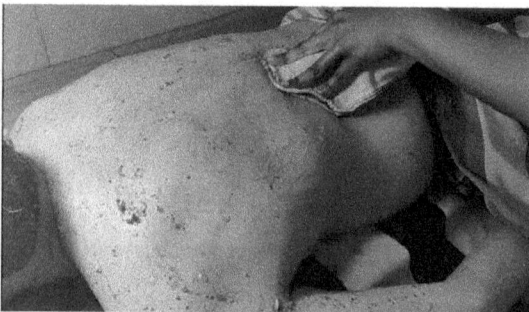

Step 2: Once you are done with scrubbing, take hot beverages as normal. You can take the herbal teas which have tremendous benefit in healing tissues. Also, add the special juices to your drink. Try recipe 1 (Green Juice). The details of recipe preparation and application are already described in the chapter 13 for nutritional facts.

Step 3: You can continue with your breakfast after beverages. Add a healthy salad and soup to your meal. The recipe 1 (Red beans) for salad and recipe 1 (Bone broth) for soup will work best. While eating make sure you support your lower back with a brace or wrap a towel around it so that it is supported.

Step 4: After about an hour of your breakfast, the first movement you need to do is to relax your spine lying down in a comfortable position and release stiffness in back muscles with gentle massage. Always do your massage with herb-infused oils. It will give you best results.

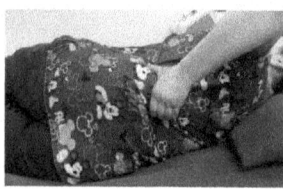
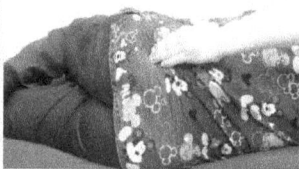
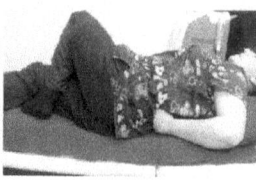
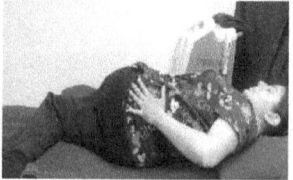

Also, you will feel pain in your lower legs and thigh because of any nerve compression. Release your stiffness in your legs also with gentle massage.

A 24-HOUR HOME REMEDY GUIDE TO YOUR BACK PAIN

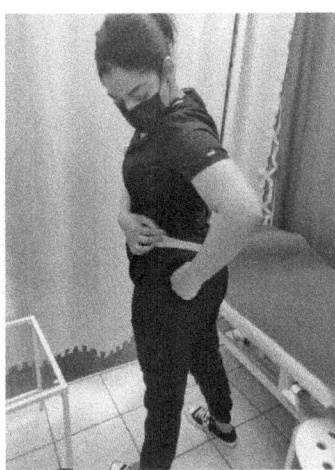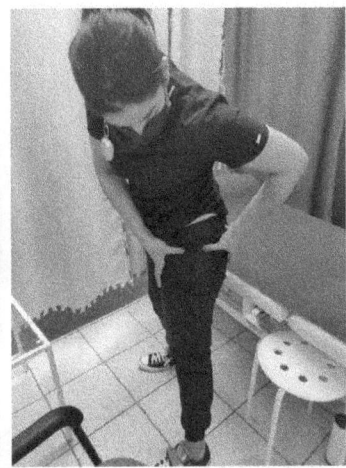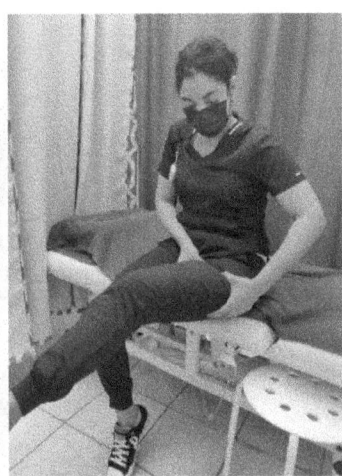

Use recipe 1 which contains sage, thyme, mint and chia seeds and recipe 2 which contains turmeric, basil, garden cress seeds and mint from chronic lower back pain section. The details for recipes and application are already described in chapter 8 (herbs and herbs infused oils).

Step 5: After massage, you will feel more relaxed. Start with gentle stretches in your lower back and leg muscles which will make the back muscles more flexible. Stiffness will be gradually released. Stretches which work best for this condition are hamstring stretch, calf stretch, Figure of four stretch, Child pose, forwards bending in standing, side stretch in standing and sitting.

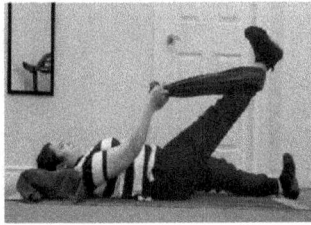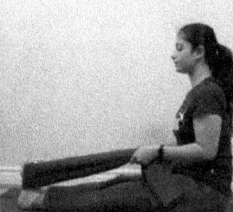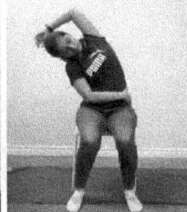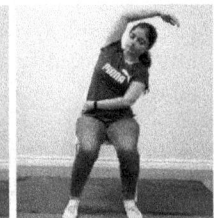

You must feel a slight pull on the tight muscle. Gradually when the muscle loosens up it will feel better. Hold each stretch for 30 seconds and repeat it for 3 times. For stretching of the legs, repeat it on both the sides. The procedure and other details have already been described in the chapter for General stretching.

Step 6: After stretching you will feel relief in your symptoms to 50%. Start with mobility exercise to your spine and legs. This will help in alignment as well as improve the range of motion. Exercises which will be helpful in this condition are knee to chest, cat and cow, lumbar rotations in sitting as well as lying down, prone extension on elbows, prone extension on hands, bridging. Initially when you start there will be restricted range of motion and attempting this exercise will cause a discomfort.

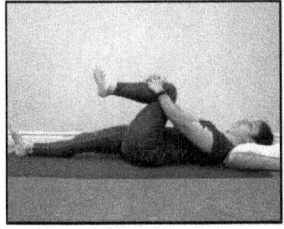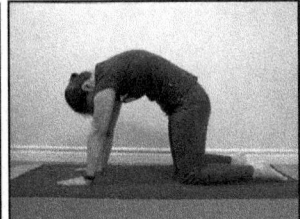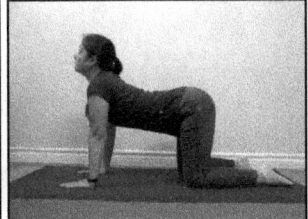

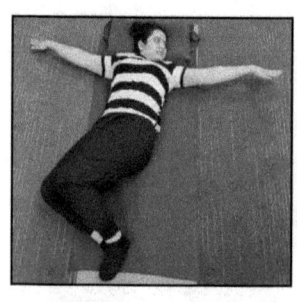 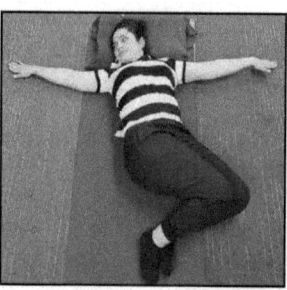 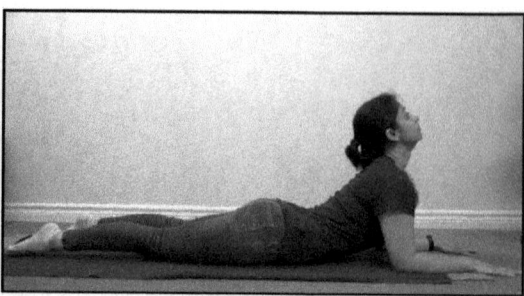

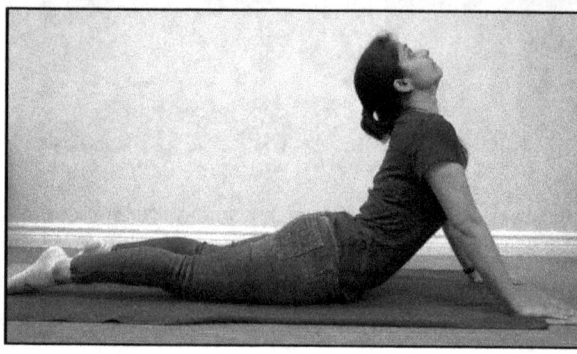 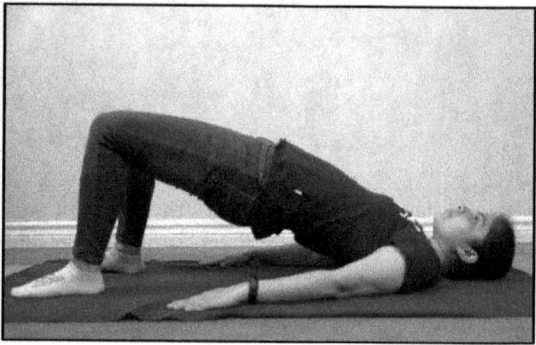

Don't stop the exercises and continue until you reach the full range. Repeat each movement for 10 times. The detail about the exercises is already described in chapter General mobility exercises.

Step 7: After this, relax yourself and use the heat or contrast compress with heat-cold compression to reduce the stiffness and pain of muscles.

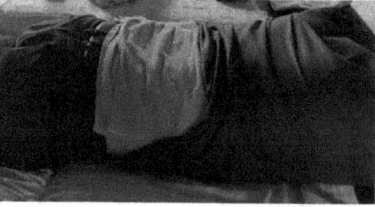

It can be applied directly to the lower back area for 10-15 minutes. Repeat the application of heat or contrast therapy 3-4 times a day. Details of application are described in the chapters for Heat and Cold therapy.

Step 8: Add on unloading exercises to the lower back. This will relive the compression forces on spine. It can be done by self-distraction exercises which are Self-lumbar traction in sitting, standing and leaning, chair unloading.

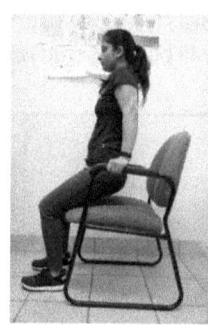 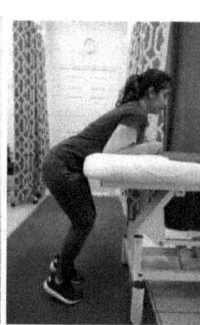 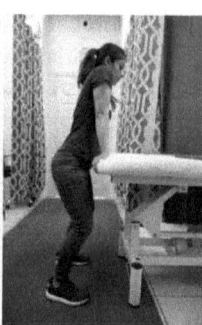 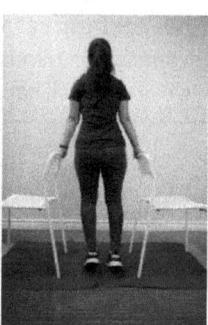

Step 9: Repeat only stretches, mobility exercises and distraction in initial days. Once the pain and symptoms ae subsided or manageable start with strengthening exercises as there is degeneration of bones and leads to instability of spine and weakness of muscles. Exercises suitable for this condition are, Buttock squeeze,

adductor squeeze, heel squeeze, Abdominal crunches, modified plank, straight leg raise, side leg raise. For the exercises you need to refer chapter General Strengthening exercise.

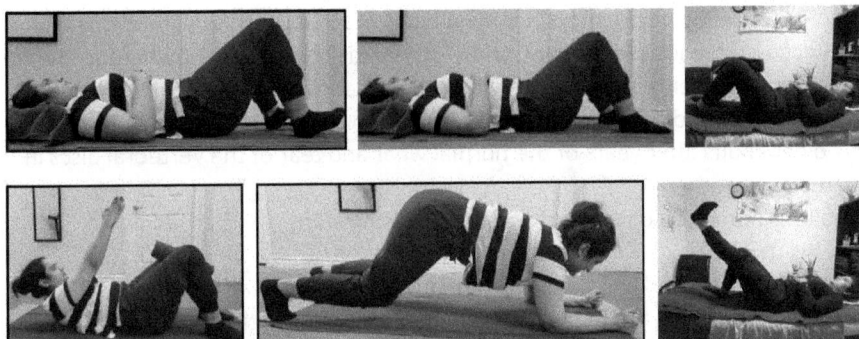

Once you start with exercises you will feel discomfort in the muscles, but don't worry that is just because we are strengthening the weak muscles. Gradually this discomfort goes away. Make sure you hold each exercise for 10 seconds and repeat it for 5-6 times initially.

Step 10: Take a balanced diet which should include food rich in vitamins, omega 3, and magnesium in your diet. Green leafy vegetables like spinach, kale, swish charred, collard greens can be consumed. The recipes which is useful are described in chapter Nutritional facts and benefits of balanced diet. There are different sections including recipes for soups, salads and juices which you can include at least one in your daily diet.

Step 11: You can use homemade pastes on your back to relieve the severe pain. These patches work on relieving stress and reduces the inflammation. The details and application are given in chapter Herbal poultices (paste) recipes under the section lower back pain.

Step 12: Use proper resting position and make sure your back is in a relaxed position. These positions are used while resting or when you have applied the patches.

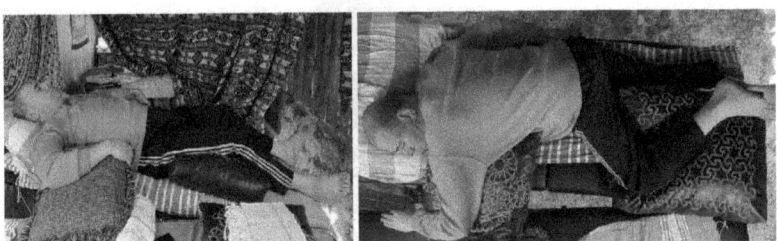

Step 13: At the end of the day, indulge yourself in foot soak and body soak with herbs. This will relax your body senses and rejuvenate it. The recipes and application are already described in chapter Body and foot soak recipes for relaxation.

Step 14: Use can also do the inhalation therapy with herbal recipes which will help reduce the stress. Before sleeping apply herbal oil to your lower back and wrap it with a linen cloth. This helps in pain relief.

TAKE AWAY MESSAGE: "Back is mainly due to degeneration of spine which is an irreversible process. These stretches and exercise will help preventing the degeneration process to occur further and improve muscle strengthening.

CHAPTER 29: SCOLIOSIS

Before screening yourself or another for scoliosis, it is important to know the different types of scoliosis your case may be and how it was caused. The most diagnosed scoliosis subtype is idiopathic scoliosis which has no known cause. However, the other main types of scoliosis include functional, neuromuscular, and degenerative. Functional scoliosis is brought on by other existing issues elsewhere in the body, like having muscle spasms or one leg being shorter than the other. Neuromuscular scoliosis is caused by neurologic and/or muscular disorders and requires the most attention by a doctor because of its severity. Degenerative scoliosis affects older adults after years of the normal wear and tear of the vertebral discs in the back.

To conduct a scoliosis home screening, perform the following steps,

- Stand with arms extended and palms held together, then bend at the waist as if touching their toes. Ask someone to examine the back both from behind and from the front, looking for any signs of asymmetry.

   Is one side of the rib cage higher than the other?
   Is the lower back uneven?
   Does one hip appear higher than the other?

- Postural changes are one of the most common visual indications of scoliosis that are apparent before the spinal curve becomes visible. Observe the individual's posture in the standing straight positions. If you see indications of one shoulder being higher than the others or signs that the hips are imbalanced.

- The clothes check - Sometimes the fit of clothing can be a telltale sign of scoliosis. Assess the situation for uneven hemlines, such as shirt sleeves or pant legs hanging lower than the other.

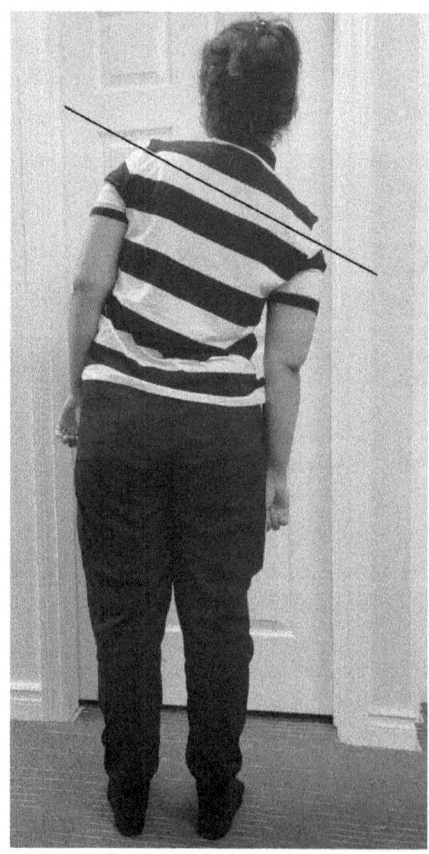

- Walking test – Ask someone to observe the walk and look for abnormalities such as a slight limp, one leg being shorter than the other or any indications that the body seems to tilt to one side.

If you find any changes in the above-mentioned test, there is a chance you are developing a scoliosis which needs to be addressed. But here are some guidelines you can follow to correct your spine as well as relieve your back pain.

Step 1: Before starting activity, you can use the skin scrub to reduce the stress of on your skin and muscles, which will increase the blood circulation of that part and soothes your skin. It also helps in relieving tension. Choose the scrub depending upon your symptom present either it can be neck, upper back or lower back. You can get the recipes for scrub in the chapter earlier.

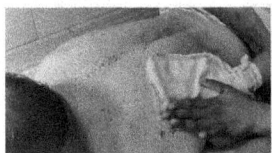 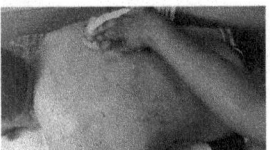 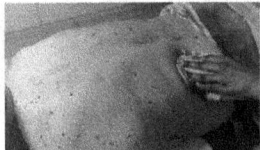 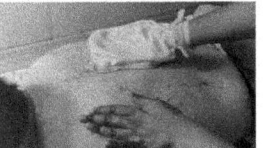

Step 2: After this, take a sip of hot herbal teas and caffeinated drinks. This will help reduce the effect of stress and make you able to carry out your routine activities as normal.

Step 3: Start stretches and mobility exercises, which will help improve your range of motion of and will also make the muscles more flexible. Stiffness will be gradually released. Stretches are done on the side which is tight, or you are leaning. The stretches useful in case of neck and upper back scoliosis are neck posterior stretch, neck diagonal stretch, neck side stretch, corner stretch, thoracic stretch with chair.

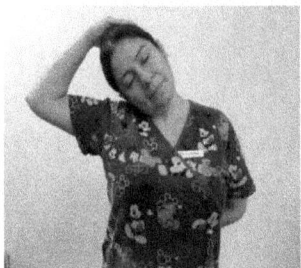 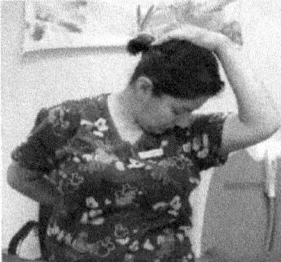 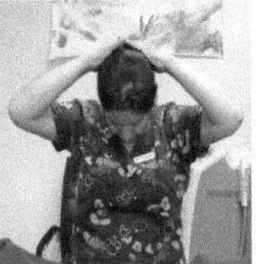 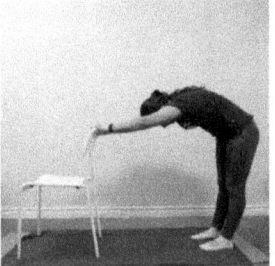

In case of thoraco-lumbar scoliosis do the side stretch in sitting or standing, child pose, cat and cow stretch, hamstrings stretch sitting and supine, figure of four stretch.

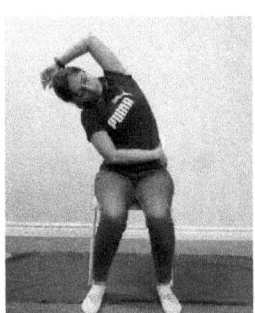 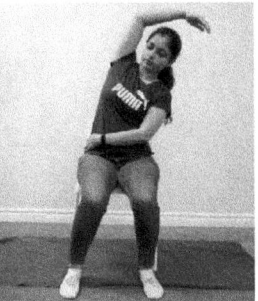 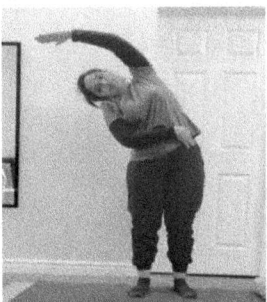 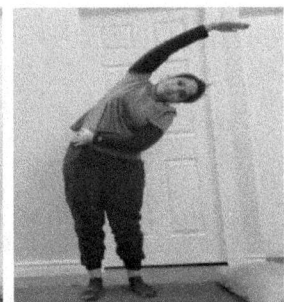

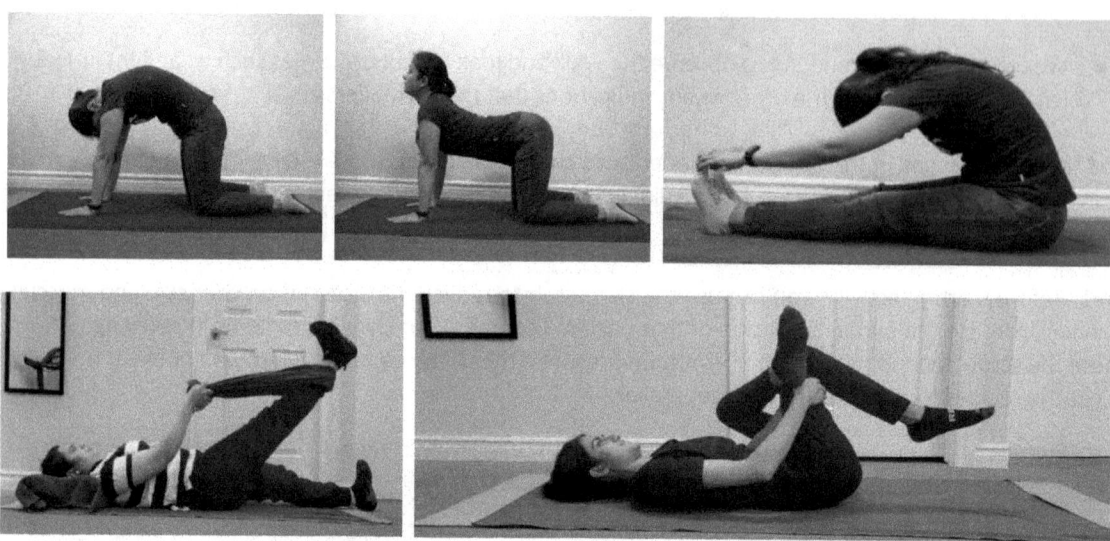

A few tips to keep in mind before you get started! "Aim to hold each stretch for at least 10 seconds and preferably 30 seconds or longer. The pain-relieving benefits will increase the longer you hold these stretches. Don't forget to breathe! It may sound silly but focusing on using your breath can help you cope with any feelings of discomfort."

Step 4: Once you are relaxed, release your stiffness on the tight side with massage. This works best with infused herbal oil recipes. The details for all the recipes are mentioned already in the chapter.

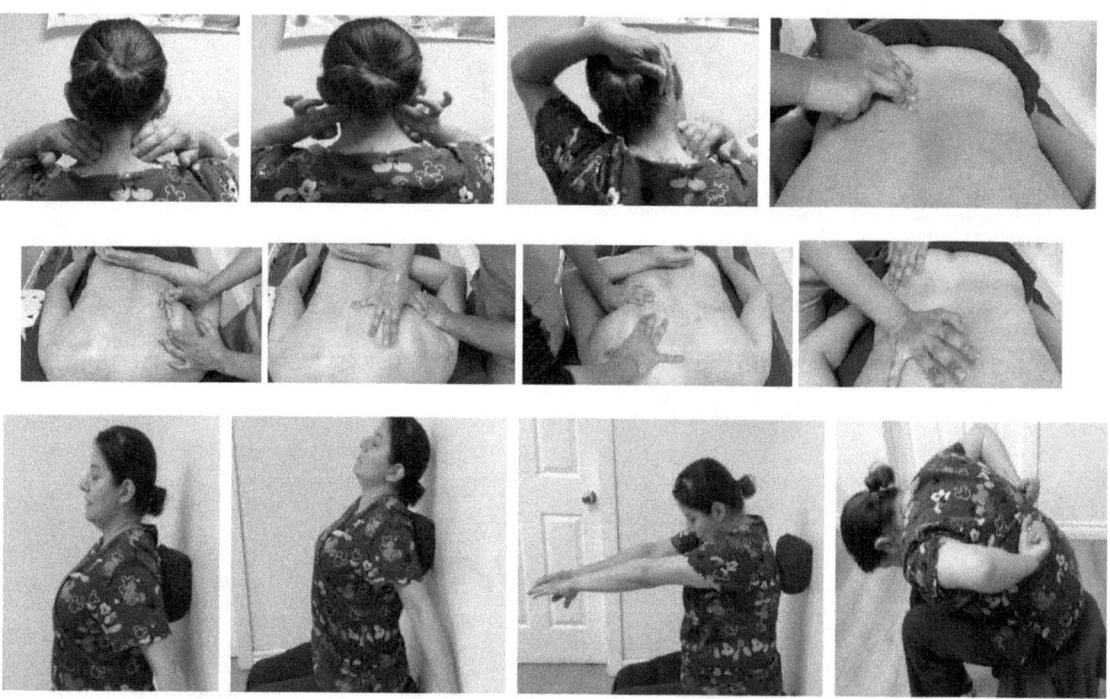

Step 5: After this, relax yourself and use the heat or contrast compress with heat-cold compression to reduce the stiffness and pain of muscles.

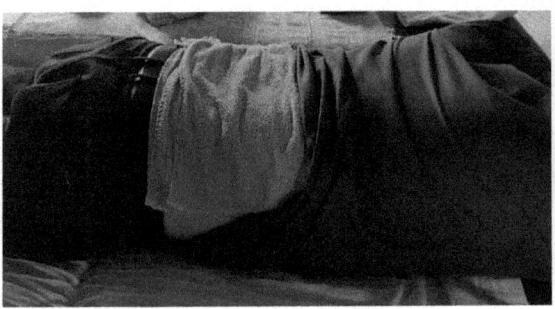
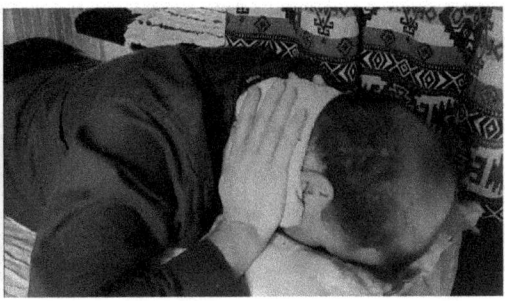

It can be applied directly to the neck, upper back, or lower back area for 10-15 minutes. Repeat the application of heat or contrast therapy 3-4 times a day. Details of application are described in the chapters for Heat and Cold therapy.

Step 6: At this point you will feel relief in your symptoms and the tissues will be completely relaxed. Start with gentle mobility exercises to correct the spinal curvatures. Mobility exercises you can do are neck movements, bridging, pelvic tilts, seated thoracic extensions, back extensions on elbow or hand.

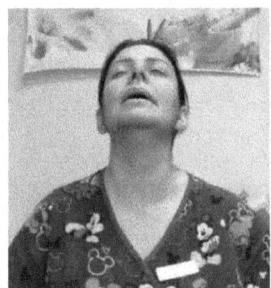
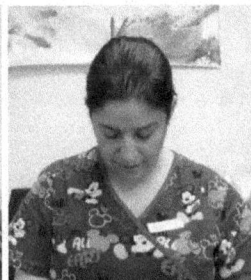
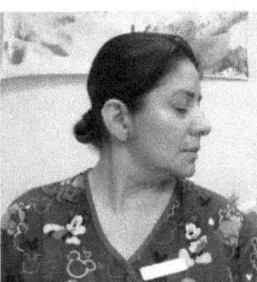
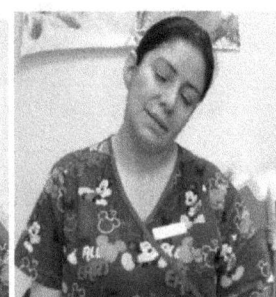

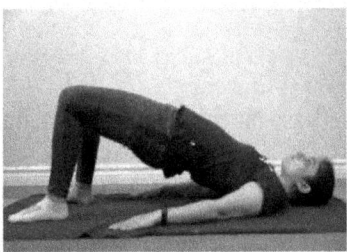
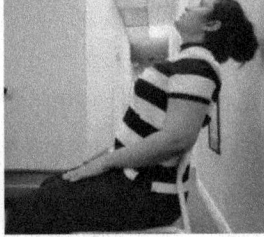
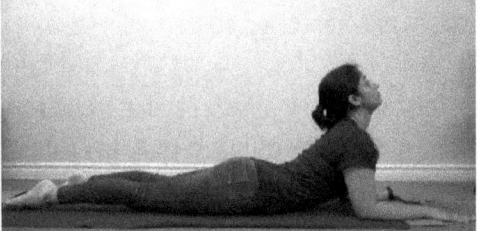

Step 6: Once your symptoms are relieved to 50%, start with the strengthening exercises. As there are imbalance between the muscles of spine, there must be proper strengthening to align the spine in neutral position. The exercises which are beneficial in this condition are – chin tucks, neck isometric, backward shoulder shrugs, pelvis stabilizing in neutral position, Arm lift in four-point kneeling, leg lift in four-point kneeling, Alternate arm and leg raise, abdominal curl ups, modified and straight leg planks.

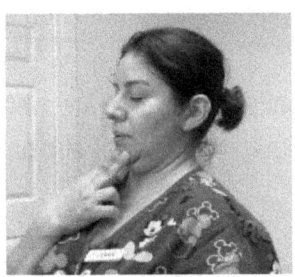
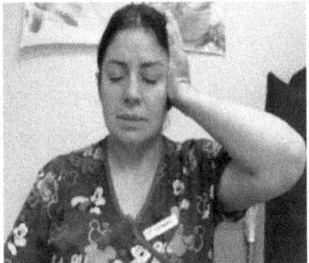
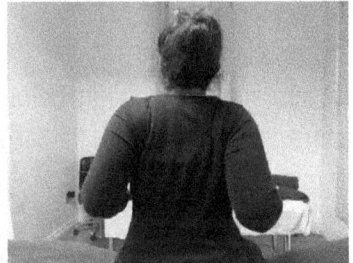

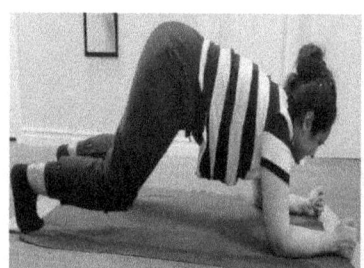
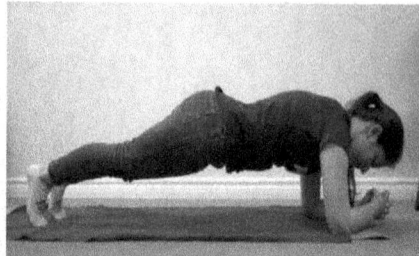
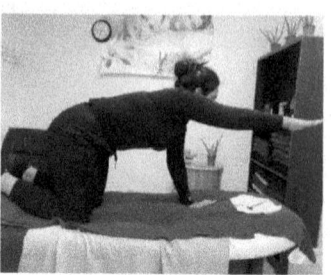
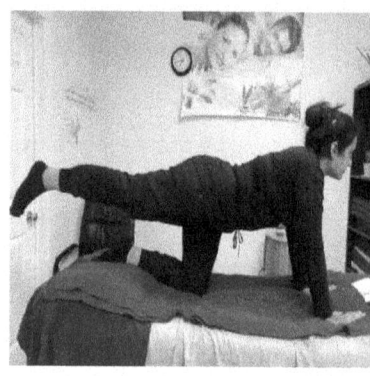
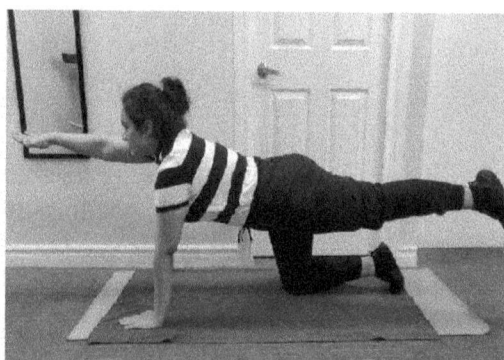

The detail for the exercise is already described in the chapter before. Once you start with exercises you will discomfort in the muscles, but don't worry that is just because we are strengthening the weak muscles.

Step 7: Take a balanced diet which should include food rich in vitamins, omega 3, and magnesium in your diet. The recipes are mentioned above.

Step 8: You can use homemade patches to your skin to relieve the severe pain. These patches work on relieving stress and reduces the stiffness. Apply the patches on the stiff muscles or the side which you are leaning.

Step 9: Use proper resting position and make sure your spine is aligned and you are taking weight equally on your buttocks while sitting. When standing, stand with equal weight on both feet. Also, to correct spinal alignment use pillow on the opposite side of leaning and lie down. You can be in this position for 10 minutes every day.

Step 10: At the end of the day, indulge yourself in foot soak and body soak with herbs. This will relax your body senses and rejuvenate it.

Step 11: Use inhalation method with herbs which will relax the senses of body and will promote overall tissue healing. Before going to bed apply herbal oil to the stiff area and cover with a linen. This will also promote in faster relief of symptoms.

Step 12: "TAKEAWAY MESSAGE" This condition is usually due to poor postural alignment. It can be structural (irreversible) or function (correctable). Posture correction is an important chunk while doing any of the daily living activities.

Numbness or tingling is an unpleasant sensation in which there is a reduced or absent feeling in the skin or a "pins and needles" sensation. The most common reason for numbness or tingling is a problem with nerve function because the nerve itself is injured; something is pressing on the nerve.

What causes numbness or tingling?
Paresthesia happens because of pressure on a nerve. When that pressure is gone -- you uncross your legs, for example -- the feeling goes away. But in some cases, it doesn't go away. Or if it does, it comes back regularly. That's called chronic paresthesia, and it can be a sign of a medical condition or nerve damage. Several things can cause chronic paresthesia, including:
- An injury or accident that caused nerve damage
- A stroke or mini-stroke -- when blood flow to your brain is cut off and causes damage
- Radiculopathy -- a compressed nerve root
- Neuropathy -- nerve damage
- A pinched nerve (often in your neck, shoulder, or arm) from injury or overuse
- Sciatica -- pressure on the sciatic nerve (which goes from your lower pelvis to your buttocks and legs), a common problem during pregnancy that typically causes numbness and pain in your back or legs

How do you feel in paresthesia or numbness?
You'll usually feel paresthesia in your hands, arms, legs, or feet. But it can happen in other areas of the body as well. People with paresthesia could feel sensations like:
- Burning
- Prickling
- Itching
- Tingling

If you are feeling this than always find the root cause of the compression. Follow this stepwise approach to treat your condition,

Step 1: As you wake up take a sip of hot herbal teas and caffeinated drinks. This will help reduce the effect of stress and make you able to carry out your routine activities as normal.

Step 2: Start with the stretches for the nerve. Nerve stretches which will relieve the symptoms of "pins and needles". Initially when you stretch there will be lots of discomfort so don't worry. Start gradually up to your tolerance level. For upper body nerve compression, you can stretch the nerves as follows - If you have the pain radiating down to your arm or hands use the nerve stretches. If the pain is radiating down to your thumb, index and middle finger stretch median nerve.

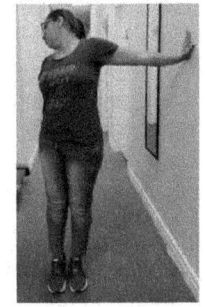

If the pain is radiating down to your pinky finger do the ulnar nerve stretch.

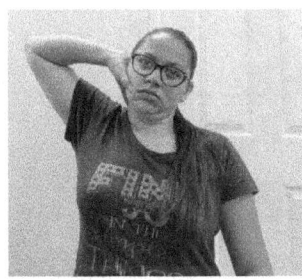 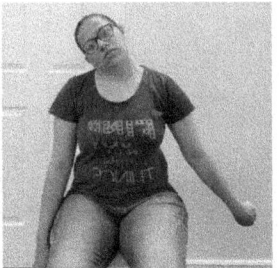

And if it is going on dorsal part of hand do the radial nerve stretch.

For nerve compression at lower back and legs. Stretch the sciatic nerve. It is the most common which is compressed.

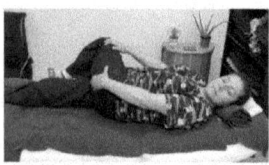 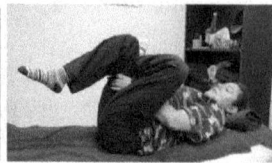 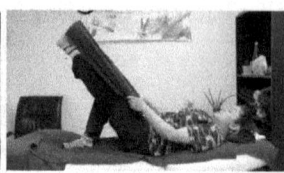 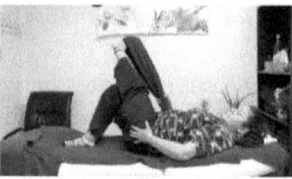

You must feel a sharp stretch along the whole course of the nerve. It will pain initially, but don't panic. Gradually when the muscle loosens up it will feel better.

Step 3: Once you are relaxed, release your stiffness with massage. This works best with infused herbal oil recipes.

Upper body nerve massage:

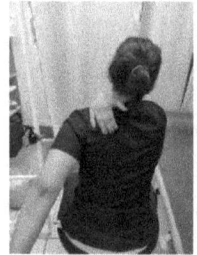 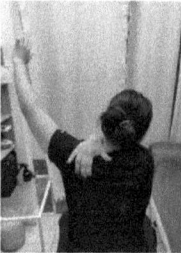 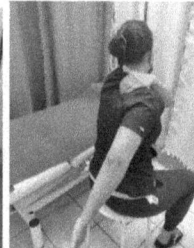 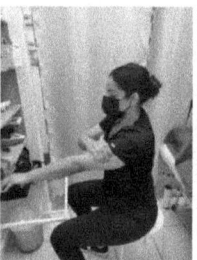 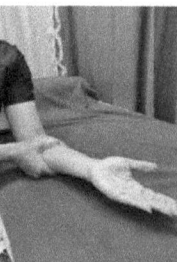 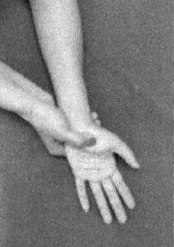

Sciatic massage:

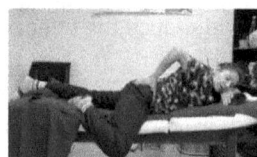 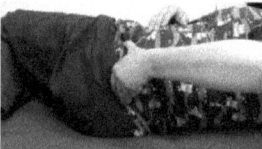 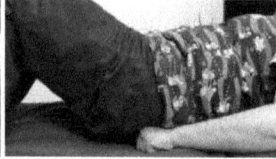 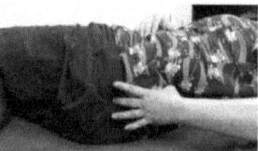

Step 6: Once your symptoms are relieved to 50%, start with the strengthening exercises. Focus right now should be on strengthening of the muscles which are weak because of the specific nerve compression.

For upper limb weakness the exercises are backward shoulder shrugs, standing shoulder crunches, shoulder flexor, abductor and rotator strengthening.

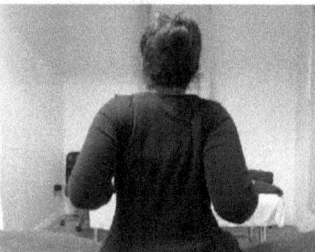 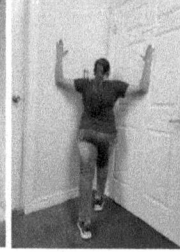 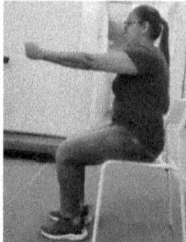 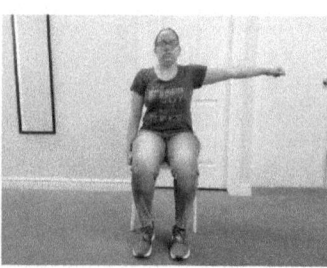

For lower limb weakness the exercises are buttock Squeeze, adductor squeeze, heel squeeze, abdominal crunches, straight leg raise, side leg raise, clam shells

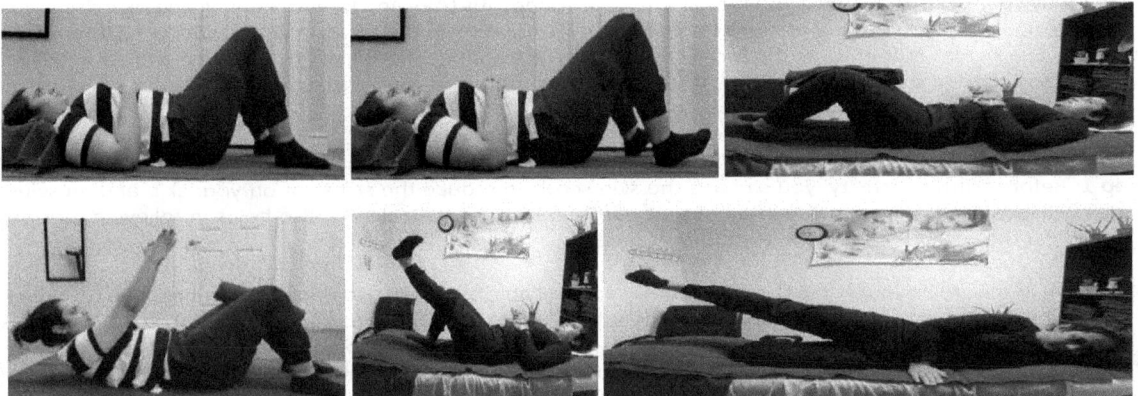

Once you start with exercises you will discomfort in the muscles, but don't worry that is just because we are strengthening the weak muscles. Gradually this discomfort goes away.

Step 7: Take a balanced diet which should include food rich in vitamins, omega 3, and magnesium in your diet. The recipes are mentioned above for salad, soups and juices.

Step 8: You can use homemade patches to your skin to relieve the severe neck pain and back pain. These patches work on relieving stress and reduces the inflammation.

Step 9: Use proper resting position and make sure your back is in a relaxed position. These positions are used while resting or when you have applied the patches.

Step 10: Again, you can use the herbal teas to relieve your stress due to pain. The recipes are already described above in step 4.

Step 11: At the end of the day, indulge yourself in foot soak with herbs. This will relax your body senses and rejuvenate it. Also use inhalation method with herb to relieve all the senses of body.

Step 12: "TAKEAWAY MESSAGE"
Lumbar and cervical degeneration usually compresses the nerve making the muscles weak. Therefore, you need to focus on improving your strength and mobility.

CHAPTER 31: ANKYLOSING SPONDYLITIS AND ITS MANAGEMENT

Back pain is typically one of those aches that worsens when you bend or walk and feels better when you rest or recline. That's not the case with ankylosing spondylitis. This inflammatory disease causes pain and stiffness in your lower back and hips — especially in the morning or after prolonged periods of not moving. Here's why your back hurts when you have ankylosing spondylitis (AS), and how stretching and exercise helps relieve symptoms. It is a form of arthritis that causes inflammation in the joints in your spine, or vertebrae. As the disease progresses, it impacts the sacroiliac joints (which connect the base of your spine and your pelvis), and can lead to severe and chronic pain, stiffness, and discomfort in your lower back and hips.

You need to follow this step wise approach to keep yourself active,

Step 1: Before starting activity, you can use the skin scrub to reduce the stress of on your skin and muscles, which will increase the blood circulation of that part and soothes your skin. It also helps in relieving tension. You can get the recipes for scrub in the chapter before.

Step 2: After this, relax yourself in the way you are comfortable and then use the heat compression to reduce the stiffness and pain of muscles. Usually, the condition develops after a long time of initial onset so always choose heat therapy. It can be applied directly to the neck, upper back, and lower back area for 10-15 minutes. Repeat the application of heat therapy 3-4 times a day. Details of application are described in the earlier chapters.

Step 3: Followed by heat, start gentle stretches and mobility exercises, which will help improve your range of motion of back especially extension and will also make the muscles more flexible. Stiffness will be gradually released. You must feel a slight pull on the tight muscle. It will pain initially, but don't panic. Gradually when the muscle loosens up it will feel better. Stretches to do for this condition are corner stretch, back extension against wall, prone extensions, seated thoracic extension, quadriceps stretch, supine figure of 4 stretch, bending back, cat and cow stretch.

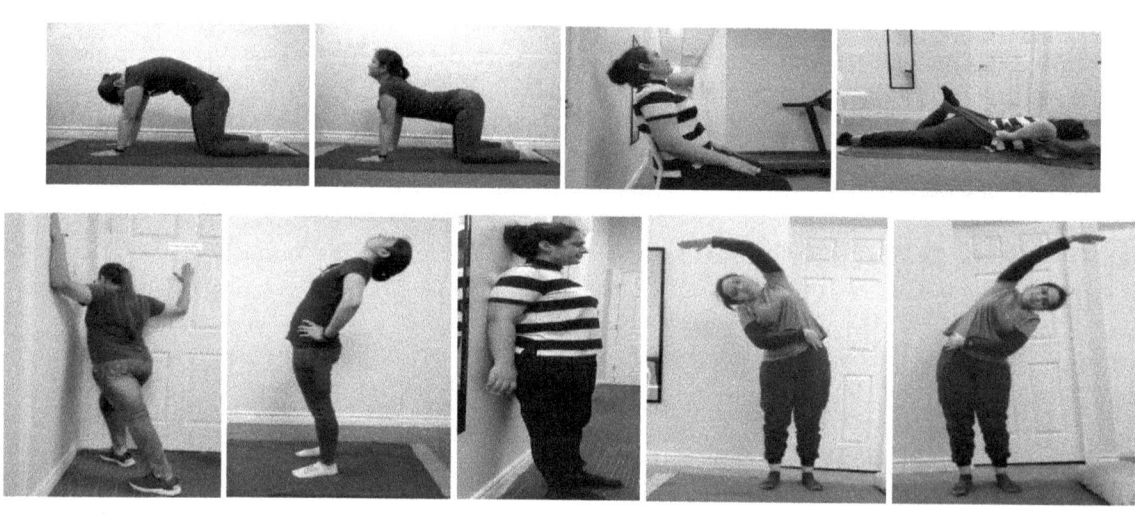

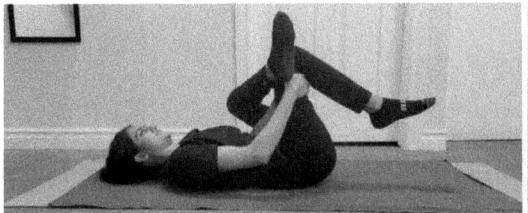 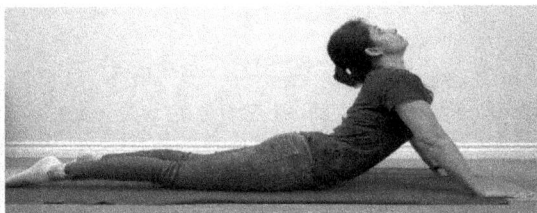

A few tips to keep in mind before you get started

Aim to hold each stretch for at least 10 seconds and preferably 30 seconds or longer. The pain-relieving benefits will increase the longer you hold these stretches.

Don't forget to breathe! It may sound silly but focusing on using your breath can help you cope with any feelings of discomfort.

Mobility exercises for this condition are bridging, lumbar flexion with rotation, seated trunk rotations, alternate arm and leg lift. The details for the exercise are described in the chapter General mobility exercise.

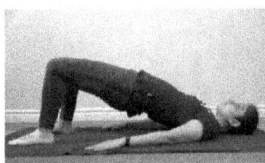 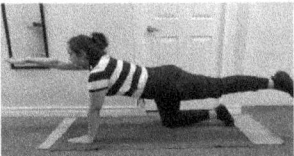 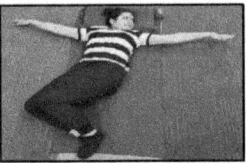 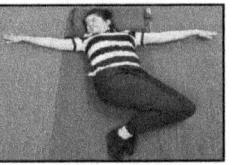

Step 4: After this, take a sip of hot herbal teas and caffeinated drinks. This will help reduce the effect of stress on your muscles and make you able to carry out your routine activities as normal.

Step 5: Once you are relaxed, release your stiffness with massage. This works best with infused herbal oil recipes. The massage techniques and recipes for herbal oil already described in the chapter above.

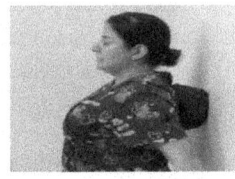 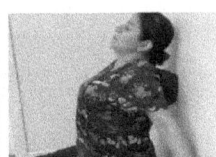 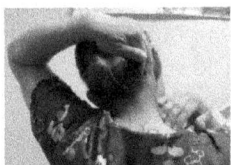 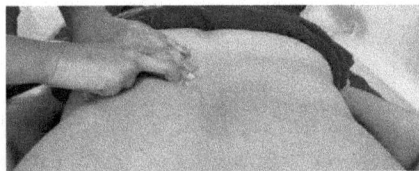

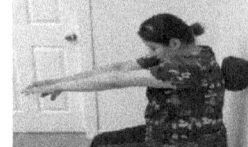 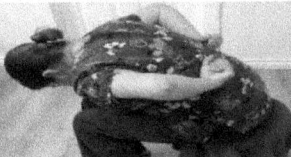 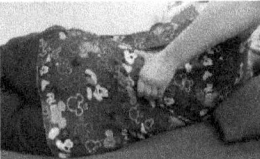 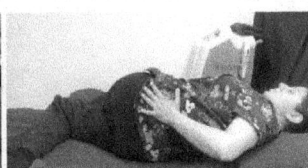

Step 6: Add breathing exercise for your schedule. In this condition, because of slouched posture breathing pattern will always be affected. Stand up with your feet hip distance apart and your arms out in front of you at chest height. Your palms should face up. Slowly breathe in and let your arms move up into a U shape — think of tracing the shape of a big wine glass. Hold your breath for a few seconds. Slowly breathe out and lower your arms to the start position.

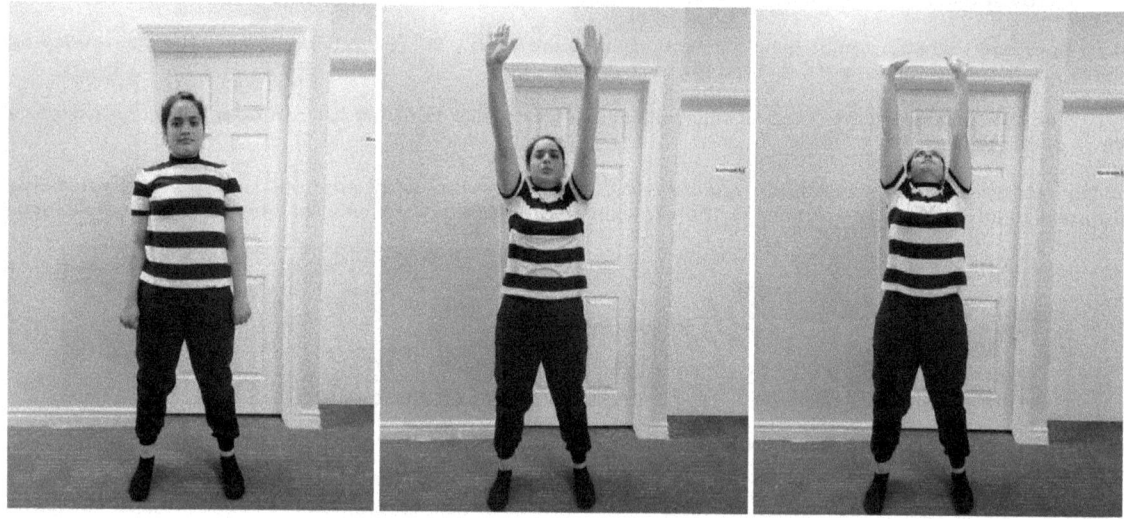

Sit comfortably with your feet shoulder-width apart. You can also do this exercise standing up. Look straight ahead, and do not allow your head to tilt back. As you take a deep breath, open your arms out to the sides and roll your arms back. Your palms will turn outward, and you will feel a stretch across your chest. Breathe normally as you hold this stretch for 15 to 30 seconds. Lower your arms to your sides and let your palms turn back toward your legs as you slowly let out your breath. Repeat 2 to 4 times. This also helps in chest expansion

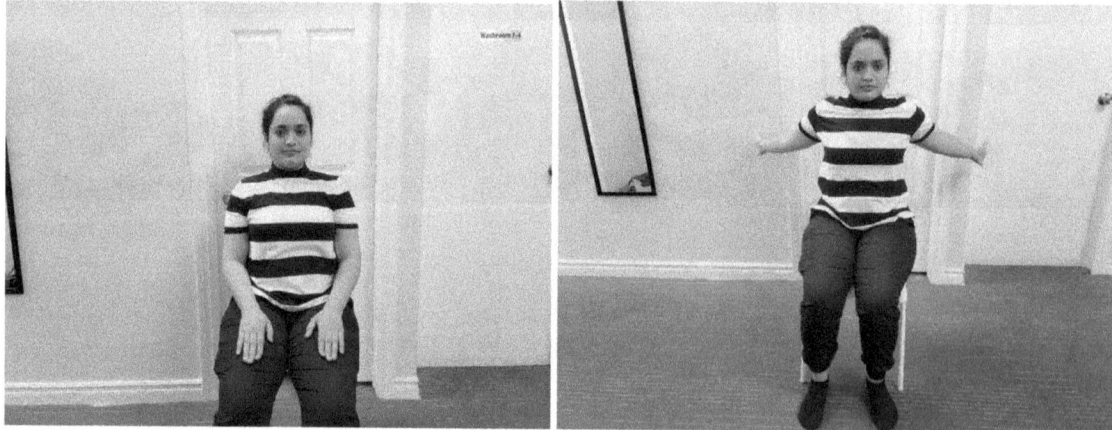

Step 7: Take a balanced diet which should include food rich in vitamins, omega 3, and magnesium in your diet. The recipes are mentioned in the chapter Nutritional benefits. At least include one recipe in your meal from the given.

Step 8: You can use homemade patches to your skin to relieve the severe pain on neck or lower back. These patches work on relieving stress and reduces the stiffness.

Step 9: Use proper resting position and make sure your spine is in a relaxed and aligned position. These positions are used while resting or when you have applied the patches or for sleeping.

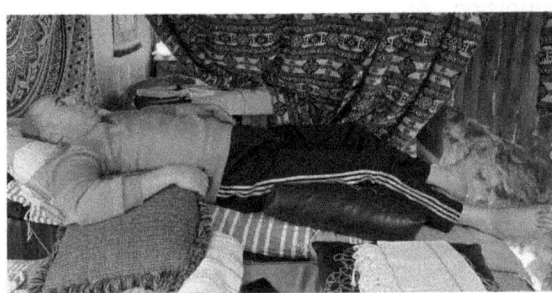 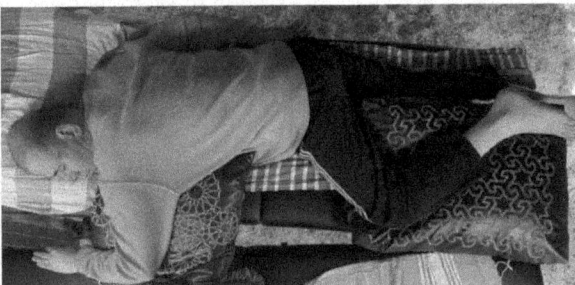

Step 10: Again, you can use the herbal teas to relieve your stress. The recipes are already described above in step 4.

Step 11: At the end of the day, indulge yourself in foot and body soak with herbs. This will relax your body senses and rejuvenate it. Also use inhalation method with herb to relieve all the senses of body.

"TAKEAWAY MESSAGE"

Ankylosing spondylitis is a chronic condition in which there is calcium deposits on the spine which makes it rigid. This will lead to poor flexibility so always focus more on mobility of the spine. Always rest your spine while doing any activities.

CHAPTER 32: SACRO-ILIAC JOINT DYSFUNCTION

About 15-30% of the time, the SI joint is a cause of chronic low back pain. Here are few questions which can rule out if your back pain is due to Sacro-iliac joint dysfunction.

- Does your back hurt at lower back where you get the dimple like impression by the joint?
- Do you avoid for sitting or standing long period of time because of pain?
- Does climbing stairs make the pain worse?
- Does travelling in vehicle making your back or buttocks pain more?
- Is it painful to stand on one leg (affected side) for a prolonged period?
- Is it painful to stand on one leg (affected side) for a prolonged period?

If you answered YES to any of the above questions, your SI joint is a potential source of your lower back pain. Here are the ways which will help you the relieve pain. Sacroiliac joint pain typically affects the lower back. It can also radiate to the buttock, hip, groin, thighs, legs and feet. In most cases, the pain affects one side of the back or one leg, but it can involve both sides. Certain activities and positions may worsen the pain, especially sleeping on the affected side and prolonged sitting, standing or walking. Transitional movements, such as rising from a seated position, can also be difficult. Initial treatments for sacroiliac joint pain typically include:

- Brief rest period. A rest period of 1 to 2 days may be advised. Resting for longer than a couple days is not recommended, as doing so may worsen stiffness and cause increased pain and generalized deconditioning.

- Supports or braces. When the SI joint is too loose (hypermobile), a pelvic brace can be wrapped around the waist to stabilize the area. A pelvic brace is about the size of a wide belt and can be helpful when the joint is inflamed and painful.

Here is a 24-hour guide to your pain which will help in reducing the pain caused by SI joint dysfunction.

- **Step 1:** Before starting activity, you can use the skin scrub to reduce the stress of on your skin and muscles, which will increase the blood circulation of that part and soothes your skin. This will help in relieving pain and stiffness and prevent your back from getting worse throughout the day. Body scrub which works best is recipe 1 (yogurt scrub) and recipe 2 (Turmeric scrub). The details of recipe preparation and application are already described in the chapter for body scrub.

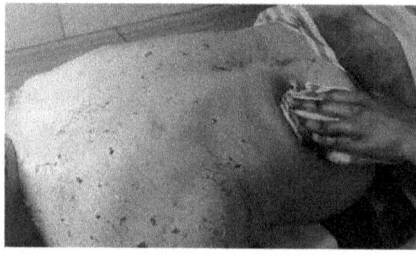
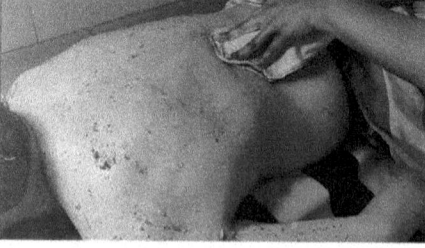

- **Step 2:** Once you are done with scrubbing, take hot beverages as normal. You can take the herbal teas which have tremendous benefit in healing tissues. Also, add the special juices to your drink. Try recipe 1 (Green Juice). The details of recipe preparation and application are already described in the chapter for nutritional facts.

- **Step 3:** You can continue with your breakfast after beverages. Add a healthy salad and soup to your meal. The recipe 1 (Red beans) for salad and recipe 1 (Bone broth) for soup will work best. While eating make sure you support your lower back with a brace or wrap a towel around it so that it is supported.

  Step 4: Resting positions: When sitting in a chair, you should aim to keep your hips neutral to avoid excess stress on the ligaments in your SI joint. Think about keeping your hips level with each other and avoid rotating more to one side. Avoid positions that hike one hip higher or put create an asymmetry in your hips, such as when you cross your legs.
  Here's how you can sit with good posture to help manage SI joint pain:
  - Sit with your chest up and your shoulder blades down and relaxed.
  - Keep your knees slightly apart and uncrossed.
  - Think about keeping both your "sit bones" in contact with your chair and the tops of your hips level.
  - If your chair doesn't support your lower back, put a pad or cushion behind your lower back.
  - You can also use a doughnut pillow under your buttocks to provide more stability and postural correction.

- **Step 5:** After about an hour of your breakfast, the first movement you need to do is to relax your spine lying down in a comfortable position and release stiffness in back muscles with gentle massage. This works best with infused herbal oil recipes. Use recipe 1 which contains sage, thyme, mint and chia seeds and recipe 2 which contains turmeric, basil, garden cress seeds and mint from chronic lower back pain section. The details for recipes and application are already described in chapter (herbs and herbs infused oils).

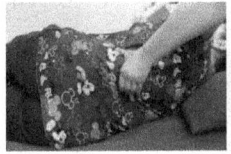 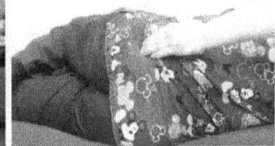 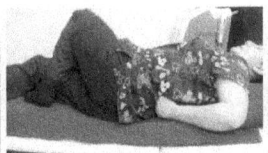 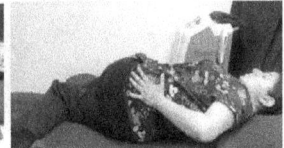

- **Step 6:** Stretching and general mobility exercises: After massage, you will feel more relaxed. Start with gentle stretches of your lower back, hips and pelvic muscles including the piriformis, glutes, and hamstring muscles. Tension in these muscles caused by sacroiliac joint dysfunction can be the primary cause of pain. Stretches which work best for this condition are figure of four, knee to chest, cat and cow, hand to knee & seated piriformis stretch. Supine figure of 4 stretch – The description of this exercise is already given in Chapter General stretching exercise.

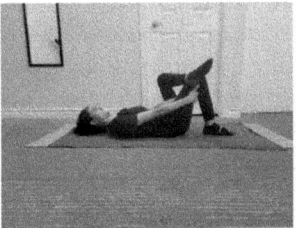 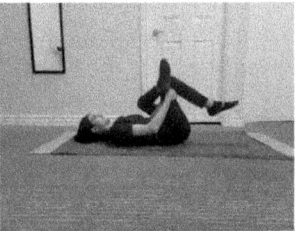

- Reclining hand to knee stretches - The description of this exercise is already given in Chapter General stretching exercise.

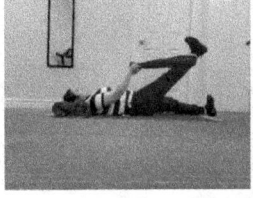 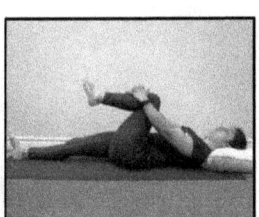

- Knee to chest stretch - The description of this exercise is already given in Chapter General stretching exercise

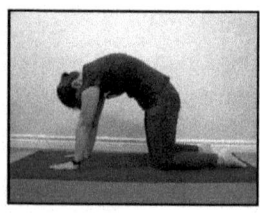 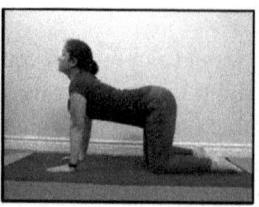

Cat and cow stretch: The description of this exercise is already given in Chapter General stretching exercise.

Seated Stretch: The description of this exercise is already given in Chapter General stretching exercise.

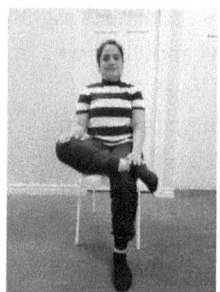 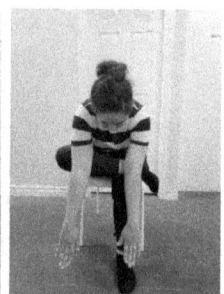

You must feel a slight pull on the tight muscle. Gradually when the muscle loosens up it will feel better. Hold each stretch for 30 seconds and repeat it for 3 times. For stretching of the legs, repeat it on both the sides.

Step 7: After stretching you will feel relief in your symptoms by 50%. Start with mobility exercise to your spine and legs. This will help in alignment as well as improve the range of motion.
Lumbar flexion with rotation: The description of this exercise is already given in Chapter General mobility exercises.

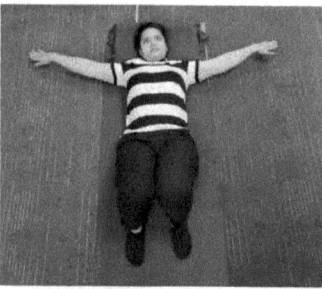 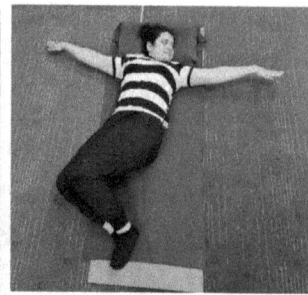 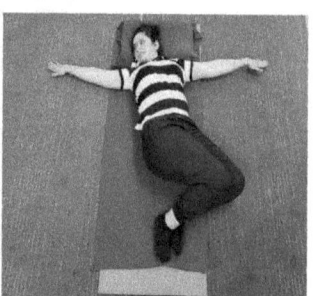

Step 8: After this, relax yourself and use the heat or cold compresses to reduce the stiffness and pain in the muscles according to your onset of pain. It can be applied directly to the lower back area for 10-15 minutes. Repeat the application of heat or cold therapy 3-4 times a day. Details of application are described in the chapters for Heat and Cold therapy.

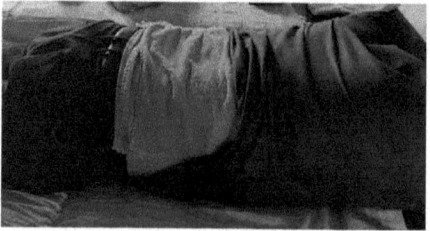

Step 9: Repeat stretches and mobility exercises in initial days. Once the pain and symptoms ae subsides or manageable start with strengthening exercises because SI joint dysfunction occurs mostly due to loose SI joint ligaments which leads to instability of spine and weakness of muscles. Better support for the joint can come from strengthening the abdominal muscles, lateral trunk muscles, and low back muscles. Exercises suitable for this condition are buttock squeeze, heel squeeze, adductor squeeze, bridging, clam shell partial sit ups and modified planks.

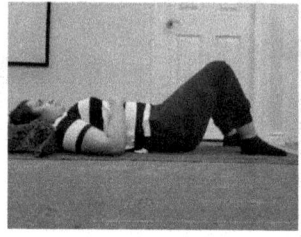 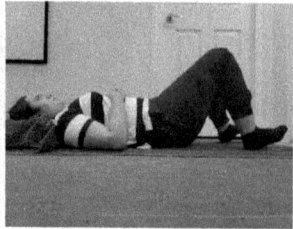 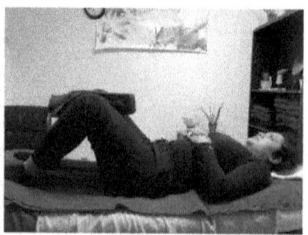

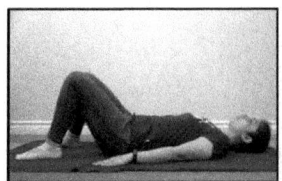 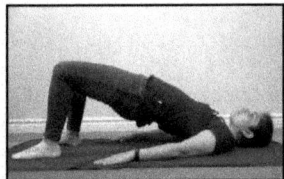 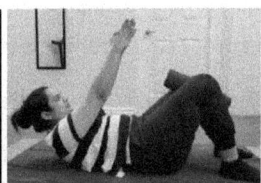 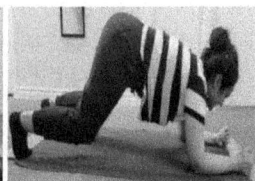

Once you start with exercises you will feel discomfort in the muscles, but don't worry that is just because we are strengthening the weak muscles. Gradually this discomfort goes away. Make sure you hold each exercise for 10 seconds and repeat it for 5-6 times initially.

Step 10: Take a balanced diet which should include food rich in vitamins, omega 3, and magnesium in your diet. Green leafy vegetables like spinach, kale, swish charred, collard greens can be consumed. The recipes which is useful are described in chapter Nutritional facts and benefits of balanced diet. There are different sections including recipes for soups, salads and juices which you can include at least one in your daily diet.

Step 11: You can use homemade pastes on your back to relieve the severe pain. These patches work on relieving stress and reduces the inflammation. The details and application are given in chapter Herbal poultices (paste) recipes under the section lower back pain.

Step 12: Use proper resting position and make sure your back is in a relaxed position. These positions are used while resting or when you have applied the patches.

If you're having SI joint pain on one side, you may want to sleep on your opposite side to take your weight off the joint. Putting a pillow between your knees and ankles can help put your hips in alignment.

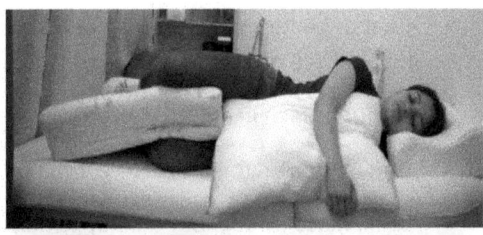

Another sleeping posture to take the stress off your SI joint is to sleep on your back with one or two pillows under your knees to put your hips in a neutral posture.

Step 13: At the end of the day, indulge yourself in foot soak

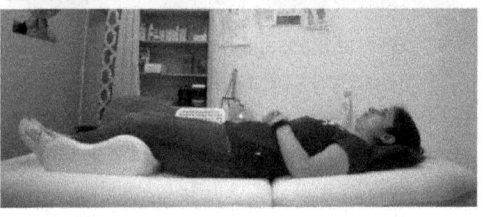

and body soak with herbs. This will relax your body senses and rejuvenate it. The recipes and application are already described in chapter Body and foot soak recipes for relaxation.

Step 14: Use can also do the inhalation therapy with herbal recipes which will help reduce the stress. Before sleeping apply herbal oil to your lower back and wrap it with a linen cloth. This helps in pain relief.

TAKE AWAY MESSAGE: Stretching the muscles around your SI joint may help reduce pain by relieving tension in your lower back. When stretching, it's better to be too gentle than too aggressive. Stretching too vigorously may cause your muscles to become tighter and worsen your symptoms.

CHAPTER 33: TAILBONE PAIN

Tailbone pain — pain that occurs in or around the bony structure at the bottom of the spine (coccyx) — can be caused by trauma to the coccyx during a fall, prolonged sitting on a hard or narrow surface, degenerative joint changes, or vaginal childbirth. Tailbone pain can feel dull and achy but typically becomes sharp during certain activities, such as sitting, rising from a seated to a standing position or prolonged standing. Defecation and sex also might become painful. For women, tailbone pain can make menstruation uncomfortable as well.

. There are three types of events that cause tailbone pain:

- **External Trauma:** A bruised, broken or dislocated coccyx caused by a fall.
- **Internal Trauma:** Trauma caused by a difficult childbirth or from sitting on a narrow or hard surface for too long.
- **Others:** Infection, abscess and tumors.

Home Remedies

Tailbone injuries are often extremely painful, so home remedies aim to control pain and avoid further irritation to the area.

- Avoid sitting down for long periods of time. When seated, avoid sitting on hard surfaces and alternate sitting on each side of the buttocks. Sit on a doughnut-shaped pillow to take pressure off the tailbone area. Also, lean forward and direct your weight away from the tailbone.

- For traumatic injuries, apply ice to the tailbone area for 15-20 minutes, four times a day, for the first few days after the injury. Details of application are described in the earlier chapters.

- Heat or heating pad. Applying heat to the bottom of the spine after the first few days of pain may help relieve muscle tension, which may accompany or exacerbate coccyx pain.

- Eat foods high in fiber to soften stools and avoid constipation.

- Don't strain on the toilet since it puts more pressure on your tailbone.

- Drink fluids throughout the day to help soften your stool.

- Gentle massage may be appropriate if your tailbone is bruised, but may not be right for a fracture. This works best with infused herbal oil recipes. Use recipe 1 which contains sage, thyme, mint and chia seeds and recipe 2 which contains turmeric, basil, garden cress seeds and mint from chronic lower back pain section. The details for recipes and application are already described in chapter 8 (herbs and herbs infused oils).

- Exercise important for tailbone pain are knee to chest stretch, Figure of four stretch, child pose, sitting glutes stretch, Pelvic tilting, bridging and planks.

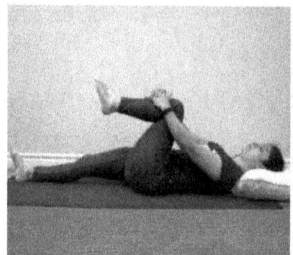
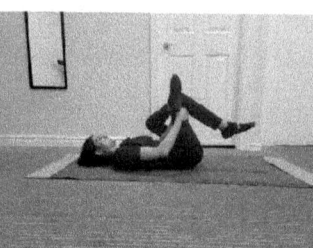
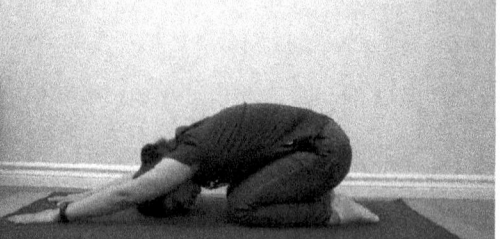

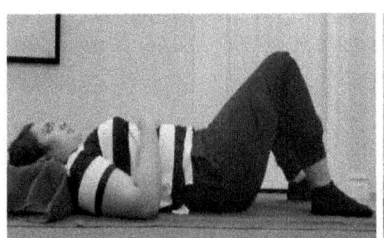 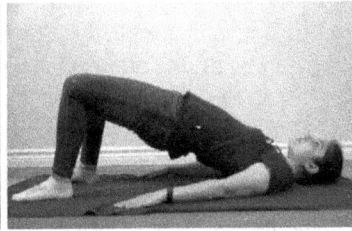 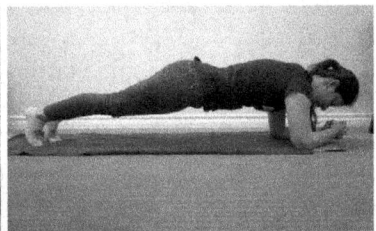

TAKEAWAY MESSAGE: The exercises above address some of the causes of tailbone pain. As with all stretches and exercises, it is crucial to remain within a range of motion that does not cause pain or injury.

CHAPTER 34: BACK PAIN DURING PREGNANCY

Nausea, back pain, pubic bone pain, weakened posture, the list goes on! Pregnancy is an incredible and rewarding journey, but your body goes through a lot of changes on the way. Back pain can come in many different forms and affect the lower back, sacroiliac joint, and upper back. The elevated relaxing hormone and your body (and the baby's body) adjusting as birth approaches contribute to your pelvis shifting and feeling different. But say "GOODBYE" to your aches and pains with this stepwise approach including stretches, exercise, diet, and other nutritional tips. This can be done during any trimester.

Stretches

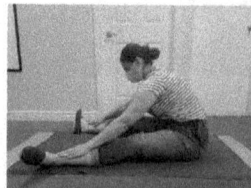

Lower back stretch - Sit on the floor, legs straight out in front of you. (If you're toward the end of the third trimester and your tummy is bigger, you can separate your legs apart, so you're seated in a "V" position, but not too wide.) Sit tall, inhale, arms reaching forward. Exhale, reaching forward from your hips till you feel a stretch at the back of your legs and lower back. Keep knees on the floor and do not slouch. Hold for 20 seconds

Seated piriformis stretches - Sit on a chair with your feet flat on the ground. Cross one foot over the other knee in the shape of the number "4." As you exhale, slowly lean forward keeping a flat back until you feel a stretch in your lower back and buttocks. Think about elongating your spine rather than curling your shoulders in toward your lap. Hold position for 30 seconds. Repeat on the other side. This stretch is helpful for those with low back or sciatic pain.

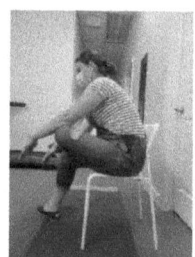

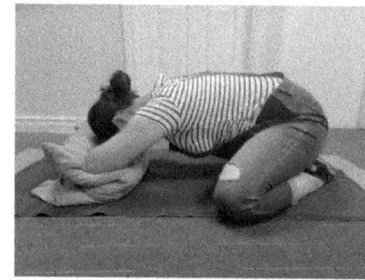

Child pose - Begin on all fours on the mat, with your knees directly under your hips. Keep your big toes touching. This will give your belly room to slide between your knees and avoid putting strain on your hips. You can also widen your toes if having them touching puts any pressure on your knees or does not provide enough room for your belly. Inhale and feel your spine grow longer. As you exhale, take your butt to your heels, and lower your heads towards the mat while tucking your chin to your chest. Rest here, with your forehead on the ground. You can also fold a blanket or use a yoga block and let your head rest on it if the ground is far away. Keep your arms outstretched. Hold this for at least 5 deep, even breaths. This resting pose is great for gently stretching those aching hips, pelvis, and thighs. You'll also stretch the spine, especially the lower back.

Bound angle pose - Sit on your mat and bend your knees, bringing the soles of your feet together in front of you. Grab hold of your toes and draw your feet gently toward your pelvis. Inhale and sit up tall on your sitting bones, not your tailbone. You don't want your pelvis tucked here. As you exhale, press your knees to the ground. Keeping your spine straight, gently begin to bend at the hips, taking your torso toward the ground. When you get as far as you can comfortably go, release any tension in your neck by dropping your chin. Stay here for 3 to 5 slow, even breaths. If possible, gently lean farther forward with each exhale, but be sure not to overstretch.

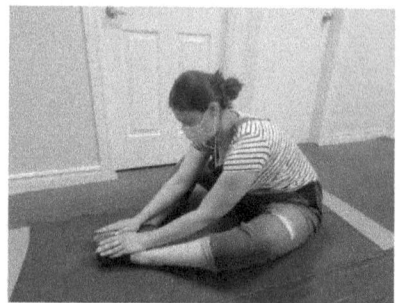

This seated pose is a hip opener. It also stabilizes and helps bring awareness to your pelvis. You'll stretch your inner thighs, back, and neck. Try it as a supported pose with a yoga or birth ball for you to lean on.

Exercises
Squats - Stand with your feet shoulder-width apart. Bend your knees and move your hips backward as if you're going to sit in a chair. Keep your knees behind your toes. Only bend as far as you feel comfortable, then return to the starting position.
Perform 10 repetitions.

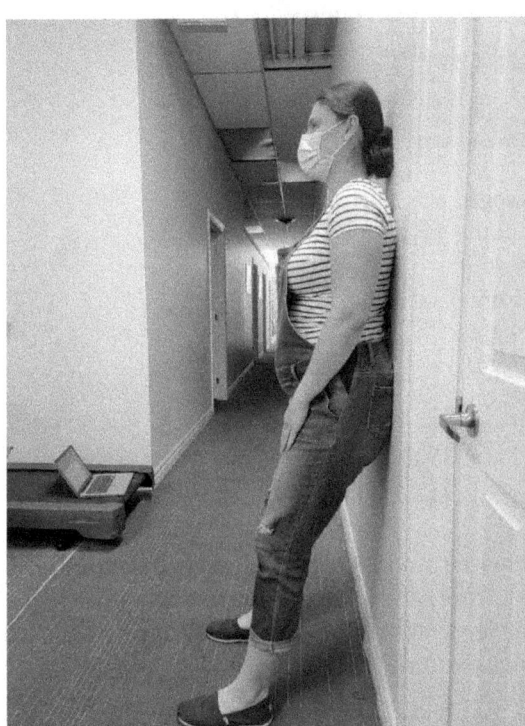
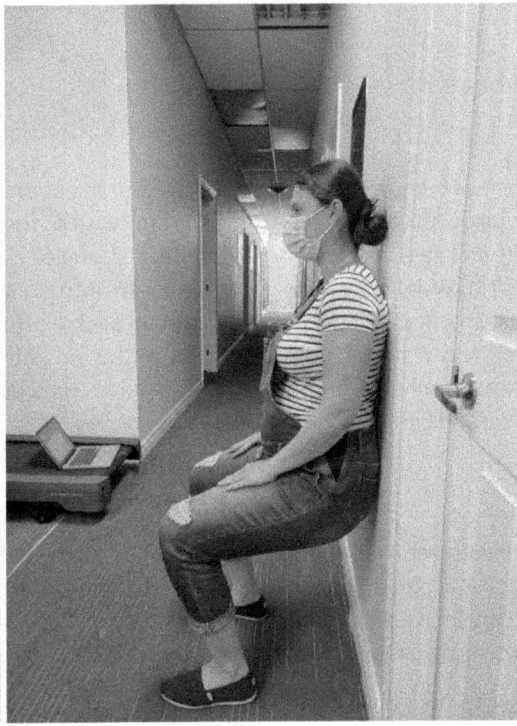

Alternate arm and leg –

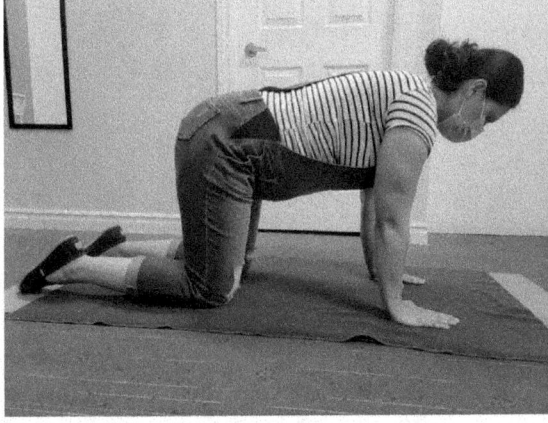
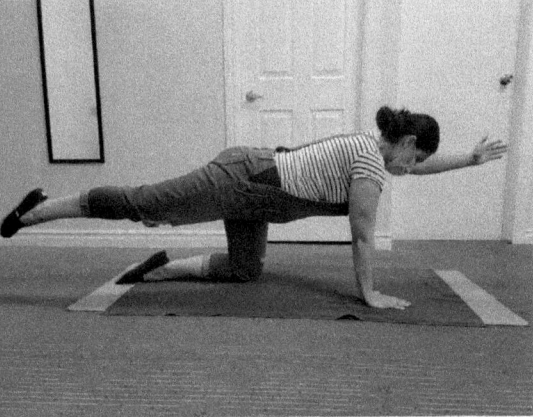

Bridging –

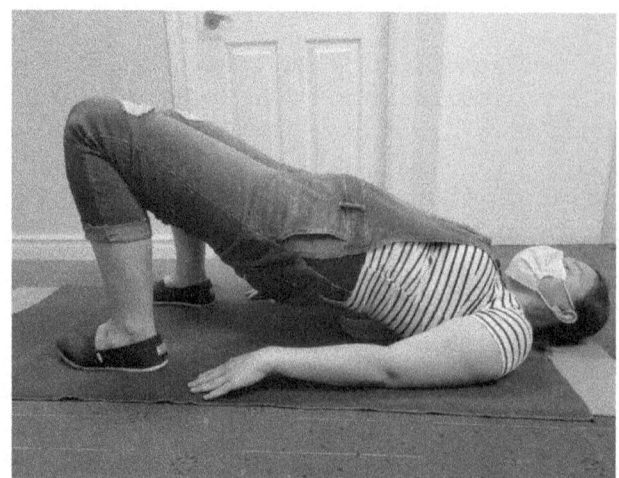

Lunges - Begin kneeling on the floor with your knees on a yoga mat or pillow for comfort. Step one foot forward so that both your front knee and hip are at 90-degree angles. As you exhale, slowly lean forward, putting weight into your front leg. Square off your hips by rotating your back hip forward until you feel a stretch down the front of the hip and thigh. Hold onto a wall or chair for balance, if needed. Hold position for 30 seconds. Repeat on the other side.

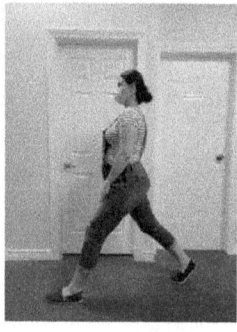 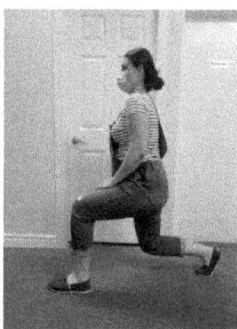

Side-lying leg raise - Lie on your left side with your shoulders, hips, and ankles in a straight line. You may place a small pillow under your side to keep your spine straight. Slowly and controlled, raise your right leg to a 45-degree angle (pain-free range of motion), then lower your leg. Perform 10 repetitions with your right leg. Switch to lying on your right side and perform 10 repetitions with your left leg.

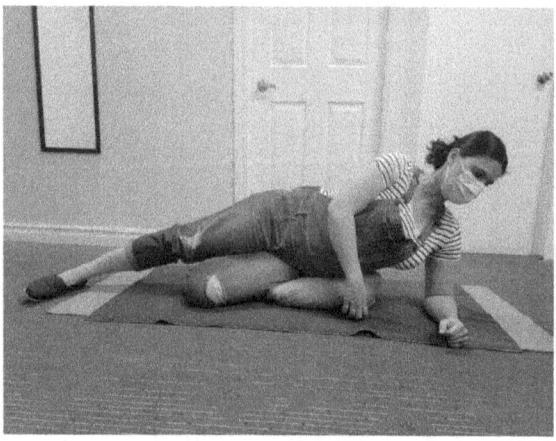 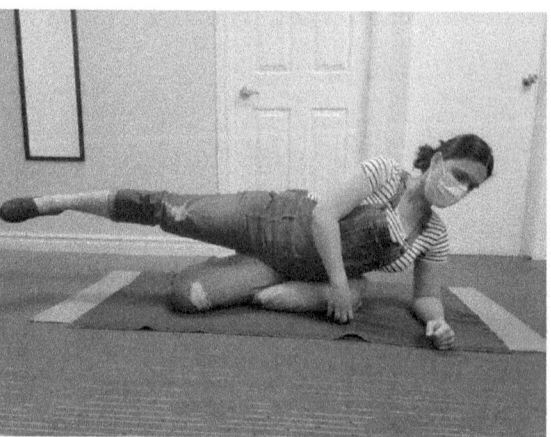

Clam shells - Lay on your side, supporting your tummy with a pillow if needed. Place your hand or a pillow under your head. Bend your knees so your heels line up with your hips, keeping your chest open. Pressing your heels together, inhale then exhale opening your top knee away from bottom knee. You should feel your hip and glute working. Try to keep your thighs relaxed. Only go a small way up if your lower back is sore. Do 10 to 20 reps each side.

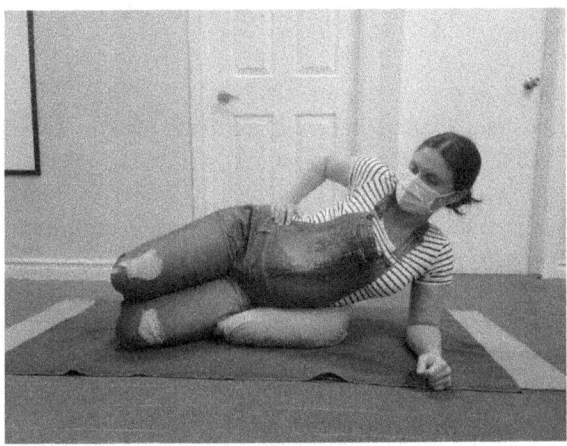 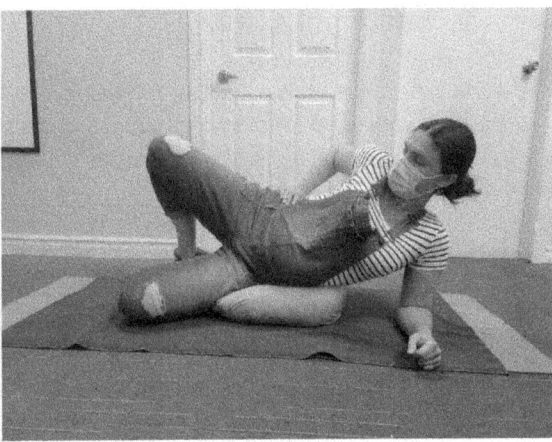

SAFETY TIPS FOR EXERCISING WHILE PREGNANT:

- After your first trimester, avoid exercising while lying flat on your back. This position causes the uterus to put pressure on a major vein called the inferior vena cava, which pumps blood back to your heart. Impeding this blood flow can make you dizzy, short of breath or nauseated.
- Exercise in a safe environment and avoid uneven terrain. As you gain weight during pregnancy, your center of gravity will shift and can affect your sense of balance.
- Wear supportive shoes.
- Avoid overheating and drink water before, during and after exercise.
- Do not exercise to the point of exhaustion. If you cannot talk while exercising, slow down the activity or take small breaks

CHAPTER 35: POSTPARTUM BACK PAIN

Why do you experience back pain after pregnancy?

Most women who experience postpartum back pain develop the symptoms due to pregnancy-related changes in the musculoskeletal system that persist after delivery. In some cases, women may undergo bodily trauma during childbirth that directly
involves the lower back and pelvic bones, joints, and/or soft tissues, causing additional pain and discomfort.

Loose ligaments and joints - During pregnancy, your body produces a hormone called relaxin. This hormone is responsible for making your bones and joints more mobile and loose throughout the pregnancy. As a result, the muscles, and joints of your lower back are very loose and flexible. This makes them prone to sprains and strains after delivery.

Weakened abdominal muscles - Many cases of back pain are related to weak abdominal muscles. Your spine is kept in normal anatomic position by the muscles of your core and low back. Unfortunately, pregnancy often causes a weakening of the abdominal muscle. That's because your abdominal muscles are stretched and separated as they accommodate the growing uterus. With a weak core, it's easy for your low back to pick up the slack and get overworked.

Postural misalignment - After the second trimester, a pregnant uterus is heavy enough to shift your center of gravity forward. As a result, your pelvis tends to tilt anteriorly. This anterior tilt is a common culprit for low back pain because it places your low back in a constantly arched position.

How to manage your pain?
Proper body mechanics. Keep these tips in mind throughout the day.
- Stand and sit up straight.
- Pay attention to your body position when feeding your baby, whether you're nursing or bottle-feeding.
- Choose a comfortable chair with armrests and use lots of pillows to give extra support to your back and arms. If you're breastfeeding, consider buying a breastfeeding pillow that goes around your middle. Also try using a footstool to keep your feet slightly raised off the floor.
- Learn to position yourself properly while nursing, and always bring your baby to your breast, rather than the other way around. Also try different breastfeeding positions. If you have tense shoulders and upper back pain, the side-lying position may be most comfortable.
- Always bend from your knees and pick up objects (and children) from a crouching position to minimize the stress on your back.
- Let someone else do the heavy lifting, especially if you had a C-section.

Step 1: Starts with waking up in the morning and scrubbing your stiff back. This will help in relieving pain and stiffness and prevent your back from getting more worse throughout the day. Body scrub which works best is recipe 1 (yogurt scrub) and recipe 2 (Turmeric scrub). The details of recipe preparation and application are already described in the chapter for body scrub.

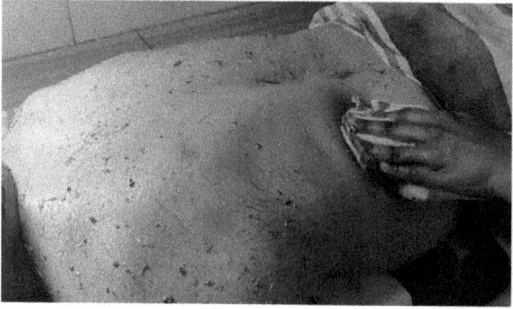 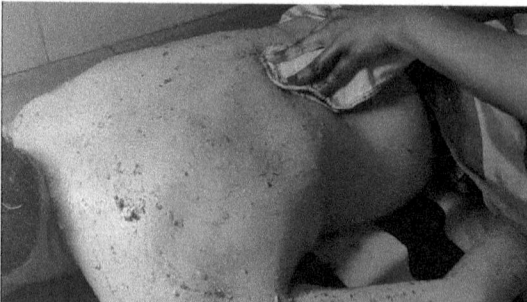

Step 2: Once you are done with scrubbing, take hot beverages as normal. You can take the herbal teas which have tremendous benefit in healing tissues. Also, add the special juices to your drink. The details of recipe preparation and application are already described in the chapter for nutritional facts.

Step 3: You can continue with your breakfast after beverages. Add a healthy salad and soup to your meal. While eating make sure you support your lower back with a brace or wrap a towel around it so that it is supported.

Step 4: After about an hour of your breakfast, the first movement you need to do is to relax your spine lying down in a comfortable position and release stiffness in back muscles with gentle massage. Always do your massage with herb-infused oils. It will give you best results.

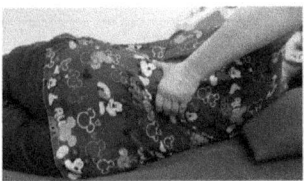 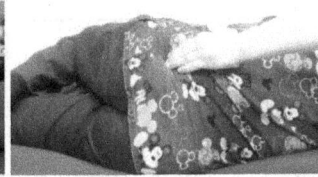 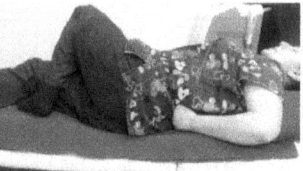

Use recipes from chronic lower back pain section. The details for recipes and application are already described in chapter (herbs and herbs infused oils).

Step 5: After massage, you will feel more relaxed. Start with gentle stretches in your lower back and leg muscles which will make the back muscles more flexible. Stiffness will be gradually released.

Stretches which work best for this condition are hamstring stretch, calf stretch, Figure of four stretch, Child pose, forwards bending in standing, side stretch in standing and sitting.

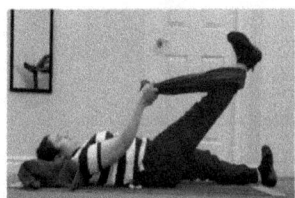 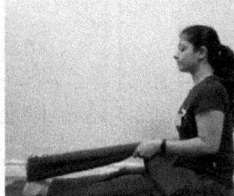 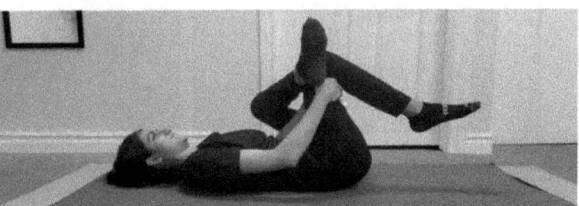

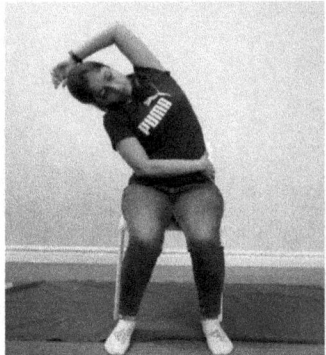 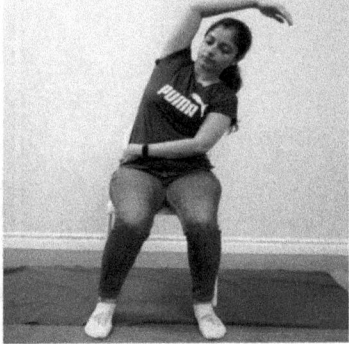

You must feel a slight pull on the tight muscle. Gradually when the muscle loosens up it will feel better. Hold each stretch for 30 seconds and repeat it for 3 times. For stretching of the legs, repeat it on both the sides. The procedure and other details have already been described in the chapter for General stretching.

Step 6: After stretching you will feel relief in your symptoms to 50%. Start with mobility exercise to your spine and legs.

Exercises which will be helpful in this condition are knee to chest, cat and cow, lumbar rotations in sitting as well as lying down, prone extension on elbows, prone extension on hands, bridging. Initially when you start there will be restricted range of motion and attempting this exercise will cause a discomfort.

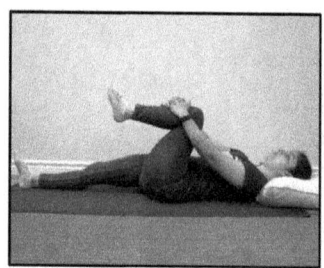
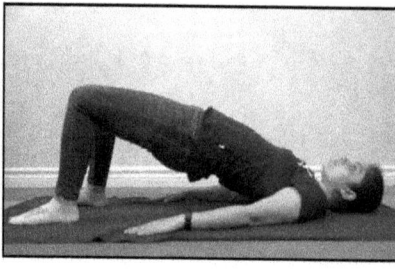
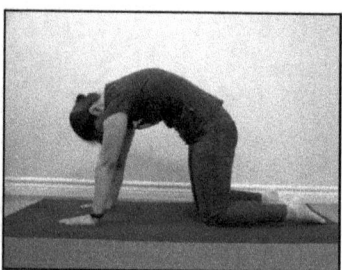
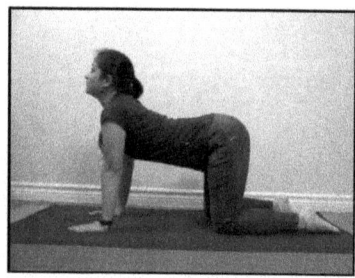
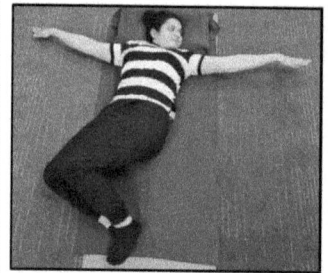
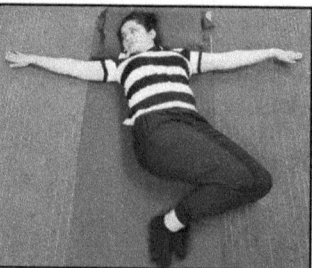
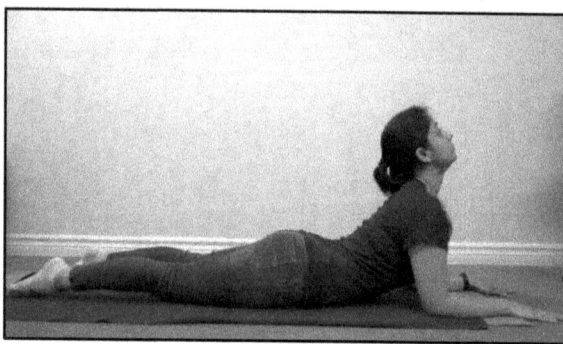
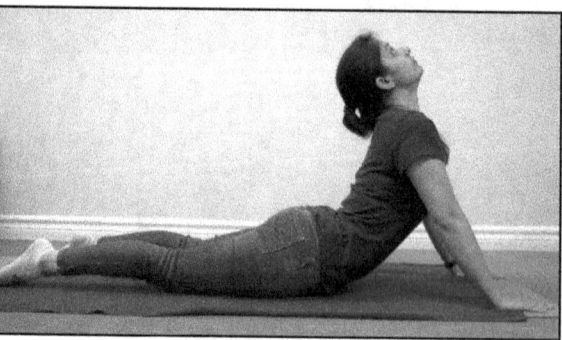

Don't stop the exercises and continue until you reach the full range. Repeat each movement for 10 times. The detail about the exercises is already described in chapter no General mobility exercises.

Step 7: After this, relax yourself and use the heat or contrast compress with heat-cold compression to reduce the stiffness and pain of muscles.

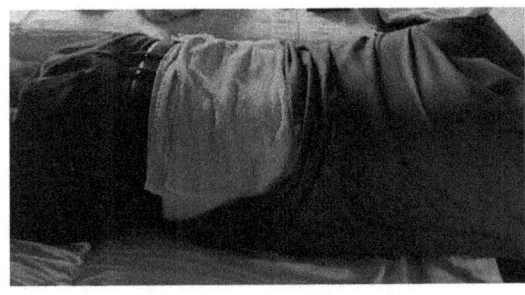

It can be applied directly to the lower back area for 10-15 minutes. Repeat the application of heat or contrast therapy 3-4 times a day. Details of application are described in the chapters for Heat and Cold therapy.

Step 8: Repeat only stretches, mobility exercises and distraction in initial days. Once the pain and symptoms ae subsided or manageable start with strengthening exercises as there is degeneration of bones and leads to instability of spine and weakness of muscles.

Exercises suitable for this condition are, Buttock squeeze, adductor squeeze, heel squeeze, Abdominal crunches, modified plank, straight leg raise, side leg raise. For the exercises you need to refer chapter General Strengthening exercise.

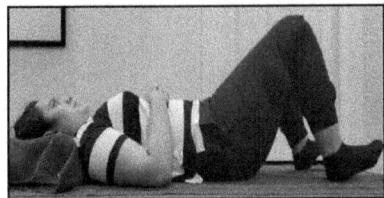
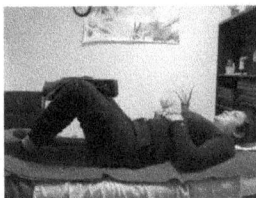
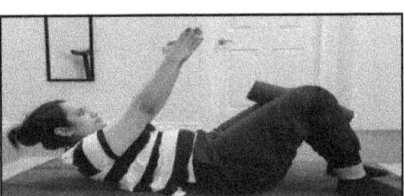
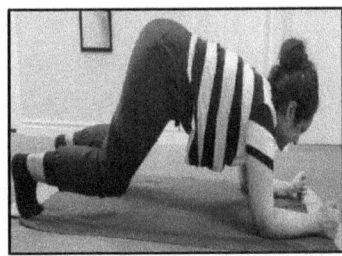
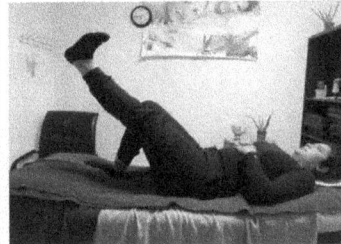
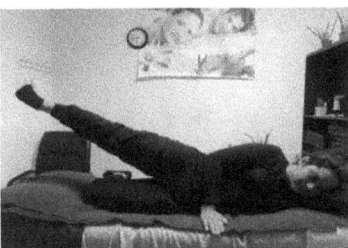

Once you start with exercises you will feel discomfort in the muscles, but don't worry that is just because we are strengthening the weak muscles. Gradually this discomfort goes away. Make sure you hold each exercise for 10 seconds and repeat it for 5-6 times initially.

Step 9: Take a balanced diet which should include food rich in vitamins, omega 3, and magnesium in your diet. The recipes which is useful are described in chapter Nutritional facts and benefits of balanced diet. There are different sections including recipes for soups, salads and juices which you can include at least one in your daily diet.

Step 10: You can use homemade pastes on your back to relieve the severe pain. These patches work on relieving stress and reduces the inflammation. The details and application are given in chapter Herbal poultices (paste) recipes under the section lower back pain.

Step 11: Use proper resting position and make sure your back is in a relaxed position. These positions are used while resting or when you have applied the patches.

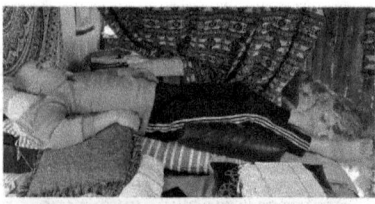
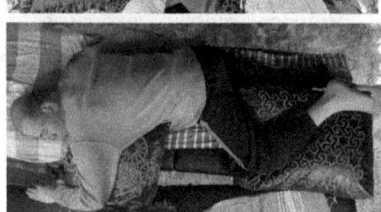

Step 12: At the end of the day, indulge yourself in foot soak and body soak with herbs. This will relax your body senses and rejuvenate it. The recipes and application are already described in chapter Body and foot soak recipes for relaxation.

Step 13: Use can also do the inhalation therapy with herbal recipes which will help reduce the stress. Before sleeping apply herbal oil to your lower back and wrap it with a linen cloth. This helps in pain relief.

CHAPTER 36: BACK PAIN DUE TO IRRITABLE BOWEL SYNDROME

People with irritable bowel syndrome (IBS) frequently mention a seemingly unrelated symptom which is lower back pain, especially during the night. This could be an unrelated pain, or it could be "referred pain." Referred pain is felt someplace other than where it originates. In the case of IBS, that pain comes from the gut. It's often due to constipation, gas, or bloating. The intestines are located at the front of the spine and can exert pressure on the vertebrae. A condition that causes pressure on the spine can cause lower backache in combination with bowel problems and problems with bladder control.

For people having IBS with back pain, the good news is, "Treating your IBS may also help to ease back pain without specifically targeting your back. Typical treatment options include exercise, massage, dietary and lifestyle changes.

Step 1: Start with stretches and mobility exercises, which will help improve your gut muscles to function properly. The movements of colon will be smooth with the stretches and movements.

Gradually when the muscle loosens up it will feel better. When you do the movements make sure you don't pull your more as it can aggravate the symptom.

The stretches helpful in this condition are knee to chest, child pose, cat and cow stretch.

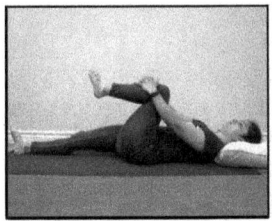
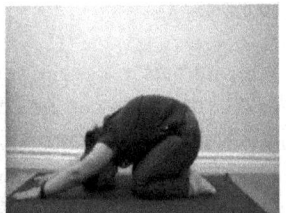
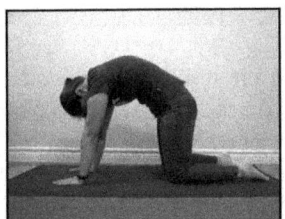
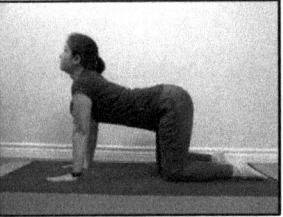

The mobility exercises helpful are bridging, back extension in prone and standing.

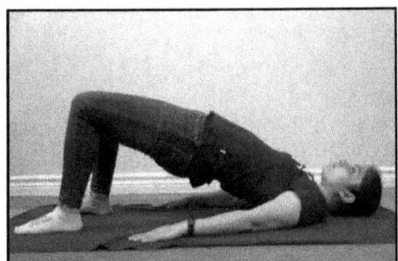
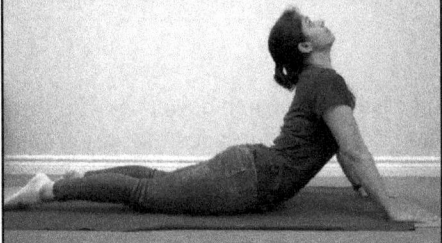
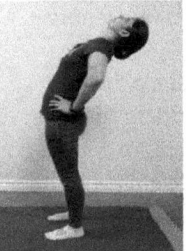

Details for each stretching exercises are given in chapter General stretching exercises and mobility exercises are already described in the chapter General mobility exercises.

Step 3: After this, take a sip of hot herbal teas. This will help reduce the effect of constipation or gas in the bowel and make you able to carry out your routine activities as normal. Avoid caffeinated drinks.

Step 4: Once you are relaxed, massage the abdomen for improving the movement of your colon. This will help the food pass easily down the tract and eventually relieve the back pain. This works best with infused herbal oil recipes. Start from right side and take it to the left side as shown in the image below.

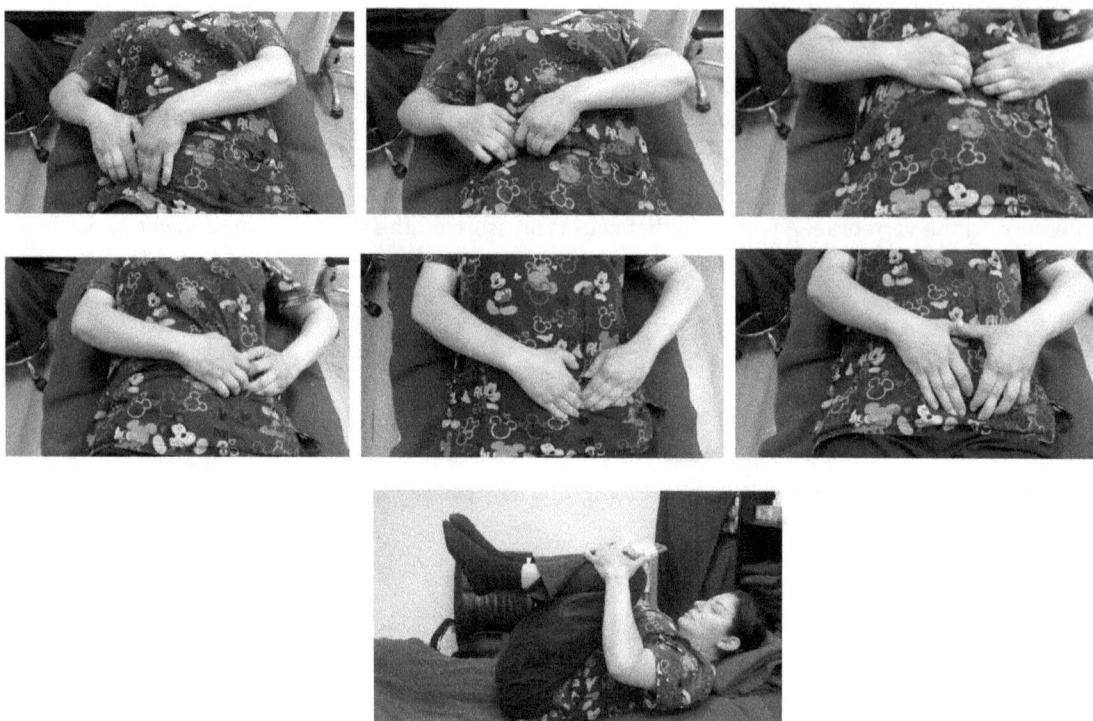

Step 6: Take a balanced diet which should include food rich in vitamins, omega 3, and magnesium in your diet. Green leafy vegetables like spinach, kale, swish charred, collard greens can be consumed. The recipes are mentioned above. The most important thing is avoiding junk food and dairy products.

Step 7: Again, you can use the herbal teas to promote gut movements. The recipes are already described above in step 3.

Step 8: At the end of the day, indulge yourself in foot soak or body soak with herbs. This will relax your body senses and rejuvenate it.

When to see a doctor?
See your doctor if you have a persistent change in bowel habits or other signs or symptoms of IBS. They may indicate a more serious condition, such as colon cancer. More-serious signs and symptoms include:
- Weight loss
- Diarrhea at night
- Rectal bleeding
- Iron deficiency anemia
- Unexplained vomiting
- Difficulty swallowing
- Persistent pain that isn't relieved by-passing gas or a bowel movement

Dietary changes:
- Increase fiber in your diet — eat more fruits, vegetables, grains, and nuts.
- Add supplemental fiber to your diet.
- Drink plenty of water — eight 8-ounce glasses per day.
- Avoid caffeine (from coffee, chocolate, teas, and sodas).
- Limit cheese and milk. Lactose intolerance is more common in people with IBS. Make sure to get
- calcium from other sources, such as broccoli, spinach, salmon, or supplements.

CHAPTER 37: BACK PAIN DUE TO ACIDITY

Acidity, also called acid reflux, is a condition that is characterized by heartburn and is felt around the lower chest area. The food we eat goes into our stomach through the esophagus. The gastric glands in your stomach create acid, which is necessary to digest the food. When the gastric glands create more acid than needed for the digestion process, you can feel a burning sensation below the breastbone. This condition is commonly known as acidity. Your digestive tract produces gas and eliminates it either through the mouth, via belching, or the rectum, via flatulence. However, gas occasionally produces intense pain that makes the entire abdomen feel full and tender. This pain can radiate to the back, causing back pain and bloating.

How does acid reflux lead to back pain?
Since back pain is not typically considered a direct symptom of acid reflux, it stems from other symptoms. Back pain that happens during acid reflux is often due to heartburn. Heartburn causes burning in the chest and neck. This can spread to the back and cause pain between the shoulder blades, or even spread to the lower back. Stress caused by recurrent acid reflux can also cause back pain.

How to treat back pain with acid reflux?
Typical treatment options include exercise, massage, dietary and lifestyle changes. Here are some exercises if you have an attack of acid reflux and giving you back ache.

Get two chairs and place them apart so that you can still reach them with your hands. Place a soft mat or similar between the chairs, kneel on it, and lay your palms on the seats. Make sure that your arms and back do not form a straight line. Your upper body should be positioned lower than your arms. Now move your upper body to the ground, so that you feel the stretch in your chest and shoulders. Leave your elbows stretched the whole time. Hold this position for two to three minutes.

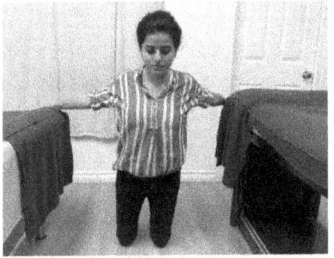

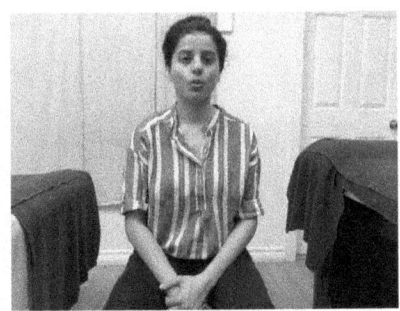

Stand up straight and relaxed or sit down comfortably on a chair. Take a deep breath and blow all the air out with great force until you feel there's no air in your lungs left. Once you have exhaled completely, close your mouth and nose with your fingers. Now make a move as if you're trying to suck in fresh air, even though your mouth and nose are closed. Perform this breathing movement if you can do so. Now breathe back in normally. Perform this exercise a few times in a row to relax your chest muscles.

Sit upright on a chair and grab our pain releaser or fascia-fit mini foam roller. Now place the mini ball at the xiphoid process under the sternum as shown on the picture and roll in small, precise, and spiral-shaped movements along the left and right costal arch. Roll a little lower with each pass and then back to the middle of your chest Always look for sensitive areas. Found one? Remain here and relax the tense tissue by rolling. Work on each side for about four to five rounds until the muscles and fasciae are fully relaxed.

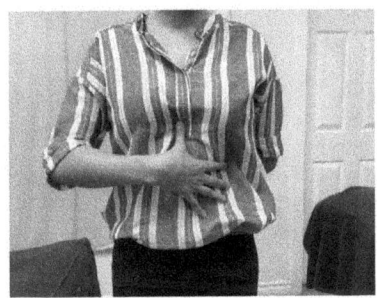

CHAPTER 38: BACK PAIN DUE TO FLAT FOOT

Flat feet are characterized by no arch; the entire sole of your foot touches, or nearly touches, the ground when standing.

Why do you feel back pain if you have flat feet?

Your musculoskeletal system is a fully integrated structure, and each section is connected by joints. Since flat feet cannot adequately absorb shock, they confer this responsibility to other joints, particularly the knees, hips, and low back. That's because without arch support, your feet tend to roll inward, causing over pronation. This, in turn, affects your walking and places excessive stress on your ankles and knees. Your ankles can generally handle the change in balance since they can roll in many directions. Knees, however, are designed to bend forward and back, not side-to-side. When you over pronate, your knees are forced in a direction they're not designed for. With your knees functioning poorly, the impact may make its way up to your hips, which need to compensate for the poor positioning of your knees. And on it goes until it reaches your low back. Poor positioning of the major joints in your lower body ultimately reaches your back and causes back pain all because of flat feet.

Self-test to evaluate if you have flat foot: There is a quick, simple test that you can do at home to see if you have fallen arches:
1. Wet your feet
2. Stand on a flat, hard surface, such as a floor or concrete pad (you need to be able to see your footprint) or walk in soft soil or sand
3. Look at your footprints. If you see a footprint that shows the heel and ball of your foot with a thin, curved imprint running along the outside, then your foot structure is normal. If you can see the imprint of your entire foot, then you probably have fallen arches.

In addition to low back pain, some people may also get tired, achy, or swollen feet, along with limited range of motion in the ankle and toes. That's because people with flat feet don't have arch support so they're saddled with the full force of your body's weight every time they stand.

How to get relief from this?
Heel stretches: Stand with your hands resting on a wall, chair, or
railing at shoulder or eye level. Keep one leg forward and the other leg extend behind you. Press both heels firmly into the floor. Keeping your spine straight, bend your front leg and push yourself into the wall or support, feeling a stretch in your back leg and Achilles' tendon. Hold this position for 30 seconds. Do each side 4 times.

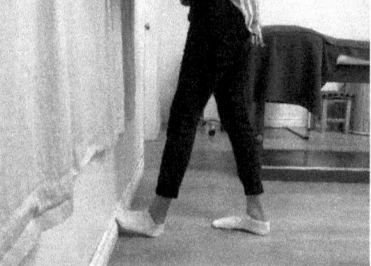 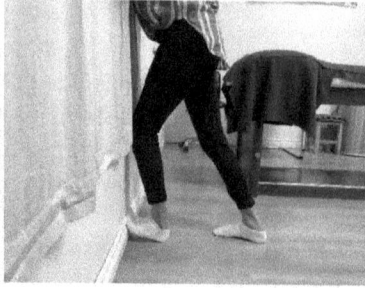 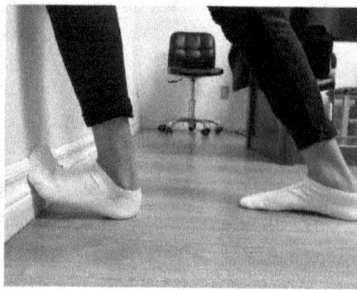

Arch lifts - Stand with your feet directly underneath your hips. Making sure to keep your toes in contact with the floor the entire time, roll your weight to the outer edges of your feet as you lift your arches up as far as you can. Then release your feet back down. You'll work the muscles that help to lift and supinate your arches. Do 2–3 sets of 10–15 repetitions.

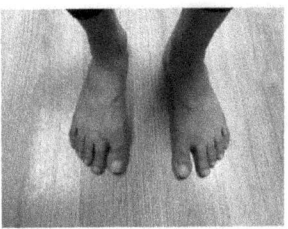 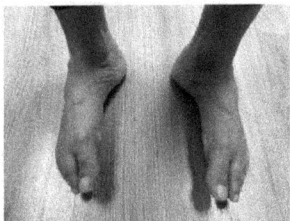

Stair arch raises - Stand on steps with your left foot one step higher than your right foot. Use your left foot for balance as you lower your right foot down so your heel hangs lower than the step. Slowly lift your right heel as high as you can, focusing on strengthening your arch. Rotate your arch inward as your knee and calf rotate slightly to the side, causing your arch to become higher. Slowly lower back down to the starting position. Do 2–3 sets of 10–15 repetitions on both sides.

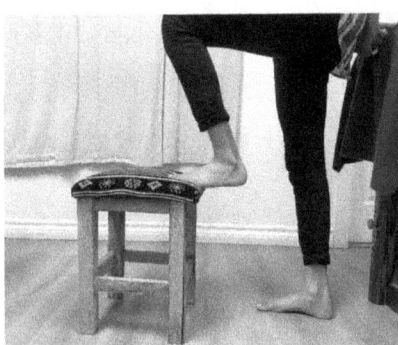 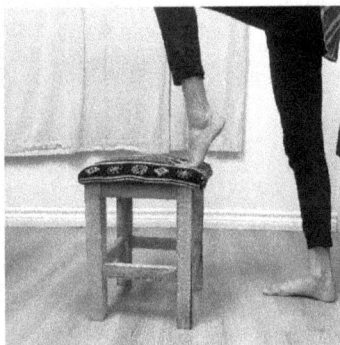

Towel curls - Sit in a chair with a towel under your feet. Root your heels into the floor as you curl your toes to scrunch up the towel. Press your toes into your foot. Hold for a few seconds and release. Make sure to keep the ball of your foot pressed into the floor or towel. Maintain an awareness of the arch of your foot being strengthened. Do 2–3 sets of 10–15 repetitions.

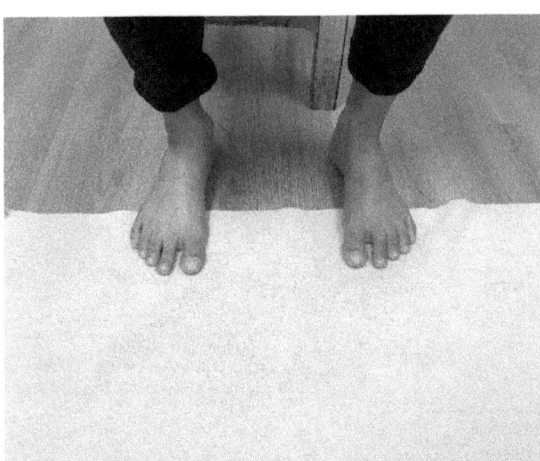 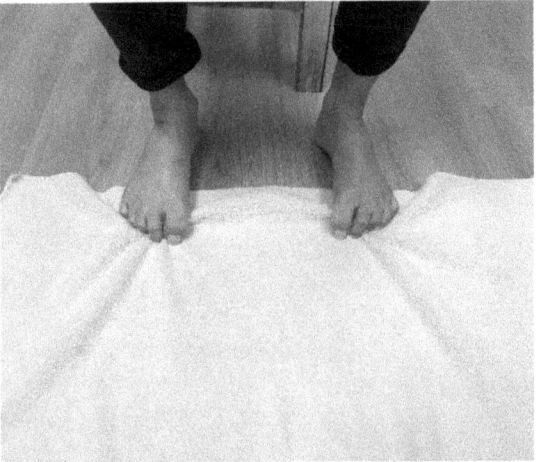

Toe raises - For variation you can try doing this exercise in standing yoga poses such as Tree Pose, Standing Forward Bend, or Standing Split. While standing, press your right big toe into the floor and lift your other four toes. Then press your four toes into the floor and lift your big toe. Do each way 5–10 times, holding each lift for 5 seconds. Then do the exercise on your left foot.

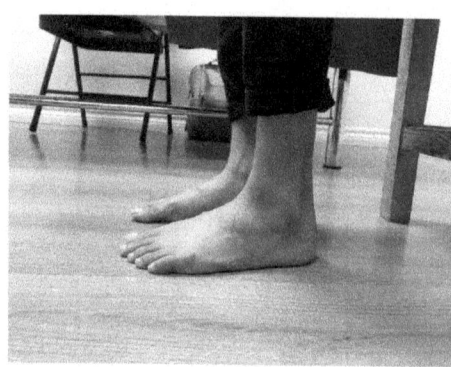 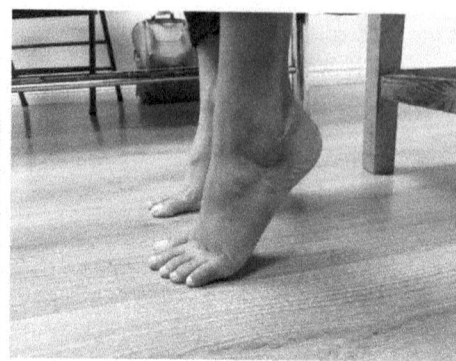

Also, with these exercises you need to stretch and strengthen your back as well which are already mentioned in the chapter before. Continue massage at your lower back with herb-infused oil. The technique for massage is already described in the chapter for Massage techniques. Also follow the herbal paste, diet recipes, foot soak, body soak and inhalation with these steps. The details are already described in the chapter above.

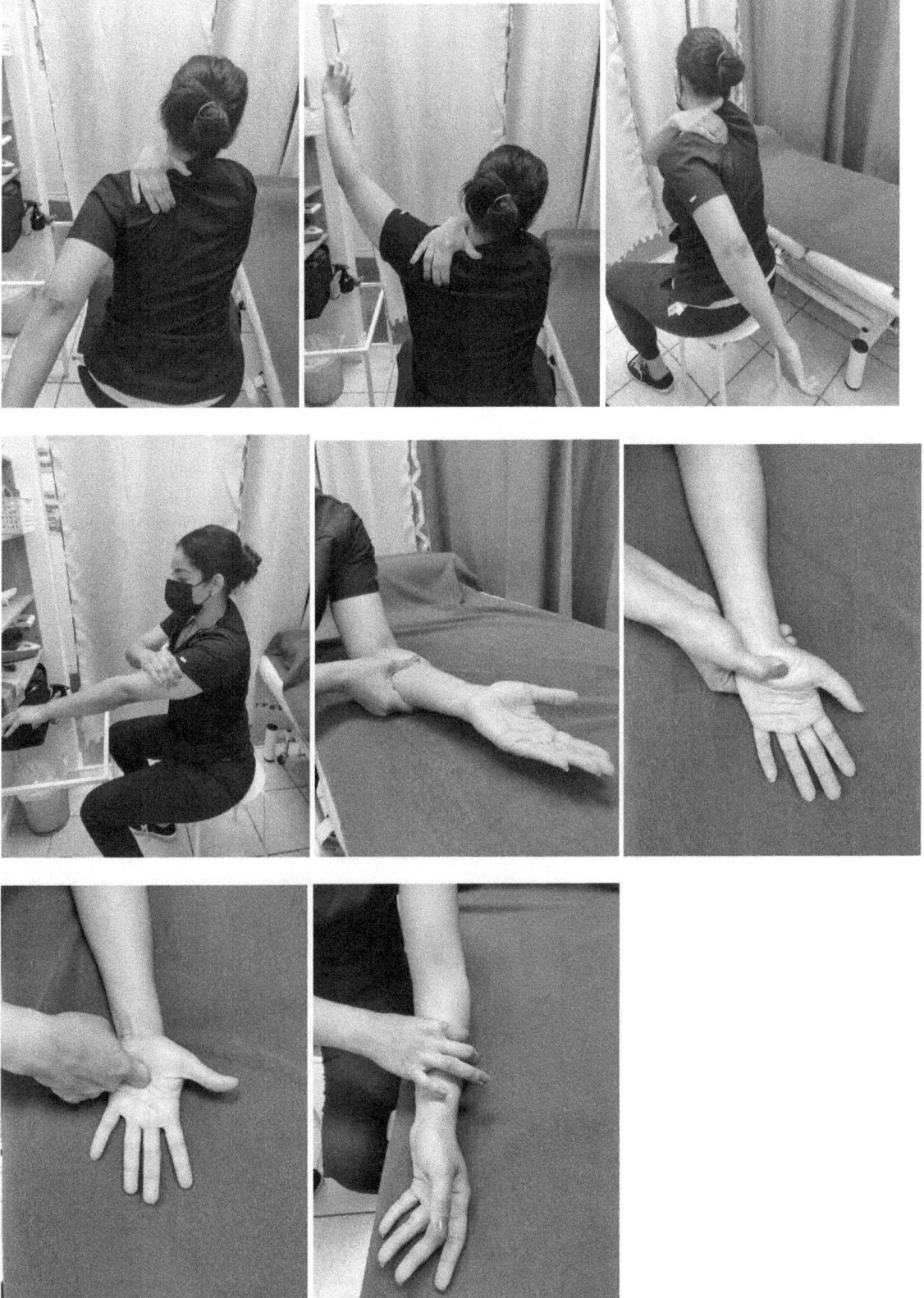

Step 6: Once your symptoms are relieved to 50%, start with the strengthening exercises. Focus right now should be on strengthening of the muscles which are weak because of the specific nerve compression.

For upper limb weakness the exercises are backward shoulder shrugs, standing shoulder crunches, shoulder flexor, abductor and rotator strengthening.

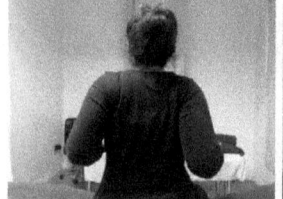 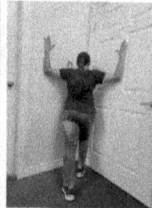 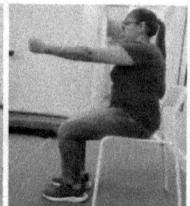 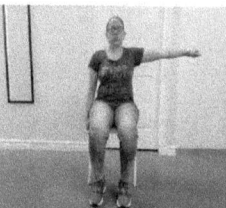 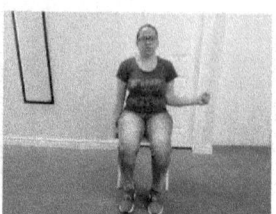

Once you start with exercises you will discomfort in the muscles, but don't worry that is just because we are strengthening the weak muscles. Gradually this discomfort goes away. For details refer to chapter General strengthening exercises.

Step 7: Take a balanced diet which should include food rich in vitamins, omega 3, and magnesium in your diet. The recipes are mentioned above for salad, soups and juices.

Step 8: You can use homemade patches to your skin to relieve the severe neck pain and back pain. These patches work on relieving stress and reduces the inflammation.

Step 9: Use proper resting position and make sure your back is in a relaxed position. These positions are used while resting or when you have applied the patches.

Step 10: Again, you can use the herbal teas to relieve your stress due to pain. The recipes are already described above in step 4.

Step 11: At the end of the day, indulge yourself in foot soak with herbs. This will relax your body senses and rejuvenate it. Also use inhalation method with herb to relieve all the senses of body.

CHAPTER 40: BACK PAIN DUE TO KIDNEY STONE

Because your kidneys are located toward your back and underneath your ribcage, it may be hard to tell if the pain you're experiencing in that area is coming from your back or your kidney. The symptoms you're having can help you figure out which is the source of the pain.

How to differentiate between the two pains: The location, type, and severity of the pain are some of the things that will be different depending on whether the pain is from a problem in your kidneys or your back. Location of the pain: Kidney pain is felt in your flank, which is the area on either side of your spine between the bottom of your ribcage and your hips. Kidney pain is felt higher and deeper in your body than back pain. It usually occurs in one side of your body, but it can occur in both sides. Muscle pain may affect one or both sides, but nerve pain usually only affects one side.

Type of pain
Kidney pain is usually sharp if you have a kidney stone and a dull ache if you have an infection.
It won't get worse with movement or go away by itself without treatment. Whereas back pain due to involvement of muscular structures feels like a dull ache. If a nerve has been injured or irritated, the pain is a sharp burning sensation that may travel down your buttock to your lower leg or even your foot.

Radiation of the pain
If you're passing a kidney stone, the pain may fluctuate as the stone moves. Sometimes the kidney pain spreads (radiates) to your inner thigh or lower abdomen. Whereas back pain from a muscle usually stays in the back and nerve pain may spread to your lower leg.

Things that make it better or worse
Typically, nothing makes the pain better until the problem is corrected, such as by passing the stone. Whereas back pain from muscular or spinal structures may get worse with movement or if you sit or stand for a long time. It may get better if you switch positions or walk around.

Accompanying symptoms for kidney pain
If you have a kidney infection or a kidney stone, you may also experience:
- fever and chills
- nausea and vomiting
- cloudy or dark urine
- an urgent need to urinate
- pain when you urinate
- a recent infection in your bladder

When to see a doctor?
Once you've determined whether your pain is coming from your back or your kidneys, consider seeing your doctor for evaluation and treatment. You should always be seen if you think you have a kidney infection or kidney stone.

Kidney Pain Treatment
To treat your kidney pain, your doctor first needs to find its cause. They may use one or more tests to find out the cause of your pain. These tests include:
- Urine tests to check your pee for blood, protein, too many white blood cells, and other signs of specific kidney problems
- An ultrasound or CT scan to look for kidney stones or other physical problems in the kidneys and urinary tract

Once your doctor diagnoses the cause of your kidney pain, they can decide on the best treatment plan for you.

There is no quick fix for getting rid of kidney stone pain. The only solution is to have a physician prescribe pain medications and sometimes fluids while just giving yourself time to pass the stone. However, there are antibiotics for kidney infections as well as home remedies. The home remedies include using heat to the area where you have discomfort, keeping yourself hydrated and taking over the counter pain meds when needed. The best advice to keep kidneys healthy is to exercise, keep hydrated especially in warm weather or when exercising, maintain a healthy weight, and quit smoking

CHAPTER 41: PROPHYLACTICS

Prevent Injuries
- Focus on good posture.
- Good posture can help prevent back pain.
- Try not to slouch when standing and sitting.
- Sit up straight with your back against the back of your chair and your feet flat on the floor. If possible, keep your knees slightly higher than your hips.
- Stand tall with your head up and shoulders back.
- If you can, switch between standing and sitting so you aren't in the same position for too long.
- To help keep your back feeling healthy, choose comfortable, well-cushioned shoes. Cushioned soles reduce the impact when you're walking on hard surfaces. This helps protect your back, hips, and knees.

Healthy Habits
- Watch your weight. Staying at a healthy weight lowers your risk of back pain. If you are overweight, losing weight in a healthy way can reduce the strain on your back.
- Get enough calcium and vitamin D. Getting enough calcium and vitamin D can help keep your bones strong and prevent osteoporosis. Osteoporosis makes your bones weaker and more likely to fracture (break).
- Spine fractures from osteoporosis are a leading cause of back pain.

Can you think of housework activities that you have been doing wrong?

I know it can be easy to get caught up, rushing around the house to get everything done but one thing to remember is to be kind to yourself and take 20-minute breaks throughout. If you start feeling any signs of pain, walk, stretch and rest your back. Don't allow yourself to get so busy checking a chore off of your to-do list that you forget the safe way to move your body. Start using these tips right away to keep your back safe.

IDEAL POSITIONS TO DO THE ACTIVITY

LIFTING: Do not attempt to lift by bending forward. Bend your hips and knees to squat down to your load, keep it close to your body, and straighten your legs to lift. Never lift a heavy object above shoulder level. Avoid turning or twisting your body while lifting or holding a heavy object.

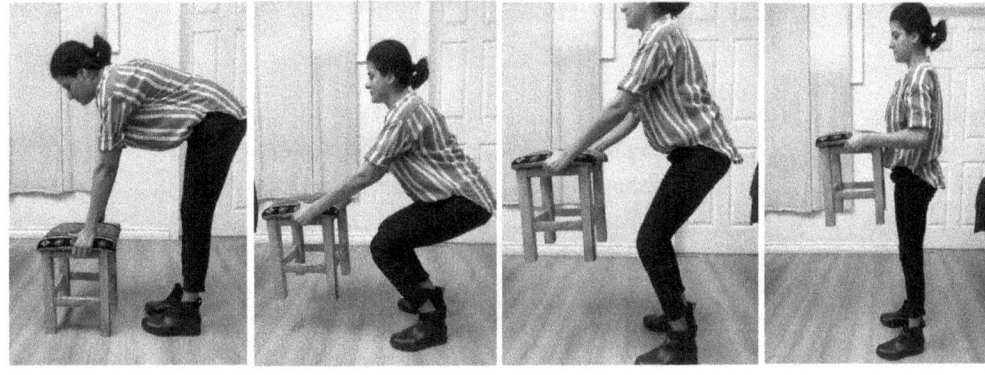

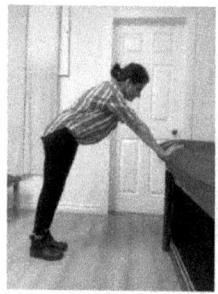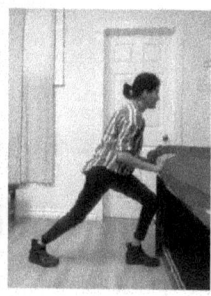

PUSHING: Stand close to the object that you wish to push. Keep your back straight, maintaining small curve in lower back. Crouch with feet apart and push with your legs. Lean forward with chest and shoulder against the object. Do not push with arms or shoulders.

PULLING: Position feet apart with one in back of the other. Stand close to object keeping back straight, maintaining small curve in lower back. Crouch and pull objects toward you, using your own body weight.

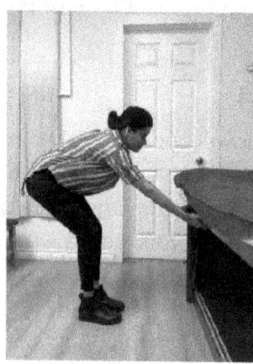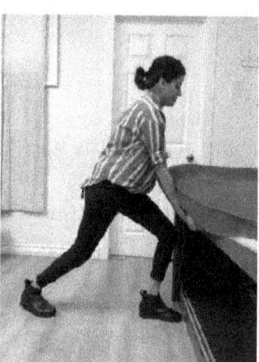

REACHING: Stand as close to object as possible. Feet should be apart for additional stability. Avoid straining to reach object, use a ladder or step stool if needed. If object is above your head, raise or lower it slowly. Overhead lifting is dangerous and should be avoided.

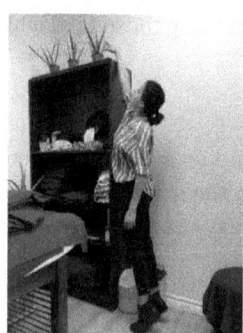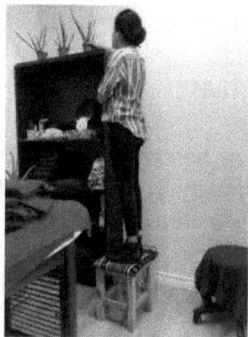

PUTTING CLOTHES IN LAUNDARY: When loading the washing machine, keep your back straight! Pick up the entire basket (via squatting, not bending) and hold it in front of you at waist height, while loading the clothes. You can use one leg to help hold the basket between your body and the front of the washer. Another option is to do your squats for the day and squat down several times (without bending your back forward) to pick up the clothes out of the basket. Another option is to carefully lift the entire basket and pour all the clothes into the washer. Just remember to keep your back straight as you lift and lower the basket.

SHIFTING WET CLOTHES TO DRYER: When taking wet clothes out of the washer, lift one leg back behind you as you lean forward and try to keep the straight position of your spine as you reach down. This is the same technique golfers use when picking up a golf ball. Then stand upright with feet spread apart. Squat with your back straight and toss the clothes into the dryer. Be extra careful not to twist your back during the transfer of clothes from washer to dryer.

TAKING OUT CLOTHES FROM DRYER: To remove clothes from the dryer, either squat, kneel or sit on a step stool in order to keep your back straight. Don't forget to keep your back straight as you lift the full laundry basket (via a squat). And do not twist your back to turn with the basket. Just take small steps whenever you need to turn.

USING VACCUM CLEANER OR MOP: one of the most common mistakes people make is reaching out with their arms while bending at the waist over and over again. Bending over in awkward positions can place a lot of strain on your muscles – especially in your back! To help fix this... the key is to keep your hips and shoulders moving towards the work.

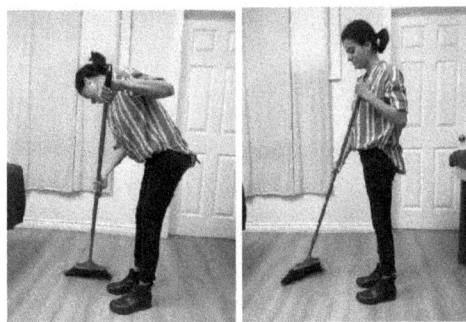

BRUSHING AND DOING DISHES: hip hinge when you are at the sink washing dishes or brushing your teeth: Place your feet about 12 inches apart. Keep your back straight (in its neutral position). As you bend your knees, move your hips backward. Fold over by sliding your hips down and back. The hip hinge works because the hip is not as limited in its motion as the spine.

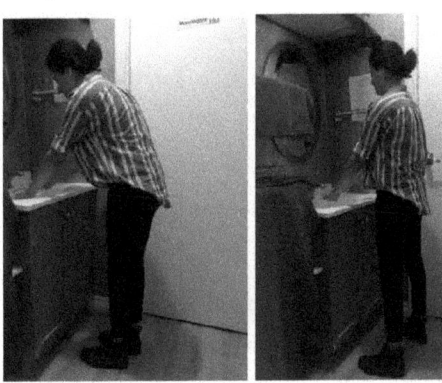

MAKING THE BED: Making the bed involves bending, reaching and pressures. If you position yourself up against the bed, you'll be able to use the bed for support and positional stability. Then use one arm to prop your weight as you reach and work with the other arm. Switch sides regularly unless that causes pain. (It may if you have a sacroiliac joint or other problem that affects one side more than the other.

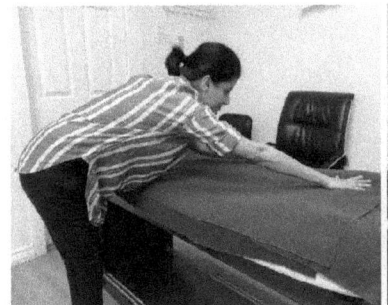 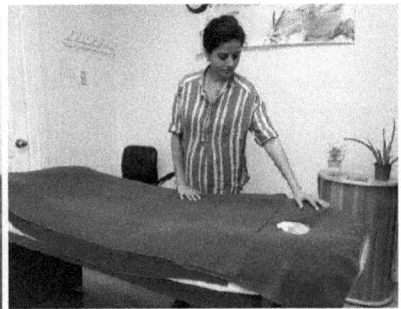

DESKTOP WORK: View your computer screen with a straight neck. Put your keyboard and mouse or touchpad at a comfortable height in front of you. Sit back in your chair. When sitting, rest your feet flat on either the floor or a foot support. Avoid prolonged standing for computer work.

DRIVING: Driving long distances can put a strain on your low back. Follow these tips to help keep your back feeling good, even on the longest trips. Move your seat forward so you don't have to bend to reach the steering wheel. Put a rolled towel, small pillow, or other lumbar support behind your lower back. Take a break every hour on long trips to get out of the car and walk around.

CPSIA information can be obtained
at www.ICGtesting.com
Printed in the USA
BVHW091158041121
620621BV00003B/10